Communication Disability
and the Psychiatry of Old Age

Communication Disability and the Psychiatry of Old Age

Edited by

Karen Bryan and Jane Maxim

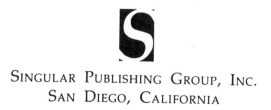

SINGULAR PUBLISHING GROUP, INC.
SAN DIEGO, CALIFORNIA

Published and Distributed in the
United States and Canada by
SINGULAR PUBLISHING GROUP, INC.
401 West A Street, Suite 325
San Diego, CA 92101, USA

British Library Cataloguing in Publication Data
A catalogue record for this book is available from the
British Library.

ISBN 1-897635-24-9

Singular Number 1-56593-747-3

Printed and bound in the UK by Athenaeum Press Ltd,
Gateshead, Tyne & Wear

Contents

Chapter 3:   37

Language, cognition and communication in the older mentally infirm
Jane Maxim and Karen Bryan

Chapter 4:   80

Issues in service provision: a management perspective
Sue Stevens

Chapter 5:   100

The team approach to working with the elderly mentally ill
Kim Zabihi and Karen Bryan

Chapter 6:   122

A survey of service provision to the cognitively impaired elderly in the USA
Danielle Ripich and Elaine Ziol

Foreword

The disproportionate increase in the elderly segment of the population has created a tremendous need for information about age-related neurologic and psychiatric conditions and their effects on communicative and cognitive functions. This book, *Communication Disability and the Psychiatry of Old Age*, is an exceptional response to that need. Professionals will find state-of-the-art information about age-related dementing diseases, their effects on communication and other aspects of cognition, assessment and treatment. To understand the various dementing diseases and the neurobehavioural sequelae requires knowledge of many disciplines and the contributors to this book have reviewed the now voluminous literature, synthesising it to form a highly readable text. Because of the quality of the scholarship of the contributors, readers can be confident in the information presented. Emphasised throughout is the perspective of the speech–language therapist and it is this emphasis that makes this book unique. Certainly it contains the most comprehensive treatment to date of the role of the speech–language therapist in diagnosing and treating dementia patients and their families. The book will provide health professionals and family carers with an understanding of the contributions that the speech–language therapist can make to the team of professionals who serve dementia patients. The emphasis on the perspective of the speech–language therapist does not detract from its value for other professionals, however, because the book is comprehensive in its coverage of the common dementing diseases, their diagnosis, approaches to service delivery, and even includes chapters about supporting the caregivers of these patients. Another valuable focus of the book is on the communicative functioning of dementia patients and certainly the importance of communicative functioning in the care and lives of elderly patients can hardly be overstated. Understanding age-related dementing diseases is life work for clinicians and caregivers and this fine contribution by Jane Maxim and Karen Bryan will provide every reader with greater insights.

Professor Kathryn A. Bayles

Preface

This book has its origins in two events. The College of Speech and Language Therapists convened a working party to investigate service provision to people with dementia and the findings were published in 1993 as a position paper. Some contributors to that report are also contributors to this book. Second, in 1993, we organised a course on research in the dementias and service provision to this clinical population. Both these events demonstrated that clinicians had great difficulty accessing information which would help them in setting up a service to this group of elderly clients. Specific interest groups are one valuable source of information but, equally, it was obvious that there were innovative, dynamic services in existence which were not known to the profession. Successful outcomes in clinical audit are not necessarily easy to translate into research outcomes and this fact may preclude writing up a service for a refereed journal. Papers on service provision issues do not have a natural forum, because professional publications do not usually have the space to print such articles in the detail required to be useful to a service provider. In fact, we need to write more about how we cope with the realities of everyday clinical life and how we evaluate whether a service is successful or not. This book sets out to give some information on what can be done to provide a service in the area of the psychiatry of old age. It is, we hope, a book that clinicians and students can turn to when they want examples of what is and can be done despite the constraints under which most clinicians work.

Karen Bryan
Jane Maxim
August 1995

Contributors

Linda Armstrong BA, BSc, PhD, MRCSLT, PGCertACS(Elderly) is an honorary lecturer in the Department of Speech and Language Sciences, Queen Margaret's College, Edinburgh.

Karen Bryan BSc, PhD, MRCSLT is a lecturer in speech and language pathology in the Department of Human Communication Science, University College London.

Jane Maxim Dip CSLT, MRCSLT, MA, PhD is a senior lecturer in speech and language therapy in the Department of Human Communication Science, University College London.

Niki Muir dipRCSLT is a freelance speech and language therapist specialising in acute and general psychiatry and care of the elderly.

Charlotte Painter BSc, MRCSLT is a speech and language therapist in Camden and Islington Community Health Services NHS Trust and currently works in an out-patient rehabilitation unit.

Bryce Pitt MD, BS, FRcPsychology is professor, psychiatry of old age, St Mary's and the Royal Postgraduate Medical Schools.

Deirdre Rainbow BSc, MRCSLT is a speech and language therapist in Camden and Islington Community Health Services NHS Trust specialising in the care of the elderly.

Danielle Ripich PhD is professor in speech and language pathology in the Department of Communication Sciences, Case Western Reserve University, USA.

Susan Stevens dipRCSLT is a speech and language therapist specialising in the care of the elderly and is manager of the speech and language therapy services at Charing Cross and Hammersmith Hospitals, London.

Kate Swinburn MA, PG Dip, MRCSLT is a research speech and language therapist at Hammersmith Hospital, London.

Barbara Tanner BSc, MLing, MRCSLT is a speech and language therapist specialising in old age psychiatry at Jocelyn Solly House, Macclesfield.

Sandra Walker MPhil, dipRCSLT, RegMRCSLT is deputy head of speech and language therapy services at the Victoria Infirmary NHS Trust,

Glasgow with responsibility for neurological services, including dementia and Parkinson's clinics, and former adviser to the RCSLT on the elderly.

Kim Zabini BSc, MSc, MRCSLT is a speech and language therapist specialising in care of the elderly at the Marjory Warren Medical Centre, West Middlesex University Hospital, London.

Elaine Ziol MHS is a research associate in the Department of Communication Sciences, Case Western Reserve University, USA.

Acknowledgements

We would particularly like to thank the contributors who met their deadlines and produced such excellent material. Special thanks go to the librarians in the Department of Human Communication Science, University College, who have responded to our many requests for help and to our colleagues who have been generous in their support when we have had deadlines to meet.

Chapter 1: Population, Health Care Issues and the Context of Care

KAREN BRYAN AND JANE MAXIM

Introduction

It is estimated that one in four people over the age of 65 has some form of psychiatric disorder. Depression is a common disorder in the elderly (Pitt, 1982) and it is important that it is recognised and treated (see Chapter 2). The other common psychiatric disorder associated with old age is dementia. In fact the term dementia refers to a group of disorders which should be referred to as 'the dementias'. Thus dementia is a heterogenous term covering a number of forms of presentation and disease progression. Definitions of dementia vary, but the Royal College of Physicians Committee on Geriatrics (1981) proposed the following definition:

> The global disturbance of higher cortical functions including memory, the capacity to solve problems of everyday living, the performance of learned perceptuo-motor skills, the correct use of social skills and control of emotional reactions, in the absence of clouding of consciousness.

Dementia therefore describes a clinical syndrome of generalised cognitive impairment in an alert patient (Rossor, 1987). There are a wide variety of causes, but the following features are common to them all:

- progressively acquired cognitive impairment, i.e. there must be evidence of deterioration from a previous level. This should distinguish a dementing process from existing learning difficulties;
- normal level of alertness as opposed to a person being drowsy or overtly agitated, which may distinguish dementia from a confusional state;
- acquired cognitive impairment evident across a range of functions. This may distinguish dementia from focal deficits such as dysphasia.

Figure 1 gives an overview of pathology (adapted from Rossor, 1987 and Cummings and Benson, 1992).

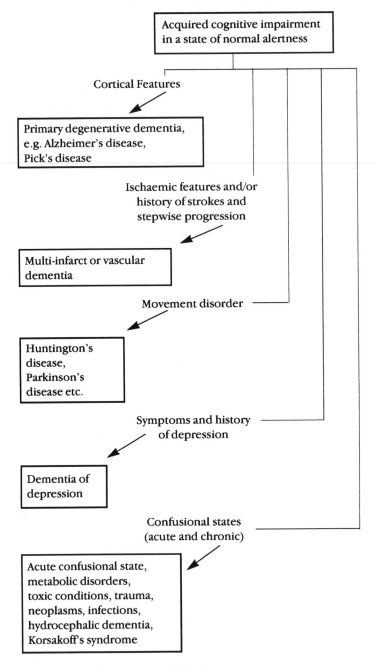

Figure 1: Diagnosis of dementia – aetiologies

To say that a client has dementia is obviously insufficient. It is essential to describe the cognitive impairment and the behavioural sequelae involved and to give an indication of the severity, onset, progression and any fluctuation in the disorder. These disorders and their associated language manifestations are discussed in Chapter 7, and psychiatric disorders associated with old age are discussed in Chapter 2.

All psychiatric disorders associated with ageing have the potential to disrupt the ability to communicate in some way. This may be directly through loss of language ability, for example, in Alzheimer's disease, or indirectly, for example, in depression as a secondary consequence of lack of interaction. Management of communication disorders must be considered within the context of the services provided to care for the elderly mentally ill.

The context of care for the elderly with psychiatric disorders

Access to specialist services for older people appears to be variable. A Royal College of Physicians report (1994) examined the need for equity and quality of care for elderly people. They described three models of (acute) care for the elderly:

- *The traditional model*: patients enter geriatric services via selection from non-geriatricians, largely general practitioners and inexperienced accident and emergency staff.
- *The age-defined model*: all medical patients over a specified age (this varies from 65 to 85 years) are assigned to geriatric services.
- *The integrated model*: physicians with special responsibility for the elderly serve as members of multi-consultant teams and take equal part in acute medical emergency work and are also responsible for providing specialist geriatric services including rehabilitation, long-stay day hospital, outpatient and community liaison work.

There are advantages and disadvantages to all three models. The important point here is that these models imply differing rates and routes of access for elderly people to specialist services. Underlying this is variability in the amount of resources which are allocated specifically to the elderly. If we then consider access for elderly people to psychiatric services for the elderly, the same set of possibilities is applicable.

Services include those that are provided for other client groups such as general medicine and services geared to the elderly such as geriatric medicine, as well as those specifically aimed at meeting the needs of this client group such as psychogeriatric services (see Moriarty and Levin, 1993 and Miller and Morris, 1993 for a general overview of services).

There is a further access to care issue concerning acute versus community provision. In general, specialist services remain focused within hospital settings so that elderly people who are not admitted to hospital, for example those with very slow progression of cognitive difficulty without accompanying physical illness, may not get access to specialist services or may have practical difficulties such as with transport if they are referred.

As speech and language therapists, we have to consider both the overall service provision to elderly clients with psychiatric disorders and how we operate within this provision, as well as the services provided by our own profession. Wattis and Martin (1994) stated that the clinical function of a comprehensive service for the elderly has four main constituents:

- assessment and communication;
- community treatment and support;
- acute inpatient treatment;
- long-stay residential/nursing care.

This partly addresses the questions of:
Who provides the service?
How do we provide it?
Where do we provide it?

These questions can be applied to any professional service, be it medical, paramedical or social. In addition, speech and language therapists (or indeed any other professionals) need to consider how they cooperate with other services and provisions and how communication between the various carers is coordinated. The multidisciplinary team and the speech and language therapist's role within it are discussed in Chapter 5.

Community provision

Many changes to the service provision for the elderly with psychiatric disorders have been brought about by the community care initiatives and policies of the 1990s (see Chapter 11) so that service provision has become much more varied. This may be seen as beneficial in that local services can be tailored to meet local needs, but can also raise questions about variations in the levels of provision. Dixon et al. (1994) discuss whether there is equity of provision across fundholding and non-fundholding general practitioners. Their survey suggested that fundholders are more generously funded. Such an anomaly would be important to elderly people with mental illness as the GP is usually the first contact with health and other services. Equity across primary (GP) and secondary (hospital) care is also questioned (Majeed et al., 1994).

In 1993 the NHS Management Executive (Mawhinney and Nichol 1993) identified seven principles of purchasing health care as a guide for commissioning health care:

- listen to patients;
- identify health targets;
- ensure that patient care contracts relate to what purchasers want to achieve;
- make better use of available information about effectiveness and outcome measures;
- use contracts to involve providers in health promotion;
- use local clinical audit;
- establish challenging efficiency targets.

Access to rehabilitation is also variable for the elderly. Again, the Royal College of Physicians (1994) recommend that:

- commissioning bodies should ensure that rehabilitation beds are used for this purpose and not as a convenient waiting area while social needs are addressed;
- adequate physiotherapy, occupational therapy, speech and language therapy and social work support should be provided within rehabilitation units to enable them to treat patients quickly and effectively.

Access to services such as rehabilitation is a key issue within private care provision for the elderly mentally ill. Only about one-third of nursing care beds for the elderly are provided by the NHS, with this number likely to decline further if current policies are continued. In NHS accommodation, medical standards and care are subject to constant scrutiny: for example, the Royal College of Physicians' guidelines on high-quality care for long-stay patients (1992). Despite such guidelines, provision of services, including speech and language therapy, is very variable across the UK. Unfortunately there is no statutory responsibility for private nursing care provision to provide services such as rehabilitation at all, unlike the USA, where rehabilitation is a statutory requirement, backed up by adequate legislation. Thus many elderly mentally ill people, particularly those with dementia, will not have access to services such as speech and language therapy or at best will have limited access, for example, an assessment-only service. A further consequence of this situation is that health workers in the private sector do not have support and information from specialist services in dealing with difficult and stressful problems such as difficulty in communicating with residents.

Health care outcomes

A further issue is that of healthcare outcomes which are currently much in favour for measuring the effectiveness of healthcare and in planning and purchasing future services. However, a note of caution needs to be sounded for groups such as the elderly mentally ill. The complexity as well as the progressive nature of the disorder in these clients is such that measurement of outcome is difficult, with results being dependent upon many factors. Orchard (1994) stated that:

- outcomes are multidimensional;
- most outcomes are qualitative;
- assessments of outcomes will be affected by timing;
- subgroups of diseases may have differing outcomes;
- outcomes may not be attributable to specific treatments.

This can be illustrated by considering an example of a client admitted to a psychogeriatric unit. MR is an 82-year-old man who was found wandering in the street. His wife had died six months before this and he had never previously cooked, cleaned, etc. He had little or no contact with other people as his mobility was restricted by joint pain and urgency of micturition which caused him to avoid leaving the house. When admitted to hospital he was dehydrated and confused. Here the problems were multifaceted and treatment consisted of medical treatment for a bladder problem, rehabilitation to improve orientation, mobility and self-care skills and improvement in nutritional status. No one single factor could be said to have 'cured' him and the most significant outcomes were qualitative, in that he felt better and functional, and he was able to return home with a package of support from community-based services.

Audit of services for the elderly mentally ill is discussed in detail in Chapter 12.

Speech and language therapy provision

This book does not specifcally aim to inform therapists about how to 'do therapy' with this client group. Rather we focus on how the service is provided and what speech and language therapists do within this framework. We know that services vary tremendously (RCSLT, 1990) and this will naturally determine to a large extent the nature of the work performed by the therapist. Chapter 3 discusses the ways in which speech and language therapy services for the elderly with mental illness can be organised from a management perspective and considers matters such as how to set contracts and how to administer clear guidelines on issues such as patient compliance.

Much of the work described here focuses on information giving and training for carers and relatives of the elderly clients. The basis for speech and language therapy services for this client group in the UK appears to be diagnostic and information-giving/training based. Relatively few elderly clients with mental illness appear to receive 'traditional' one-to-one or small-group therapy (see Chapter 10 for further discussion). The current emphasis is on 'management' of the communication disorder rather than 'treatment' *per se*. Whether or not this is correct and whether or not there is a correct balance between therapy and management are continuing issues for debate within the speech and language therapy profession.

Particular aspects of the speech and language therapist's work are specifically highlighted. These are not intended to be exhaustive, but are aimed at emphasising the areas in which speech and language therapy can have a particularly important role, as well as providing a detailed description of the work currently being undertaken. Speech and language therapy has a particularly important role in changing care behaviour in nursing and residential homes and in enabling care assistants to achieve effective work practices in communication. Assessment is discussed in Chapter 9, Chapter 11 discusses working with carers and Chapters 6 and 7 examine service provision in the USA and the UK. Wherever possible client examples are given.

Specific therapy techniques or programmes can essentially be considered as falling into two categories:

- those that are applicable to other acquired neurogenic disorder client groups, for example therapy for dysphagia, dysarthria and functional communication. Here therapists have expertise from their experience with other neurogenic disorders although the way that this treatment is given might need to be adapted to the co-occuring problems that these clients may have, such as difficulty with short-term memory, reduced attention span and orientation problems.
- those therapies which are specific to this group. An example is the work with clients who have multi-infarct or vascular dementia, as described in Chapter 10.

An overview of the few treatment studies which are published is included in Chapter 3 along with a detailed description of how language and communication can break down in the psychiatric disorders associated with old age.

Social factors in ageing

In addition to medical models of psychiatric disorders in the elderly, there has been a recent move to consider these problems as psychosocial problems. In other words, to look at the psychological problems that arise from the illness and how these affect both elderly individuals with a psychiatric disorder and their carers (Miller and Morris, 1993). This allows the complexities of the deficits and people's reactions to them to be examined.

A specific example of such a theory is that provided by Kitwood

(1990) and called the Dialectal Model of the Dementing Process. Kitwood examines the relationship between neurological and social-psychological factors and looks at how the reaction of society to an elderly person who first shows signs of reduction in mental activity or efficiency contributes to the cycle of decline.

Psycho-social models of dementia have led to greater awareness of the strains that arise due to a dementing illness for both such clients and their carers (Morris, Morris and Britton, 1988; Rabins, Mace and Lucas, 1982). In addition the central role of the carer in 'community care' has led to awareness of the potential burden for the carer (Gerritsen and van der Ende, 1994) and the need to include education and sufficient support for the carer in the client's management plan.

The elderly population

As in other developed countries, the population in the UK is ageing. In addition the composition of the elderly population is changing, with increased numbers of over 75s and over 85s. In 1951:

- 10.9% of the population were over 65;
- 3.5 % were over 75 ;
- 0.5 % were over 85.

In 1991 it was estimated that:

- 15.8 of the population were over 65;
- 7% were over 75 ;
- 1.6% were over 85 (Henwood, 1992).

This represents a total of more than 13.5 million people over the age of 65, with the numbers expected to rise for the remainder of the century.

Where do the elderly live?

The numbers of places in residential care have also increased from 244 800 in 1970 to 498 300 in 1990 (Laing and Buisson, 1990). This needs to be put into perspective, though, as this number represents only 3.7% of the over-65 population. Therefore the vast majority of elderly people remain in their own homes. Given the closure of long-stay hositals in the 1990s, the proportion of elderly people remaining at home might be expected to rise still further in the near future.

What has changed within the residential care sector is the relative provision of the various sectors. In 1976 local authorities provided around 70% of all residential care. By 1986 local authorities were providing less than half of the total volume, whilst the private sector had increased its share to 40% of the market (Wistow and Henwood, 1991). Since 1986 these trends have become more marked.

What levels of care do the elderly need?

Studies which look at the levels of care needed by elderly people in residential care give differing results but generally indicate that levels of dependency are high. Pattie and Heaton's (1990) study in York showed that the following percentages of elderly people were classed as maximum dependency:

* 84% of those in hospital care;
* 22% of those in part III homes;
* 19% of those in private residential homes;
* 50% of those in private nursing homes.

Estimates of disability also vary according to factors such as sampling methods. The numbers of elderly women with disability are higher than those of men, but this is partly due to the larger numbers of women in the population. For example in the over 85s, 752 men per thousand are disabled whilst 852 women per thousand are disabled.

Of those living in private households, 37% of over 60s are classed as disabled and 32% of over 75s. Of these people, for the over 60s:

* 14% have communication problems;
* 13% have problems in intellectual functioning;
* 7% have eating problems.

For the over 75s:

* 20% have communication problems;
* 19% have problems in intellectual functioning;
* 3% have problems with eating.

For the elderly living in communal establishments (i.e. in care) of the over 60s:

* 52% present with communication problems;
* 68% have problems in intellectual functioning;
* 15% have problems with eating.

In the over 75s:

* 46% have communication problems;
* 67% have problems in intellectual functioning;

- 16% have problems with eating.

Details of these figures and breakdowns per population groups can be found in the OPCS survey of the prevalence of disability among adults (Martin, Meltzer and Elliot, 1988).

How does ageing affect communication?

Language changes associated with normal ageing are apparent in elderly people. These are normal features of ageing and need to be distinguished from pathological features of language. Maxim and Bryan (1994) give a detailed description of these changes including extensive linguistic analysis.

Attitudes to communicating with older people

Recent studies in sociolinguistics have shown that the way in which other people (i.e. younger ones) communicate with older people is in part responsible for the perceived 'deficits' in the language of the elderly (Coupland, Coupland and Giles, 1991). For example, when an older individual is perceived as having some diminished capacity such as a hearing loss then the younger adult may resort to simplified speech or baby talk. Older people may in turn perceive this as a reflection of their reduced status in relation to others. The value of communication to older people is frequently emphasised, with recognition of the need to ensure that the elderly have sufficient opportunities to experience communication and that carers and professionals are able to communicate effectively with their relative or client (Dreher, 1987; Gravell, 1988).

Communication within residential settings for the elderly is also being studied. Lubinski (1995) described the impoverished nature of communication in nursing homes and outlines the role for speech and language therapists in remediating this disability.

What uses do the elderly have for communication skills?

Studies have shown that the elderly watch on average over 30 hours of television a week with television consumption increasing up to the age of 70. They prefer programmes which provide information rather than pure entertainment. They also listen to, on average, two hours of radio a day with an emphasis on news and current affairs programmes (Nussbaum, Thompson and Robinson, 1989). The elderly are also reported as spending on average 80 minutes a day reading, although the time spent reading reduces with age. Within this decreasing time, the time spent on newspaper reading increases with age (McEnvoy and Vincent, 1980).

These studies are further evidence to support the notion that a wide range of communication skills are both preserved and utilised by the elderly. The value of communication to the elderly cannot be over-emphasised. Nussbaum, Thompson and Robinson (1989) state that, although successful ageing is a very complex phenonenom dependent upon many psychological factors, maintaining communication is of vital importance in achieving successful ageing.

Empowerment and the elderly

The concept of empowerment is complex and involves extending one's ability to take effective action on one's own behalf, but does not end there. Strategies might range from the provision of information about particular health services, through to democratic control of decision-making bodies (Meade and Carter, 1990).

Often the right of elderly people to retain some control over their lives is overlooked. Organisations and individuals who work with the elderly often find it easier to do things for them, rather than enabling them to be more independent and to make choices for themselves. This is partly due to stereotypical, ageist attitudes towards the elderly, where inactivity and illness are regarded as the dominant characteristics of older age. In fact, research confirms the continuing physical and mental competence of older people with potential for lifelong development (Muir Gray, 1988).

Initiatives such as health courses, health shops and health shows indicate that elderly people can develop a role for themselves in the planning of services and facilities (Meade and Carter, 1990). Professionals who are involved in initiating and directing health care services for the elderly need to ensure that the elderly themselves are properly represented in the decision-making process.

Methodological issues in research

Investigations into language functioning in the elderly can be difficult to organise, with considerable methodological problems. The older population is not heterogenous so that issues such as age range, gender, culture, education and environment need to be addressed in terms of planning research, but also in interpreting the results. For example, Holland (1990) asks 'what norms are appropriate for judging language-disordered patients in long-term residential units?'.

Approaches to research with the elderly involve a variety of methodologies. The traditional ones are:

* group studies;
* single case studies;
* longitudinal studies which allow language breakdown to be charted

over time in the same subjects;
- cross-sectional studies which sample a population, for example subjects with Alzheimer's disease at early, middle and advanced stages of the disease process

For therapy or intervention studies with the elderly, randomised control trials are widely accepted. Here groups of subjects with a particular disorder are randomly assigned to different treatment groups or control groups. This allows the value of different interventions to be proven and is widely accepted in medical research.

Treatment given to target populations allows the value of therapy interventions to be assessed and yields essential information about who will benefit from the intervention and under what circumstance. This is important information for prioritising of services. Other methodologies are now emerging.

Action research is a relatively new methodology which developed primarily in the social science field. The emphasis is on doing research under normal working conditions to inform and develop clinical practice (Hart and Bond, 1995). Action research can be:

- *experimental*: e.g. carrying out an intervention in two different environments;
- *organisational*: e.g. altering practices within a residential home;
- *empowering*: e.g. allowing clients to determine the services that they want;
- *professionalising*: e.g. study of multidisciplinary input to elderly people in the community or the evaluation of professional input into a setting such as a residential home.

The emphasis within action research is on working within the current situation and involving existing staff so that there is an emphasis on research implementation. The study of changing practices for speech and language therapists outlined in Chapter 8 is a good example of this type of research. The need for research implementation within the health service is widely recognised (Haines and Jones, 1994). It is therefore important that a variety of methodologies are accepted by all professionals and researchers, so that research is carried out and published which addresses the issues that are relevant to professionals such as speech and language therapists.

Conclusion

Many of the issues which are currently being debated in relation to health care generally are pertinent to health care provision specifically for the elderly mentally ill. Such elderly people are likely to have difficulties with language and/or communication. This in itself may lead to a deterioration in the quality of life for these people and for their carers. Speech and language therapy services are therefore an important constituent in health care provision for this group of clients. But such services have to be considered within the context of overall health care provision and resource allocation for the elderly mentally ill. The remaining chapters of this book explore the older mentally ill client group and the management of communication disabilities currently offered by speech and language therapy services. In many respects the services and practices described here represent examples of good practice which may not be representative of service provision in all parts of the UK, but these services are all provided within existing NHS resources.

Chapter 2:
Psychogeriatric Assessment And Management

BRYCE PITT

Introduction

Psychogeriatrics (the psychiatry of old age) has developed as a consequence of the remarkable ageing of the world through the 20th century. At first this phenomenon was confined to the more developed countries – North-west Europe, North America, Australasia – but it is now apparent in Southern Europe and the more prosperous Asian nations (Japan, Singapore), and the less developed countries are following suit; indeed, the greatest increase in the aged population in the next 25–50 years is expected in those countries (United Nations, 1979). The major factors are good public health and birth control.

In Britain in 1900 people over 65 formed 5% of the population; now they account for 16%. Over the next 20 years the younger old (65–75) will increase little, but the old old (85+) will increase by 40% (OPCS, 1987). Life expectancy for a male baby is now 75 years, and for a female almost 80 years. This is good news for those approaching retirement, but funding pensions presents governments with a problem. Further, old age can, of course, be accompanied by illness and infirmity, physical and mental, and the burden of care falls heavily on family carers and a not wholly willing state.

Britain pioneered specialist psychogeriatric services in the 1960s, and still leads the world in the scale and breadth of their provision: every health district in the country has at least one consultant in the specialty. This is attributable to the existence of a National Health Service.

Epidemiology

Epidemiological studies of psychiatric disorder in old people are important not only to point to possible causes but to measure the likely need for services. They enable service providers to know how common the various disorders are and who is most at risk: for example, dementia is more likely to be found among the octogenarian residents of an old

14

people's home than among the newly retired, depression among those who have been recently bereaved or have been taken ill than in those who still have their partners and are fit, alcoholism in old soldiers more than elderly nuns.

The most useful (and rarest, because they are costly and time-consuming) measure incidence and outcomes – how many new cases arise over a certain period and what becomes of them – by measuring morbidity in the same population on two separate occasions, with an interval of some years. Most, however, are cross-sectional prevalence studies, looking at how things are here and now. If one study is to be comparable with another then both need to be reaching the same population ('knocking on doors', though laborious, is more thorough than using electoral rolls or GPs' lists) including those who, because of infirmity, are no longer at home but in some form of institutional care. There needs to be agreement on the screening instruments to be used, and, having thus identified a possible case, on the criteria for diagnosing a case as such. Despite all these provisos, most epidemiological studies of psychiatric disorder in old age have reached rather similar conclusions.

It appears, then, that one in four people over the age of 65 (Kay et al., 1964) has some form of psychiatric disorder (usually mild). It is questionable that this is a higher morbidity than in younger people, but certainly dementia looms ever larger with increasing age: the prevalence has been estimated as doubling every five years over the age of 65 (Jorm, 1990). Ageing largely, but not exclusively, accounts for this. If one in five octogenarians has dementia, then four out of five do not have dementia, and the term 'senile dementia' is not wholly apt. Old people are much more liable to delirium when seriously ill than younger people (Lipowski, 1989), but, as this is a transitory disorder, it does not feature in community prevalence but is represented in hospital incidence studies.

Delirium and dementia are organic mental illnesses, arising from pathology of the brain, temporary or permanent. The major functional mental illness of later life, as in younger people, is depression. Some studies have found the least depression in older people (Regier et al., 1988), but this does not accord with the high first admission rate to psychiatric units in later life (Department of Health & Social Security, 1985), nor with the high suicide rate in older people, who, in Britain, account for 15% of the population and 25% of the suicides: a classic study of suicide in older people on the south coast (Barraclough, 1971) concluded that the great majority were suffering from depression.

Schizophrenia rarely arises in old age, except as the variant paraphrenia which afflicts about 1% of those over 65. However, there are many 'graduate' schizophrenics who have grown old with their illness, and, after not coping with their release from the mental hospital which had so long given them asylum, come the way of old-age psychiatry.

Anxiety states, it has been recently realised (Lindesay, Briggs and Murphy, 1989), are not a lot less common in older people than young; as many as 10% may be housebound by fear of falling. Overall, though, neurotic illnesses appear to decline with ageing, as do substance abuse and personality disorder – at least, as far as admissions to psychiatric wards are concerned. Alcohol abuse in late life – either continuing from earlier life or developing secondarily to loneliness or depression – is more likely to lead to admission to general hospital wards, because of accidents or such complications as neuritis and cirrhosis. Drug abuse in older people is rarely illicit, but may take the form of overuse of physician-prescribed hypnotics and tranquillisers. Personality disorder may arise from an intensification of introversion: the solitary becoming reclusive, the thrifty miserly, whilst hoarders may be submerged in the chaos known as Diogenes' syndrome (Clark et al., 1975).

Organic mental illnesses: delirium

The term 'organic' indicates that the mental illness is known to result from malfunction of the brain: from infection, intoxication, deficiency of oxygen and other vital substances, damage or deterioration. Delirium results from the first three of these factors. It afflicts about 15% of people over 65 admitted to general hospital wards, and another 10% during their stay (Rockwood, 1989). It is an acute syndrome of cognitive impairment, disturbances of thinking and comprehension, perceptual abnormalities, emotional and sometimes behavioural disturbance, developing over the course of hours or a couple of days, usually in association with physical illness.

The *cognitive* features include:

- disorientation for time, place and/or person;
- impairment of recent memory;
- 'clouding of consciousness' (generally reduced, but sometimes heightened alertness);
- inattention;
- speech and language impairment (dysarthria, dysphasia, disconnected words and phrases and occasional incoherence). Mistress Quickly remarked of the dying – and delirious – Falstaff that 'sometimes 'a babbled of green fields'.

Disturbances of *thinking* and *comprehension* include:

- *delusions*, often paranoid and based on misunderstanding of the situation, e.g. feeling imprisoned rather than in hospital.

Perceptual abnormalities are part of a state like a waking dream. They include:

- *hallucinations*, classically *visual* (insects, strange people, shadowy presences) but sometimes *auditory* (voices) or a sensation of being crawled over (*formication*);
- *distortions* of sounds, distances and time;
- *illusions* (misperceptions, e.g. seeing patterned curtains as swarming ants).

Emotional disturbances include:

- perplexity;
- anxiety;
- depression and euphoria;
- anger;
- apathy;
- lability: rapid changing from one of the above to another.

Behavioural disturbances include:

- *agitation and restlessness*;
- occasionally, *aggression*;
- *tremor*, plucking at the bedclothes;
- *somnolence* as part of reversal of the sleep–wake cycle.

All these signs and symptoms fluctuate considerably in the course of the day, and most are transitory, but tend to recur, until the delirium is over.

The older the patient, the sicker, the more sensorily impaired and cerebrally impaired, e.g. by dementia, stroke or Parkinson's disease, the greater the *risk* of delirium.

Common *causes* of delirium include:

- *infections*, e.g. pneumonia, urinary tract, cellulitis;
- *stroke* and *transient ischaemic attacks* (TIAs); *head injury* (old people are very likely to fall);
- *respiratory disease*(e.g. chronic obstructive airways disease)
- *heart disease*, e.g. myocardial infarction, heart failure, arrhythmias;
- *anaemia*, especially due to bleeding, e.g. from a duodenal ulcer;
- *drugs*, e.g. whatever was last prescribed!

The *diagnosis* of delirium is by:

- *the history* (which usually has to be obtained from someone who knows the patient, if available) of the illness from which the patient is likely to be suffering and of a confusional state of recent onset;

- the *physical signs* of illness (e.g. raised body temperature, rapid pulse and respiration, local signs), and the results of laboratory and radiological investigations;
- the *mental state*.

A popular instrument to assess the mental state is the Abbreviated Mental Test Score (AMTS) (Hodkinson, 1972). Subjects are asked:

- their *age*;
- the *time* (to the nearest hour);
- an *address* (e.g. '42 West Street, Bedford') to be repeated and *recalled* at the end of the test;
- the *current year*;
- the *name* of the hospital;
- to *recognise* two people, e.g. nurse and doctor;
- their *date of birth*;
- the *year* the First World War began;
- the *name of the present monarch*;
- to *count backwards* from 20 to one.

Each correct answer scores 1. Scores of less than 7 are suggestive of cognitive impairment (provided that the subject is cooperating). Geriatricians find the AMTS useful in monitoring cognition in delirium and dementia; in the throes of delirium the score may be 1 or 2, on recovery 9 or 10.

Differential diagnosis

Delirium resembles dementia in all respects except that:

- the onset is acute;
- the history is short; there is an underlying physical illness; consciousness is often 'clouded';
- there are fluctuations between derangement and normality.

Frequently, however, delirium complicates dementia. Without an informant the diagnosis may depend upon 'waiting and seeing'.

Mania may resemble delirium in the suddenness of its onset, the rambling, disconnected speech, the labile mood and restlessness. However, the state is more prolonged and sustained, without the fluctuations characteristic of delirium, there is no underlying physical cause, no 'clouding' of consciousness and there may well be a previous history of mood disorder.

Treatment and management

Most delirious patients need to be treated in a properly resourced general or geriatric hospital, in a ward appropriate for the underlying illness. Apart from specific treatment for this illness patients need:

- *fluids* – oral or intravenous;
- *nourishment* – nutritious, high-calorie drinks until a balanced oral diet can be taken;
- *elimination* – catheterisation and a gentle laxative or enema if need be;
- *information* – reality orientation keeps patients repeatedly informed about who and where they are and what is going on; clocks, calendars and photos may help;
- *reassurance* – 'you're ill, and it's made you a bit muddled, but we're giving you treatment and you're getting better';
- *rest* – plain, well-lit surroundings, ready access to nurses, quiet, physical comfort and a regular routine all help to allay anxiety and promote rest
- *sedation* – the last resort if agitation, restlessness and lack of sleep are causing exhaustion.

Prognosis

The presence of delirium worsens the outlook for whatever is its cause. In one study (Cameron et al, 1987) 65% of the delirious, compared with only 3% of those without delirium, died. In those who survive, though, recovery of normal mental function is to be expected, though it may take weeks, and occasionally some months.

Organic mental illnesses: dementia

Dementia is the terror of old age. 'O let me not be mad!' cried poor old King Lear. It is the most devastating disorder in late life, for both the sufferers and those who care for them. There are several syndromes and causes, but the main *functions* affected are *memory, orientation, intellectual grasp, communication and personality*. Secondary manifestations such as *behaviour disorder and depression, delusions and hallucinations* are not uncommon.

Memory

Memory impairment is an early feature which becomes increasingly disabling. Old, overlearned memories are the last to go, whilst recent and new information is poorly retained, if at all. Forgetting people's names, who calls when, what to buy and when to pay bills, when to turn the oven, heater and lights on or off and mislaying things are great inconveniences, which may for a while be offset by diaries, calendars, notepads and *aides-mémoire*. Forgetting the day, date, year, time, where one is and lives and with whom and loss of insight into the fading memory are major obstacles to independent living.

Disorientation

Orientation is usually first lost for *time*, then for *place* and finally, less commonly, for *person* – not knowing who others are (the old man at the other side of the fireplace is not recognised as the husband of 50 years' standing) or, rarely, who one is oneself.

Intellectual grasp

In dementia intellect dwindles in the wake of memory, and illogical conclusions may be drawn – e.g. asked the season, with snow driving against the windows, the patient replies: 'summer'. There is a lack of foresight, e.g. to go to the lavatory before a journey, take an umbrella if it is raining or take care if paths are icy.

Communication

Difficulty in finding words is an early feature, whilst *problems with reading, writing, comprehension and verbal expression* come later, often accompanied by difficulties in recognition, e.g. that the face in a mirror is one's own, or the picture in a frame is not real (agnosia), and integrating movements, e.g. for the purpose of eating or dressing (apraxia).

Personality change

The commonest personality change is towards a self-protective withdrawal from potentially challenging social contact with others. Some (perhaps most) people with dementia, half-recognising their disability, become more mellow, compliant and willingly dependent than they were. Others (much more common among the clientele of the old-age psychiatrist!) are *difficult*, denying that they have any problem, obstinate and obstructive; disinhibited, making embarrassing remarks, sometimes stripping inappropriately or stealing in shops, verbally and sometimes physically aggressive; or apathetic, slovenly, unwilling to wash or change clothes.

Behaviour disorder

Troublesome forms of behaviour include:

- *wandering*, which may lead to the person becoming lost and being in serious danger of assault, exposure or being run over. Patients may wander because they are bored, restless, uncomfortable, used to taking a walk, seeking shops or a former home;
- *incontinence* of urine and/or faeces may arise because of lack of foresight, inability to find or recognise the lavatory, urgency or frequency because of infection (perhaps related to poor hygiene), constipation, apathy or loss of cerebral cortical control;
- *nocturnal restlessness*, 'day–night reversal', because of too little to do by day, loss of sense of time;
- *dangerous carelessness* with cookers, fires, gas, electrical equipment, or if driving.

Secondary psychiatric symptoms

- *Depression* commonly accompanies early dementia.
- *Paranoid delusions* are common in moderate dementia, e.g. blaming others for stealing what one has lost.
- *Visual hallucinations*, e.g. children (who may have to be fed!), strange-looking intruders, or tiny people off the television screen, are most common towards night.

Syndromes and their causes

Dementia after the age of 65 used to be called senile, with the implication that it was an inevitable consequence of 'not ageing well'. However, for more than 20 years it has been recognised that the brain pathology in the commonest form of dementia in old age is the same as that of the pre-senile dementia described by Alzheimer in 1907; it is characterised by shrinkage of the cortex of the brain, enlargement of the ventricles and, at the microscopic level, amyloid plaques which destroy nerve cells and neurofibrillary tangles which disrupt axons, and is commonly known as *Senile Dementia of the Alzheimer Type* (SDAT). Risk factors include:

- *age* (Jorm, 1990);
- a *family history* (especially in pre-senile Alzheimer's);
- the *apolipoprotein E4 allele* (especially in SDAT) (Hardy et al., 1993);
- *serious head injury* (Amaducci and Lippi, 1994);
- *Down's syndrome* (associated with an extra chromosome 21);
- possibly, *high levels of aluminium in drinking water* (Candy et al., 1986);
- possibly, being a *non-smoker* (though smoking kills many people before they reach the age at which they might get Alzheimer's.

The course may be rapid or slow, from 2 to 20 years, with an average of

10. Decline is pretty inexorable, though there are occasional 'plateaux' for up to a year. Incoherence, inaccessiblity, instability of gait and extreme helplessness are the final features, and death is commonly from pneumonia. The only specific treatment is with oral anticholinesterases, such as Tacrine (Chatellier and Lacomblez, 1990), which hold back deterioration for perhaps a year. Tacrine acts on the central cholinergic system, which is compromised in Alzheimer's, but causes nausea and is sometimes toxic to the liver. It is not yet licensed in the UK. Much research is now focused on preventing the laying down of amyloid by the amyloid precursor protein (Goate et al 1991).

The second most common late-life dementia is probably *vascular, or multi-infarct dementia* (MID). This typically has a more episodic course; a succession of small strokes and transient ischaemic attacks cause 'stepladder deterioration', rather than a smooth decline. *Good preservation of the personality* at first, a greater tendency to *depression, earlier speech and language problems, earlier neurological signs* and complaints of *headache, dizziness* and the occurrence of *fits* all help to differentiate MID from Alzheimer's disease. Risk factors include hypertension, smoking, diabetes, hyperlipidaemia, obesity, peripheral vascular disease and being male: all save the last are potentially remediable. Many of these features are incorporated in the Hachinski scale, based on history and clinical examination (Hachinski et al., 1975), which was designed to help differentiate the two major dementias. The task is not easy, however, not least because Alzheimer's and vascular dementia may occur together. Aspirin daily, in low dosage, helps to prevent the small infarctions whereby the disease progresses.

Rivalling MID for second place in the late-life dementias is the recently recognised *Lewy body disease* (LBD) (Perry et al., 1989). Lewy bodies abound in the basal ganglia of those who suffer from Parkinson's disease, but in this dementia they are found in the cortex of the brain. Dementia may follow the development of Parkinson's disease (as in Steele Richardson Olszewski syndrome), but in Lewy body disease dementia – in some ways like a prolonged, subacute delirium – precedes any signs of the movement disorder. LBD runs a swift course to demise and is characterised by an excess of adverse reactions to neuroleptic drugs such as haloperidol.

Other dementias, rarer in later life, include:

- *Pick's disease*, which at first affects the frontal lobes, causing a personality change before memory or intellectual loss;
- *Huntington's chorea*, a hereditary combination of a moderate dementia with a severe movement disorder;
- *alcoholic dementia*, as well as a specific memory disorder, *Korsakoff's syndrome* (following *Wernicke's encephalopathy*, due to

acute thiamine deficiency) in which there is allegedly a pure memory disorder, with extreme confabulation;
- *semantic dementia*, in which dysphasia is followed by dementia;
- *dementia pugilistica*, the ultimate fate of too many boxers;
- *traumatic dementia*, following severe head injury;
- *Creutzfeld-Jakob disease*, a spongy encephalopathy (like the notorious bovine spongy encephalopathy, or BSE, in cattle), possibly attributable to the action of a variant of a virus called a prion in those with hereditary susceptibility;
- *AIDS dementia*, or *HIV encephalopathy*;
- *syphilitic dementia* (which used to account for one in 20 admissions to psychiatric wards).

Most dementias are as yet irreversible. The few *reversible* causes include:

- benign *brain tumours*, e.g. *meningiomas*;
- *subdural haematoma* ('a clot on the brain') following head injury;
- *hydrocephalus*, often following head injury or subarachnoid haemorrhage, suggested by the onset of dementia, incontinence and unsteady gait, and sometimes remediable by a shunt carrying cerebrospinal fluid to a large vein or the peritoneal cavity in the abdomen;
- possibly *hypothyroidism*, as one manifestation of 'myxodematous madness' (Asher, 1949).

Differential diagnosis

The *differential diagnosis* of dementia is by:
- the *history*, from the patient in the early stages, from others later, of gradual cognitive decline, usually starting with memory failure;
- the *mental state*, including a cognitive test such as the AMTS (Hodkinson, 1972) or the Mini Mental State Examination (MMSE) (Folstein, Folstein and McHugh, 1975). This very popular test, known internationally, includes five questions on orientation in time, five on orientation in place, the registration and recall of three words, taking seven away from 100 five times or spelling 'WORLD' backwards, repeating 'no ifs, ands or buts', naming a pencil and watch, obeying verbal and written instructions, writing a sentence and copying a design of interlocking pentagons. A score of less than 24/30 suggests significant cognitive impairment, though allowances should be made for the patient's likely intelligence, education and cooperation. A sometimes revealing complementary test requires the patient to draw a clock (Shulman, Shedletski and Silver, 1986). The ability to draw a circle, place the numbers and set the hands at a particular time are all

noted. It has been found (Stevens et al., 1992) that in early dementia the Boston Naming Test (BNT) (Kaplan, Goodglass and Weintraub, 1983) may be a more sensitive 'screen' than the MMSE;

- *physical examination and laboratory investigations*, e.g. to identify raised blood pressure, anaemia, cardiological (such as arrhythmias) and endocrinological abnormalities (such as diabetes or hypothyroldism), neurological signs (such as homonymous hemianopia, increased muscle tone and extensor plantar reflexes in MID) or malignant disease, or to exclude all of these in the diagnosis of Alzheimer's disease;
- *imaging, with computerised axial tomography (CT) or magnetic resonance* (MRI), to demonstrate focal abnormalities such as infarcts or tumours, or cortical atrophy and ventricular enlargement;
- *the state of living*, including appraisal at home, the activities of daily life and social circumstances;
- *time and review*: what is unclear now will become more obvious after some months.

The main disorders from which dementia must be distinguished are:

- *delirium* (see above);
- *depression*: depressed older people commonly complain of a bad memory which, on testing, is no worse than that of others of their age; being depressed they conclude the worst from memory lapses which are quite normal. Severely depressed older people, however, may show 'pseudodementia' (see below);
- *other mental illness*, e.g. schizophrenia: schizophrenia rarely arises in old age except in the form of paraphrenia (see below) which is unlike dementia. Large numbers of patients with chronic schizophrenia, however, have now left hospital without necessarily having fully recovered, and where they neglect themselves, talk to themselves or show thought disorder they may appear to be demented. However, their behaviour shows that they are correctly orientated in place, and their condition does not progress;
- *communication disorders*, e.g. deafness, dysarthria, dysphasia, dyslexia and being foreign to the language;
- people with *learning difficulties*, who may find it hard to cope when their elderly parents die. Again, the disorder is not progressive – unless dementia complicates the picture, as in the susceptibility of those with Down's syndrome to Alzheimer's;
- those of a *waggish disposition* who don't take cognitive testing seriously!

Treatment and management

The management of dementia where there is a significant informal (usually family) key carer differs somewhat from where there is none. If there are any specific treatments, such as thyroxine for hypothyroidism, a shunt for hydrocephalus, neurosurgery for brain tumours and subdural haematoma, Tacrine for some people with early Alzheimer's, they may be given, but certain general principles most often apply:

- *early identification* (e.g. by screening the 'over 75' population with the AMTS);
- *assessment*, initially at home, by the GP and the specialist pschogeriatric multidisciplinary team (psychiatrist, psychologist, social worker, occupational, speech/language and physiotherapist, community psychogeriatric nurse);
- matching a *key worker* in the team to a *key carer* (if any);
- *supporting* patient and carer by regular visiting, social services (meals on wheels, home help, attendance allowance, information – much is available from the Alzheimer's Disease Society, carers' groups, day centres and hospitals, respite admissions to hospital or Homes;
- involving the patient in *plans for future care*, e.g. making an enduring power of attorney, so that a trusted relative or friend can take over financial affairs when and if necessary;
- *rehabilitation* by occupational, speech/language or physiotherapy where appropriate, and *environmental aids* such as wall calendars, *aides-mémoire*, simplifying the use of the telephone, cooker, central heating, etc.;
- *psychological approaches*: *reality orientation therapy* aims to correct the patients' orientation by giving 'bites' of information repeatedly; *reminiscence therapy* informs them of who they are by reminding them who they were; *validation therapy* validates their feelings (e.g. about being a parent) without correcting their wrong ideas that they have to provide for their children;
- *pharmacological approaches*, e.g. sedation (possibly benzodiazepines or thioridazine) for the restless, tranquillisers (such as haloperidol for the paranoid and aggressive, hypnotics (e.g. temazepam or chlormethiazole) for those who are up all night, antidepressants (lofepramine, paroxetine, perhaps) for the depressed: all carry the risk of side-effects, none can be counted upon to be always effective, but they have a place in relieving distress in patients and those who care for them;
- *'tender, loving care'* to provide patients with nourishment, warmth, clothing, activity and entertainment so that they may live as full and satisfying lives as possible;
- *institutional care* if and when the patient's and/or carers' welfare demands it, in *sheltered housing, residential or nursing home, or hospital*, according to need.

Two final points need to be made:

- Some old people with dementia are exceedingly reluctant to accept the help that they clearly need. Even though they may come to some grief in consequence (old people with dementia are over-represented in general hospital wards because of self-neglect and foreseeable accidents) coercion is as a rule inapplicable, and persuasion, often repeated, by someone who has made a good relationship with the old person is the better approach. The balance of 'rights versus risks' is especially tricky in elderly people with moderate dementia living alone at home.
- Caring for an elderly person with dementia, though often undertaken willingly, is stressful and, at worst, can cause the carer to become ill or the old person to be abused. There may at times be conflict between what the carer and the demented old person – or one carer and another – want.

These difficulties are frequently best addressed by a case conference, often convened by the case manager (social worker) and attended by all the relevant members of the primary and specialist health care team, social services, concerned members of the family, friends and neighbours and, where possible, the patient.

Prognosis

The natural history of dementia is worsening cognition, affecting all functions, and physical deterioration over the course of months (for example, Creutzfeld-Jakob disease) or many years (some cases of Alzheimer's). The course tends to be most rapid in the early onset dementias, with severe reduction in life expectancy. The decline may be steady (most cases of Alzheimer's) or irregular (vascular dementia).

Patients who live alone, without significant care from family or friends, are more likely to die or be admitted to hospital or Homes than those who have carers. Interestingly, providing extra care for those 'home alone' may increase their chances of going into a Home (O'Connor et al., 1991).

Functional mental illnesses: depression

'Functional' here means that there is no known brain disorder to account for the mental illness – though research might find one tomorrow! Depression, to a relatively minor degree, is a universal human experience, as both a normal emotional reaction to loss and an attack, for no obvious reason, of 'the blues'. There is circumstantial evidence, however, that severe depression is associated with depletion of monoamine neurotransmitters, and it only responds to medical or physical treatment.

A problem for old people who suffer from depressive illness in silence, and for doctors and others who fail to diagnose it, is that it may appear to be justified. To the young, the very fact of being old seems to explain depression, whilst the old may not feel entitled to take such a problem to the doctor. They will be 'wasting his time', told to 'snap out of it', or worse still their fears that they are 'going senile' or 'mad' will be confirmed.

Doctors can diagnose depression if put to the test (Macdonald, 1986) but tend not to do so, or not to do much about it if they do! Depression is often associated with physical illness, which may seem sufficient to account for it although many other older patients, likewise afflicted, are not depressed. Depression related to bereavement (a common event in later life, especially for women) may likewise be deemed justified, and consequently (though not very logically!) not be treated.

There may be worries about the efficacy and safety of treatment. 'May not antidepressants, with their slow action (if any) be a cure worse than the disease?' 'Are psychological therapies (supposing they were available) applicable if you can't teach an old dog new tricks?'

Perhaps the seriousness of depression is not appreciated: it carries a high mortality (Murphy et al., 1988), partly because *suicide* – old people form 15% of the population, and 25% of those who take their lives, generally because they are suffering unrecognised severe depression (Barraclough, 1971) – and partly because they fail to eat and drink, or 'give up' if they become physically ill. Those who do not die may still have their final years unnecessarily blighted, whilst their carers suffer considerable strain: living with someone who is 'helpless and hopeless', or filled with 'gloom and doom', is not easy.

Symptoms

Psychological

- *self-doubt, self-reproach, inability to converse, indecision*;
- *impaired concentration and memory, pessimism*;
- regrets;
- life seems *pointless*;
- *delusions of guilt and poverty* ('I'm the wickedest person in the world'; 'I'm infectious!'; 'I deserve to be shot!'; 'I'm ruined!').

Mood

- *gloom, despondency, misery, despair*;
- *irritability*;

- *anhedonia* (inability to enjoy anything);
- *hypochondriasis*;
- feeling *suicidal*;
- *variation* – feeling worse at the beginning (typically) or end of the day, or having good and bad days;
- *loss of feeling* – including affection.

Physiological
- *anorexia* and *weight loss*;
- *exhaustion*;
- *insomnia* – early or late ;
- *loss of sexual drive*;
- *aches and pains*.

Behavioural
- *agitation*;
- *retardation*;
- social *withdrawal*;
- *not drinking*;
- *not eating*;
- *deliberate self-harm*.

Syndromes

Depressive illness may be mild, moderate or severe; predominantly agitated or retarded ('worked up' or 'slowed up'); psychotic (with delusions) or neurotic (with prominent irritability, feeling worse at the end of the day and varying from day to day); *bipolar* (with episodes of mania) or *unipolar* (recurrences of depression only); or *masked* (by denial of feeling depressed, and a smiling face). When severe retardation or retardation predominate, there may be *pseudo-dementia*.

Causes

The *losses* of later life – physical illness and infirmity, bereavement, reduction of income, companions, mobility and life expectancy – appear to be the main *precipitants* of depression in old age.

Predisposing factors include *family* and *previous history of depression, loss of the mother at an early age*, an *obsessional* (inflexible, meticulous) *personality, marital strife* and other situations arousing anger which cannot readily be expressed.

Diagnosis

Depression or loss of enjoyment and four of the other symptoms listed above should have been consistently present for more than two weeks. Useful screening instruments for depression in later life are the *Geriatric Depression Scale* (GDS, with 15 questions to be answered 'Yes' or 'No') (Yesavage et al.,1983) and the Brief Assessment Schedule Depression Cards (BASDEC – 19 items to be declared 'True' or 'False') (Adshead, Day Cody Pitt, 1992).

Differential diagnosis

Anxiety states share with depression apprehension, hypochondriasis and sleep disturbance, but not loss of interests or the will to live: the anxious person fears the worst, the depressed feels that it has happened! Anxiety and depression, however, are often mixed. Some people are *always rather miserable*. To diagnose depression it is necessary to show that the patient used to function at a better, more optimistic level.

Pseudodementia differs from true dementia in that:

* *the history is of weeks or months* rather than years;
* the dementia is *never more than moderate*;
* *on cognitive testing*, failures are because of 'don't know 'rather than erroneous answers;
* *performance* on such testing is *worse than in real life*; e.g. if admitted to hospital, patients soon learn their way about;
* there is no *confabulation* (making up a story to fill a memory gap) or *dysphasia*;
* there may be a *previous history of depression*;
* *time and antidepressant treatment* are likely to effect a cure.

Physical illnesses, such as thyroid disease, Parkinson's and cancer, can cause debility (including weight loss and sleep disturbance) and lassitude. Hopelessness, self-criticism and sustained misery are not characteristic of purely physical illness, and if present suggest that the patient is depressed, or, of course, both depressed and physically ill.

Treatment

Simply to *recognise* depression helps its treatment. Putting a label on the disorder helps by defining its limits and prospects with treatment, and, perhaps, reducing self-blame; no one is at fault for getting depressed.

Mild depression is likely to pass in a month or less, but if it does not, *psychological* and *social* approaches are best. *Psychological* approaches are popular with patients, not least because they offer personal support. However, they take the time of trained therapists, and require commitment by the patient. Nor are they universally available, even though any trained person in a multidisciplinary team, not just the doctors, may undertake them. The commonest psychological approach is *counselling*. Increasingly, GPs have counsellors in their practices. Ideally counselling provides:

- sympathetic listening;
- helpful comments and questions to determine what is now relevant:
- encouragement and reassurance – that the depression is likely to lift, that treatments will help, that the case is far from hopeless;
- help to face any important decisions and dilemmas and to try to solve them;
- prompting to do something, even if only to make a phone call, write a letter, or go for a walk;
- advice about taking exercise, eating enough and not drinking too much alcohol.

For more intractable problems, *psychodynamic* approaches (ultimately derived from Freud, and taking account of unconscious mental processes such as unacknowledged aggression) may be appropriate, in the form of individual (one-to-one) psychotherapy, marital therapy, family and group therapy.

Where low self-esteem is especially prominent (though not of delusional intensity) *cognitive behaviour therapy* is especially helpful, in painstakingly and supportively challenging patients' self-condemnation.

Social measures include support by family, friends, neighbours, priests and other carers, informal or formal, suitably briefed; practical help with problems which may be contributing to the depression, such as bills, tax returns, housing, health care; personal services, where appropriate, such as meals on wheels, home helps; lunch clubs and day centres.

Pharmacological approaches, usually with antidepressive drugs, are indicated if the depression is moderate or severe. Antidepressives may work by increasing the availability of monoamine neurotransmitters at nerve synapses – particularly noradrenaline and serotonin. All are equally effective (though some work better for certain individuals than others), none is addictive, and all take a week or more to work.

- The *old tricyclics* (imipramine, amitriptyline, dothiepin) have anticholinergic side-effects such as dry mouth, difficulty in passing water, constipation, blurring of vision and sweating. They may cause hypotension and falls, and may be cardiotoxic. They are dangerous in overdosage – but well established and cheap.
- The *newer tricyclics* (lofepramine) have fewer side-effects, are safer, and cost rather more.

- *Monoamine oxidase inhibitors (MAOIs)* sometimes work where other antidepressives do not, but have the disadvantage that foods rich in tyramine (cheese, for example) may cause a dangerous rise in blood pressure, indicated by a very severe occipital headache and sometimes leading to fatal cerebral haemorrhage. They are also incompatible with certain other drugs, e.g. cold cures. They may also cause severe hypotension. However, with due dietary precautions patients who need these drugs are usually able to take them.
- *Serotonin specific reuptake inhibitors (SSRIs)* have had much public exposure because of the media attention to fluoxetine, better known as Prozac. It is doubtful whether Prozac is any more of a 'wonder drug' than other antidepressives, but at least it has made the public aware that antidepressives work.
- Newer drugs still include a *monoamine oxidase A inhibitor* (less likely to produce the 'cheese' reaction) and a *serotonin and noradrenaline reuptake inhibitor*.

Other drugs used in the treatment of depression include:

- *lithium carbonate*, which may augment the action of antidepressives or reduce the frequency and severity of relapses, especially in bipolar (manic) depression (see below). Blood levels of lithium must be monitored, as the difference between a therapeutic and a toxic dose is not great, and varies from one person to another;
- *benzodiazepines* may be of use in the short term, to allay anxiety and improve sleep until the antidepressive has had time to work. However, the more sedative antidepressives (e.g. amitriptyline) can often achieve this effect. Care must be taken if benzodiazepines are used for more than a month as they may be habit-forming;
- *antipsychotics* (e.g. trifluoperazine, haloperidol) may be used for psychotic symptoms such as delusions and hallucinations ('I can hear everyone saying that I'm not fit to live'), though usually these respond to antidepressives or ECT.

Electro-convulsive therapy (ECT) has, undeservedly, a terrible name, but is an invaluable treatment for the severely depressed. It relieves the agony of the worst depression (than which no other illness is more terrible) within a week or two, and saves lives. Those who campaign against it exaggerate its ill-effects (which are few and small) and have no notion of the dreadfulness of severe depression: the 'risk–benefit ratio' hugely favours the treatment. It was discovered serendipitously and we still cannot fully explain how it works – which by no means invalidates it: it was centuries before the efficacy of 'foxglove tea' in heart failure was explained by a full understanding of the key ingredient, digitalis.

The patient is anaesthetised and an electric current is passed across the temples for a split second, sufficient to cause a fit – the outward signs of which are reduced to a minimum by giving a musle relaxant with the anaesthetic. The patient recovers within half an hour and is able to continue normal daily activities. A course of treatments – usually four to 16 – is given, at a rate of two treatments per week. It is exceedingly safe, and though there may be memory impairment for some weeks, in practice the lifting of the depression more often greatly *improves* memory.

The great majority of depressed patients never need ECT, but it is indispensable for those who do. It does not prevent later episodes of depression – lithium carbonate or continuing antidepressive therapy are better for that purpose but it frequently cuts the presenting illness short.

Settings of treatment

Most patients with depression are treated at home, with visits to the GP or from a practice or community psychiatric nurse, or at out-patient clinics or day hospitals. If the patient is already in a general hospital ward, treatment is given there, with advice given by a liaison consultation from a psychiatrist. Treatment by a psychiatrist is also indicated if the GP's first-line treatments have not worked, if the patient is significantly incapacitated or agitated or retarded, not eating or drinking enough, suicidal or psychotic. Under the latter circumstances admission to a psychiatric ward is indicated occasionally under compulsion (the Mental Health Act) if the illness is severe and/or it endangers the patient: sometimes patients refuse the help they desperately need – because the illness affects their insight: 'I don't need treatment – I need to be put down!'

Prognosis

Depression tends to get better but does sometimes relapse. The milder the depression, the less this matters, though even mild depression spoils the declining years. Sometimes the depression does not lift ('refractory depression') and taxes therapeutic resources to the full. Depression carries an increased mortality – through self-neglect, as well as suicide – at all ages. This mortality is highest in old people, but as regards chronicity and relapse may be no worse than in younger people. It is still well worth identifying and treating.

Functional mental illness: mania

Mania is always associated with depression, but depression is not necessarily associated with mania. It is much the rarer mood disorder. In mania the mood is elevated to the point of euphoria and the patient is garrulous, disinhibited and overactive. Usually the illness starts in young adulthood (often, in women, after giving birth) but it may begin in old age, with or without a previous history of depression. It may be precipitated by a life event such as (paradoxically) a bereavement, or by brain damage – stroke or head injury. The classic picture of being 'madly jolly' is modified in old age,when 'miserable mania' (a mixture of depression with mania, causing irritability or peevish circumstantiality) is common.

The treatment is mainly with medication (haloperidol, lithium) sometimes under compulsion. The outlook for remission of the present episode is good, but poor for relapse within a year or less.

Functional mental illness: anxiety states

Only recently has it been realised that anxiety states are almost as common in older people as in young. The main reason why they were not identified previously was because the right questions were not asked! The commonest form is *agoraphobia* (Lindesay, 1991) causing the sufferer to be housebound. Of course, there may be other reasons for an older person to be housebound, such as reduced mobility and effort tolerance, from arthritis, angina or heart failure, but it appears that the disability is often more psychological than physical. Fears of falling, after an episode of dizziness or giddiness and (especially in inner cities) of being 'mugged' often rationalise the agoraphobia.

It must be said that as yet studies of how best to treat such anxiety states are lacking. As they usually last for years, medication with, say, benzodiazepine tranquillisers is unlikely to be helpful. It may reduce anxiety for a while, but that alone is unlikely to make the patient go out and about, and benzodiazepine dependency may well be induced. Probably graded excursions from a day hospital with, say, an appropriately trained physiotherapist have most to offer.

Functional mental illness: paraphrenia and schizophrenia

Schizophrenia is essentially an illness which begins in late adolescence or early adulthood, but may persist throughout life. 'Graduate' schizophrenics – who have retained some symptoms past the age of 65 – are coming increasingly to old-age psychiatry as the asylums close and patients' links with their former mental health teams loosen after their discharge to hostels, group homes or residential homes. For the most part the symptoms are not *florid* – having delusions or hearing voices – but *'negative'* – being apathetic, indolent, unemotional, solitary, eccentric and poorly motivated to look after themselves or their personal hygiene.

When schizophrenia presents for the first time in later life it usually takes the form of *paraphrenia*: a paranoid psychosis in which the patient – typically female, alone, hard of hearing and somewhat eccentric but without a history of frank mental illness – believes that her neighbours are spying on and talking about her in a scurrilous manner. They may be spying through holes in the wall or ceiling or by hidden television cameras and microphones, and may address the patient through hidden loudspeakers. They may be running a machine shop, stealing the patient's electricity, engaged in drug traffic or prostitution, or blow noxious gases into the dwelling. Patients may therefore insulate their walls and ceiling, have many bolts and locks, complain to the police or threaten their supposed persecutors, verbally or physically. Those accused may respond with resentment and indignation, and the situation may escalate.

Happily, paraphrenia is very treatable with antipsychotic drugs such as trifluoperazine (Stelazine) or sulpiride. The main obstacle is lack of compliance and insight: 'Why treat me? Treat them!' Much persuasion, and sometimes compulsion, is needed. Depot drugs such as flupenthixol (Depixol), which are given in an oily solution by intramuscular injection and can act for several weeks, often administered by a community psychiatric nurse, are useful aids to compliance, but carry the risk of extrapyramidal (Parkinsonian) side-effects and tardive orofacial dyskinesia – a delayed, largely irreversible neurological consequence of supersensitive dopamine receptors, causing grimacing, repetitive involuntary movements of face and tongue and, at worst, dysarthria and dysphagia. Reasoning and relocation, alas, rarely work.

Substance abuse: alcohol

Serious alcoholics are unlikely to survive into old age, but some do. Some people take to drink in old age, perhaps following bereavement or secondarily to depression from some other cause. Alcohol abuse in late life is very likely to lead to accidents, especially falls, and is associated with cirrhosis of the liver, oesophageal varices (which may bleed catastrophically) and peripheral neuropathy. It is also an important cause of states of confusion – *delirium and dementia*.

At all ages it is hard to treat the alcoholic who does not want to stop drinking. In old age, however, the drinker may depend upon others to get his drink for him. (The problem, incidentally, is not found exclusively in men!) It is remarkable how often carers who shake their heads over the drink are those who bring it in! Ambivalence is all too plain: 'Poor old chap, it's a shame to deprive him'/'It's terrible! He's drinking himself to death!'

It may help to provide support, counselling and medication to combat the underlying loneliness and depression, but very often the only answer is to cut off the supply. Not infrequently a move into the relatively secure environment of an old people's home, where some company and supervision are available, solves the problem.

Substance abuse: benzodiazepines

Old people often do not sleep long at night, though instead they catnap by day. To lie awake when trying to get to sleep, or to wake up in the small hours, is distressing and tedious, so many elderly 'insomniacs' seek a hypnotic, and, strangely, their doctors seem much more ready to prescribe a benzodiazepine sleeping tablet than the same, or a very similar, drug as a tranquilliser. Such drugs carry the risk of 'hangover' and accident-proneness far into the next day, and their effectiveness as sleeping tablets tends to wear off after three weeks. They may also cause quite marked memory lapses. Ideally, older people should be told that it is normal to sleep for fewer hours at night. A comfortable bed, warmth, quiet and an empty bladder all help sleep. It is a good idea to put any wakeful hours to some practical use – sewing or ironing or doing accounts or writing memoirs – or recreational use – reading, listening to music, watching late-night television or videos, and count on catching up on sleep by day. One old lady complained of 'early morning waking': she went to bed at 7 p.m., and woke at 10 a.m., but it was too early for her: her problem was, of course, depression.

Personality and behaviour disorders

People with psychopathic personalities lead such self-destructive lives that they may not survive into later life, or may be in prison rather than the community at large. Older people are not very delinquent, though they are occasionally charged with shoplifting or sexual misdemeanours for which there may be a psychiatric explanation such as dementia or mood disorder. It is said that with ageing people become 'more like themselves', but this seems to be truer of introvert than extrovert traits.

Those who are of a suspicious, litigious nature may become more frankly paranoid, the cautious and thrifty miserly, worriers about their health more overtly and less rationally hypochondriacal, the shy and solitary reclusive. A condition known either as the *senile squalor syndrome* or *Diogenes syndrome* is characterised by living rather blandly in extreme clutter and filth: typically there are no other signs of mental illness, though careful appraisal may identify the negative symptoms of schizophrenia, a frontal lobe dementia, substance abuse or low-grade depression.

Occasionally a formerly competent person, alone and lacking a self-justifying occupation, becomes clamorously dependent, exhausting the patience of friends, neighbours, families and doctors and other professional carers by excessive, insistent and ultimately alienating demands for instant care, cure and attention, frequently by telephone. It is sometimes helpful for a senior member of the multidisciplinary team to make a contract with such a person to meet regularly on condition that there are no calls at other times.

Conclusion

Psychiatric illness is so common in old age that all who work with older people must often meet it. Confusion, due to dementia or delirium, depression and anxiety are especially common and need to be reckoned with in management and treatment plans. Cure is sometimes possible, and it always helps to identify, and often to quantify disability – so that it is neither overlooked nor exaggerated. Old-age psychiatry services provide useful back-up, but could not begin to cope with all the morbidity. Other health care professionals, including speech and language therapists, are therefore vital agents in the recognition and care of old people with mental disorder.

Chapter 3:
Language, Cognition and Communication in Older Mentally Ill People

JANE MAXIM AND KAREN BRYAN

Introduction

A *British Medical Journal* editorial in April 1995 (Orrell and Sahakian, 1995) discussed the evidence for the 'use it or lose it' hypothesis of cognitive function and skill in old age. If we remain mentally active, does this activity help to maintain cognitive function? Several studies have concluded that education may reduce the risk of dementia (Jorm, 1990; Ott et al., 1995). The mechanisms for this protection are not clear: better premorbid intellect may indicate greater neural reserves or education might improve the ability of neuronal networks to compensate. Whatever the reason, findings from studies of learning in normal ageing are positive enough to suggest that rigorous research into maintenance and enhancement of cognitive functions in the dementias is necessary (Yesavage, 1985) and a growing body of work in this area points to possible methods of intervention.

Another BMJ editorial (July 1993) suggested that distinguishing cortical from subcortical dementia was worthwhile because treatment with dopamine agonists and levadopa might be of benefit for patients other than those with Parkinsonian symptoms. The same argument is true in the management of communication disability in the dementias. It is worthwhile differentiating cortical from subcortical dementia but it is also worthwhile trying to differentiate within the cortical dementias because research is already producing different descriptions of breakdown and retained skills within these dementias which might lead to more effective management. Whilst most speech and language therapy services do not at present have the resources to provide individual treatment programmes for clients within this group, indirect intervention may be most usefully targeted when the medical diagnosis is based on a thorough evaluation of the symptomatology.

37

This chapter will look at language function, significant cognitive parameters of language, communication disability in specific dementias and also discuss possible interventions. The only major cause of dementia not covered here is multi-infarct dementia which is discussed separately in Chapter 10. The dementias are an area of active research at present and some of the work on dementia typology reviewed here is very topical. Research on interventions, on the other hand, is proceeding more slowly. Whereas, even a few years ago, undifferentiated groups of older people with dementia were being used in research studies looking at the disease process and deficits, the same is now true of intervention studies which rarely define their population precisely. This does not invalidate their often very useful findings but it does mean that there is much further work to be done.

Why is an accurate diagnosis necessary? First, there are causes of progressive cognitive and language deterioration which are reversible or where the progressive decline may be slowed or halted (see Chapter 2). Second, research is now taking us to the stage where we can describe different patterns of impairment and retained abilities which suggest that different dementias and different stages of those dementias require different types of advice to the carers.

Why intervene with more than palliative care for those with progressive disorders? First, because quality of life may be improved for the person with dementia and, second, because quality of life for the carers may be improved. Whether the carer is in paid employment, a volunteer or is a family member, easing the distressed state and distressing behaviour of someone with dementia promotes more mutual satisfaction between that person and the carer.

To some extent, any consideration of the incidence and prevalence of the dementias is not useful in a climate where research is now changing the map of aetiologies quite quickly. Alzheimer's disease, for example, might be said to be fragmenting into a number of other diseases such as diffuse Lewy body disease, familial Alzheimer's disease and early onset Alzheimer's disease, as well as the more familiar late onset type (Rossor, 1993).

We have been selective, in this chapter, in the depth of our descriptions of certain dementias for two reasons:

- the incidence of some rare types of dementia such as normal-pressure hydrocephalus is tiny but, more importantly, for some dementias such as that in multi-systems atrophy (Robbins et al., 1992), we have not been able to find any studies which describe language functions;
- in some diseases such as Parkinson's disease, dementia is only present in a small percentage of the clinical population and the disease and interventions are well documented elsewhere.

Aphasia and the dementias

Researchers have used the term aphasia extensively to describe the language deficits in the dementias. Whilst this is a useful research term, we see little point and much to recommend not using the term in a clinical situation. Use of some syndrome-based descriptions of types of aphasia is helpful as a quick means of identifying a number of features in the dementias. For example, the language impairment seen in many people with Alzheimer's disease has much in common with transcortical sensory aphasia. Similarly, the term progressive aphasia accurately describes a group of disorders which primarily or only affect language function and in which cognitive parameters are either well retained or deteriorate at a slower rate than language functions. In the clinical arena, we would prefer to use the term language disorder secondary to dementia to differentiate what happens to language in the dementias from the aphasia secondary to a sudden focal lesion.

There are of course difficulties with even this differentiation. In multi-infarct dementia, the dividing line between that condition and one in which an individual has undergone a number of strokes which have produced an aphasia is often unclear. However, in clinical terms, management and intervention for sudden onset focal aphasias and progressive language disorders are very different, in terms of the nature of the intervention, the context in which it takes place and the likely outcome.

Intervention in the progressive aphasias, semantic dementia and Pick's disease

For the clinician working in the field of old-age psychiatry, this group of dementias deserves a special mention because a major symptom is a specific language deficit without significant or any cognitive impairment. In the case of the progressive dementias and semantic dementia, a language disorder is the main or only presenting symptom and it may be so in Pick's disease. Because language may be impaired with little cognitive deficit and the disease progression is often slow, intervention which is aimed at the individual's specific problems may be more appropriate than a more generalised communication approach.

In the research literature, there are now several excellent single-case and small-group studies which look at these specific dementias. Mesulam (1982) first used the term progressive dysphasia to describe a group of patients with a progressive language disorder. Semantic dementia was first described as such by Snowden, Goulding and Neary (1989) but we see it very much as one of the specific dementias which predominantly affects language function. Pick's disease poses another problem in the literature. Pick's patient (1892) had a language disorder as a major presenting feature and other studies have described a similar picture (Holland et al., 1985; Poeck and Luzzatti, 1988), yet the clinical descriptions of Pick's disease usually suggest that early behaviourial changes are an important feature of diagnosis. However, it is clear that some patients who are diagnosed as having Pick's disease do have a specific language impairment and may not have behaviourial changes. As Pick's disease may progress very slowly with major language change and less cognitive change, then, as with the progressive aphasias, specific intervention may be appropriate. In all these dementias, age of onset is reported as being younger than the norm in Alzheimer's disease so referral may well come from neurology rather than old-age psychiatry or geriatric medicine.

Assessing the dementias

Though current assessment tools require careful selection for use in different contexts, there is now a range of tests and profiles which can be used in a clinical context, looking at language, communication, diagnosis and description. However, for the clinician the selection process is not easy, primarily because of two factors: the clinical service being offered may well dictate the type and length of assessments that can be used and, in addition, many potentially useful tests are not adequately standardised. The standardisation process is particularly vital when working with older people because language and cognition show greater variation in the older population than in younger age groups.

In order to test specific hypotheses when looking at language and cognitive processing, researchers usually have to construct their own tests and use a normal age and education matched control group. Many of the tests being used to investigate language processing in Alzheimer's disease and semantic dementia have a cognitive neuropsychological background and are often well enough described in the literature so that the keen clinician can devise similar tests. PALPA (Kay, Lesser and Coltheart, 1992) is another source of such tests but is not adequately standardised for older people.

The assessment process and differential diagnosis of the dementias and those conditions which have similar symptoms are described in depth in Chapter 9.

Intervention strategies in the dementias

We have said that the current literature on the dementias is now divided into research looking at the nature of the impairment within each dementia type and work describing interventions which are usually not specific to a particular type of dementia. Bourgeois (1991) has produced an excellent and exhaustive study of treatments for the communication disorder in dementia. Her main finding was that the speech and language therapist (SLT) has been involved in research which has been centred on assessment, diagnosis and description of the dementias but that there is a large body of work on dementia management and intervention in communication problems, mainly produced in psychology, social science and nursing journals. Very few of the papers in Bourgeois's reference list are specific to a particular dementia and when they are, it is always Alzheimer's disease. Since then, however, the area of SLT intervention research has become more active with a subsequent increase in publications (see, for example, *Topics in Language Disorders*, Vol. 15, No. 2, 1995). Research methodology in this area is still evolving but needs to become more rigorous before evidence of effectiveness can be accepted. As in most areas of research, replications of successful studies also need to be published before interventions can be accepted as effective. Whilst some studies have used control and subject groups to look at differences in outcome, much of the research is qualitative and describes pre-treatment conditions and post-treatment behaviours. Action research which 'reflects the interplay between practice wisdom and theoretical concepts' (Hart and Bond, 1995, p. 5) is particularly suited to this area because 'it is a form of research which could marry the experimental approach of social science with social action in response to a major social problem' (Hart and Bond, 1995, p. 15). The increase in the percentage of the older population with one of the dementias must surely be best described as a major social problem, with social, economic and employment implications for the whole population.

Bourgeois (1991) has provided us with useful divisions for looking at intervention research. Below is a summary of those divisions and some of the most useful research cited within each category:

1. *Changing the communication environment* includes studies which show communication change when changes are made either to the physical environment or to what is offered within that environment:

- rearranging furniture (Melin and Gotestam, 1981);
- provision of conversational partners (Corson and Corson, 1978);
- offering group activities (Blackman, Howe and Pinkston, 1976);
- offering refreshments (Blackman et al., 1976; Quattrochi-Tubin and Jason, 1980; Carstenson and Ericksen, 1986).

2. *Control of stimulus conditions* describes studies which attempt to change specific aspects of memory, skills and behaviours by stimulus control. These studies use retraining or behaviour modification techniques:

- public announcements increase attendance at a social activity (McClannahan and Risley, 1975);

- verbal prompts are more effective than signs, loudspeakers or written invitations in increasing attendance at group activity (McClannahan and Risley, 1975; Newkirk et al., 1976; Reitz, 1978);
- orientation is improved by training residents to attend to signs (Hanley, 1981);
- diary and watch memory aids are used effectively after training (Hanley and Lusty, 1984);
- repetitious behaviour is reduced by cue card response (Smith, 1988);
- memory wallet with personal details improves communication (Bourgeois, 1990);
- responding and appropriately reinforcing individuals' communication improves orientation (Hanley et al., 1981);
- reduced stimulation may improve communication (Cleary et al., 1988).

3. *Changing the consequences of appropriate communication* looks at the effects of reinforcing appropriate communication:

- food or other similar tokens have increased group therapy interactions (Mueller and Atlas, 1972), non-delusional answers to questions (Patterson and Teigen, 1973), orientation memory (Beck, 1982), frequency and length of verbalisations (Hoyer et al., 1974);
- staff praise and conversation increase verbal initiations and interactions (Hoyer et al., 1974, MacDonald, 1978);
- reinforcement of appropriate behaviour decreases screaming (Baltes and Lascomb, 1975);
- withholding reinforcement and ignoring inappropriate behaviour decreases it (Carstensen and Fremouw, 1981; Mishara, Robertson and Kastenbaum, 1973);
- response-specific feedback improves correct orientation responses (Greene, Nichol and Jamieson, 1979);
- reinforcement may need to be continuous if it is to be effective (Lawton, 1980).

4. *Multicomponent treatment packages* have been developed to include treatments of potential benefit and improved treatment gains but the findings are often difficult to interpret because of the methodologies used:

- behaviourial training techniques improve communication skills (Lopez et al., 1980; McEvoy and Patterson, 1986; Praderas and MacDonald, 1986);
- reality orientation is a more effective intervention than nothing or minimal intervention groups (Hanley et al., 1981; Hart and Fleming, 1985);

- token economies produce more change than either treatment or non-treatment (Mishara, 1978).

5. *Group therapy interventions* are the most frequently used method of service delivery and most studies cited here are group studies. There appear to be no studies which contrast group with individual intervention.

6. *Caregivers as communication partners* looks at enhancement of communication between the caregiver and person with dementia:

- caregivers can learn to change either their own communications or those of the people in their care (Linsk et al., 1986; Linsk Howe and Pinkston, 1975; Pinkston and Linsk, 1984; Reitz 1978, Shulman and Mandel, 1988);
- there are benefits to caregivers from these changes in communication (Bandura, 1977; Linsk et al., 1975).

Working with older people who have dementia requires the ability to assess both the communication abilities of the individual and the communicative context and to act upon those findings in a way which is useful for both the person him or herself and his or her carers. It is a complex process requiring the clinician to pay attention to communication disability, functional possibilities and client context. The context in which the clinician is working may dictate the focus of intervention which in turn may be influenced by service resources rather than by client need. Conversation has become a particular focus for research by speech and language therapists. There is a growing awareness that communication can be enhanced through specific work on conversation (Erber, 1994; Kaakinen, 1995, Orange et al., 1995). Shadden (1995), for example, discusses the use of discourse analysis in residential settings. She describes one resident whose conversation changed positively along the following parameters: increase in communication efficiency, reduction in irrelevant informational units, reduction in off-topic information units, greater balance in conversational turns. Another resident in her study showed increased use of repair strategies.

Gravell (1988) stresses the need to ensure that sight, hearing and dentition are adequately compensated for, whether intervention is direct or indirect and before intervention begins. For Gravell, barriers to direct intervention are factors such as reduced or absent insight, poor cooperation, low motivation, memory loss, cognitive impairment, unmanaged sensory impairment, fatiguability, physical illness and environmental factors. But in the population with dementia, it is just some of these factors which may need direct intervention. Poor cooperation and cognitive impairment, for example, may respond to individual treatment approaches (Baltes and Lascomb, 1975; Hanley, 1986). Gravell suggests that indirect interventions may be vital in encouraging communication. Some patients benefit from indirect therapy which may gently encourage their involvement in communicative situations and can then progress to more direct therapies.

A Royal College of Speech and Language Therapists (RCSLT) survey (1990c) found that speech and language therapists in the UK differentiated between Alzheimer's disease and multi-infarct dementia patients for the purposes of intervention. Whilst assessment and advice was the most common service provided for Alzheimer's disease patients, specific therapy for dysarthria and dysphagia was used with multi-infarct disease patients, if any service was provided.

Speech and language therapy intervention in elderly mentally infirm units in the UK is a slowly developing speciality which requires evaluation of its effectiveness. The RCSLT survey (1990c) describes, for example, an innovative joint venture between a health authority and a county council, providing multidisciplinary management to elderly clients. After initial assessment, which is carried out wherever the elderly client is living at the time, each client is assigned to a key worker who is responsible for the client's individually designed care plan which includes working with the family or other carers to increase their understanding of the client's communication abilities.

What specific interventions are commonly used with people who have dementia? A survey of speech and language therapists working with clients whose diagnosis included dementia (RCSLT, 1990) found the following types of interventions:

- direct therapy intervention for focal impairments in MID;
- communication and memory groups;
- environmental manipulation and adaptation of communication strategies;
- social skills and functional communication therapy with counselling;
- monitoring and maintenance strategies;
- working with carers;
- education of other staff.

Group work which encourages the use of existing or newly acquired skills and the generalisation of these skills to more everyday communicative settings is common in the UK. In residential settings, speech and language therapists may be involved in setting up and running groups which have different aims: direct treatment groups, social groups, conversation groups and reminiscence groups. In these groups, communication might form only one of the aims of the group and the groups are often run by staff other than speech and language therapists. Clark (1995) considers that consistency in scheduling is one of the most important factors and outlines principles for group work which include preparation, the physical environment of the group, communication principles and the management of emotional and behaviourial disruptions.

Memory groups are used by speech and language therapists to improve specific memory problems and are different from reminiscence therapy which enables identification of common or individual memories and interests (Perotta and Meacham, 1981).

Wilson and Moffat (1984) describe different types of memory intervention but caution that careful assessment is necessary to differentiate organic from non-organic problems such as depression which can best be treated pharmacologically or with counselling. Borsley (RCSLT, 1990) describes a memory-line service run by a team working with the elderly mentally infirm, which has input from speech and language therapy. A telephone link provides an open referral service for any elderly person who is anxious about his or her memory function.

Environmental manipulation can encourage and facilitate communication by altering the physical environment of the older person: decreasing the effects of background noise, creating seating arrangements which encourage social proximity and good lighting which can impair communication. Powell, Hale and Bayer (1995) found that carers reported people with dementia to be more sensitive to sound than a normal elderly control group. In institutional settings, the detrimental effects of an unstimulating environment on communication are well recognised (Lubinski, Morrison and Rigrodsky, 1981; Orange et al., 1995). Increases in communicative behaviour have been demonstrated after altering ward routines in institutionalised settings (Melin and Gotestam, 1981).

Regular monitoring can be regarded as a valid intervention with this client group. It has been advocated for elderly clients with progressive diseases such as Parkinson's disease (Johnson and Pring, 1990) so that, as the disease profile changes, the effects on speech and language skills can be explained to the family or other carers. Monitoring can target advice to the family and specific therapy for the client as and when it is needed rather than just at the stage of initial diagnosis. Holland et al. (1985) illustrate the value of monitoring in a single case study of a patient with Pick's disease where the patient's means of communication and the communication strategies used by his family changed as the disease progressed. Carers need information in an accessible form which can be repeated at intervals. They need not only strategies to assist communication but clear demonstrations within a natural, familiar environment. Erber (1994) discusses the use of conversation as therapy in residential homes. He stresses that most carers need instruction, counselling and feedback to become effective in this role. Care giver burden is well recognised (Jones and Peters, 1992). Rabins (1982) reported that carers of people with Alzheimer's disease reported problems with communication and with eating meals in 73% and in 55% of the study population respectively. Aspects such as repetitive questioning are reported as being particularly stressful to carers (Quayhagen and Quayhagen, 1988). Powell, Hale and Bayer (1995) found the following aspects of communication to be distressing to carers: repetitive questioning, struggle to name place, trouble following TV programmes, difficulty in conversation, calling someone by the wrong name, inability to remember topic of conversation and repeated telling of the same story. Knight (1992) concludes that carers require education and counselling, group support and respite services. Riggans (1992) found that relatives who are primary carers of people with dementia suffer symptoms of bereavement and that emotional support is vital to allow them to continue caring. A pilot project using a telephone helpline revealed large areas of unmet need among carers of the elderly mentally ill (O'Donovan 1993). Chapter 11 considers the SLT role with carers in depth.

The cost of providing monitoring and continued support to carers both as individuals and via relative support schemes is recognised as significant but Brodaty and Peters (1991) showed that the provision of an intensive ten-day educational and support programme, with continued follow-up for the carers of dementia patients, was cost effective in terms of keeping the patients at home for longer. There was a saving on the cost of institutional care, as well significant reductions in carers' psychological stress.

Toner (1987) found that written guides for carers of people with dementia can be effective in providing useful general information. Behaviour in dementia can be distressing to the carers who may need help in understanding that behaviour is a reflection of the progressive brain damage. Whilst face-to-face discussion is often the means for communicating information, written information can usefully recall and amplify what has been discussed.

Education and training of care staff via reports, direct liaison at ward rounds, case conferences and educational programmes has now become a normal part of the SLT's remit. Speech and language therapists need to demonstrate therapeutic techniques directly. For example, in the area of feeding and swallowing, talks and videos can be helpful but a demonstration of the techniques used with a particular client may be necessary to convince busy nursing staff that these techniques can be incorporated into nursing routines. Dissemination of information on SLT intervention is vital for agencies which may be the first contact for people with dementia and which are only likely to refer when the nature of the service is explicit, e.g. general practitioners and health visitors. As an increasing number of people with dementia are living in the community, either in their own homes or in independent sector homes, it is important for speech and language therapists to work with care staff in residential homes where contracts to provide a service exist as well as providing domiciliary services. Bryan and Drew (1987) asked home managers what input they would like from a speech and language therapy service. The main request was staff training, which was then provided. The training was well received but needed to be very basic and to address the specific problems that each group of staff was experiencing. Examples of the type of input needed are given in handbooks for care assistants working with the elderly mentally infirm (Maxim and Bryan, 1989; Bryan and Maxim, 1991).

Some specific methods of intervention with this client group have been used extensively and are described below.

Reality orientation (RO) is probably the best known and most researched therapy for people with dementia and it has become a major intervention method for this group in the USA (Hussain, 1981). Because those dementias which impair cognition and memory make the person with dementia disorientated to person, place and time, reality orientation seeks to reorientate. It is used as a set of principles in some settings for groups of patients, whilst other settings have used it primarily as a tool for working with the individual. Much emphasis is placed on provision of an environment which is orientating with the use of material, memory aids and environmental changes. Formal RO is in the form of structured, regular sessions in small groups of similarly impaired people. In addition, continuous 24-hour RO and consistent use of strategies by staff are stressed as important (Holden and Woods, 1988). In contrast with other therapies, RO principles mean that the person is explicitly told when he or she displays orientation that is clearly at odds with the context (Holden, 1990).

RO can improve orientation in elderly people with dementia but it needs to be continued if gains are to be maintained (Hanley, McGuire and Boyd, 1981; Powell-Proctor and Miller, 1982; Holden and Woods, 1988). Absence of behaviourial change may be due to implementing groups only, without continuous 24-hour RO (Woods and Britton, 1985). Hanley (1986) gives a clinically illuminating account of three patients in whom the targeted use of specific RO solved particular problems. Holden and Woods (1988) describe RO in detail, suggesting appropriate assessment procedures and different methods of implementation. They stress that RO is most successful when it is used continuously by care staff or relatives. Speech and language therapists will recognise many of the communication strategies routinely used in RO because the strategies have been drawn from many sources as in Lubinski (1981) who outlines a communication programme which incorporates aspects of RO. RO requires careful planning and the cooperation of care staff if it is to be successful. Implementing such a programme in residential homes may also help to increase positive staff attitudes to elderly people (Smith and Barker, 1972; Barnett-Douglas, 1986).

Reminiscence therapy developed out of the concept of the need for a life review with approaching death (Butler, 1963), both to think about past experiences and about unresolved conflicts. Largely used as a group activity, there is now published material of high quality available (e.g. Help the Aged and Winslow Press) which makes the use of reminiscence therapy easier for the clinician. Reminiscence therapy has been found to improve behaviour if attendance is consistent (Kiernat, 1979) and when it is combined with RO, orientation and other cognitive tasks (Baines, Saxby and Ehlet, 1987). Goldwasser, Auerbach and Harkins (1987) found no effect on cognition or behaviour but depression was lessened in the RT group compared with a therapy and control group. Woods et al. (1992) describe a life review for people whose dementia is mild to moderate. The emphasis is on making such a review positive for the person and his or her carers and/or family. The fact that RT appears to be of particular benefit in helping staff to get to know residents is highlighted in a number of studies (Bender, Cooper and Howe, 1983).

Validation therapy has been developed specifically for use with people who have late onset dementia (Feil, 1992). The main aim is to listen to whatever the person with dementia is trying to communicate about his or her feelings in order to establish a dialogue and to 'validate' what is being said, rather than correcting factual errors in orientation. Feil has taken concepts and techniques from a number of psychotherapeutic backgrounds, Jungian and gestalt theories and transactional analysis (see Feil, 1985). This therapy is used in individual and group settings where participants have similar levels of severity. Groups are highly structured both for content and for environmental context with an emphasis on emotional issues, group membership and touch. Responses to the group participants always facilitate and accept what is being communicated. Agitation may be lessened in individuals who are distressed by reality approaches (Dietch, Hewett and Jones, 1989). Crying and pacing behaviours may be lessened, whilst speech, non-verbal communication and eye contact may be improved (Feil, 1992).

In a controlled trial pilot study, Morton and Bleathman (1991) found no increase in the degree of interaction of the participants although individual gains were variable and in some cases considerable. This finding suggests that VT needs to be evaluated in terms of the individual's progress rather than as a group study. Robb, Stegman and Wolanin (1986), in another small comparative study, found increases in mental status, morale and requests for communication in their VT group but these did not reach statistical significance. These studies recommend that VT be integrated into all aspects of care within the institutional context. It has potential for helping with behaviours such as crying and repetitive actions which often distress staff, as well as being symptoms of distress. VT's strength lies in its humanistic client-centred principle of validating what has been communicated by the individual but it requires careful and extensive staff training if it is to be carried out effectively (Benjamin, 1995).

Many of the interventions described in the literature have been evaluated in studies which have design and methodological problems but Bourgeois states:

> The literature reviewed supports the potential for positive outcomes from communicative treatment and treatment research for individuals with diffuse degenerative neurological disease. Although the individuals treated do not constitute a homogeneous population, the fact that positive communication outcomes were reported in such a diverse population is encouraging (1991: 840).

There is clearly a need for more systematic research in this area. There is a particular need to identify those interventions which can be applied with some success to most people with dementia versus interventions which can be applied successfully to individuals with specific difficulties.

Finally, successful intervention with the elderly communicatively disabled is crucially dependent on the speech and language therapist working as part of the care team, as opposed to accepting referrals from them. Change, according to Walker and Williams (1980), and Griffiths and Baldwin (1989) is most possible when the clinician can work directly with other professionals and carers to demonstrate strategies and to facilitate communication.

Alzheimer's disease

Alzheimer's disease (AD) is largely a disease of old age. Of the approximately 40 000 people in the UK with AD, it is estimated that about 18 000 are below retirement age (Rossor, 1993). AD is the most common form of dementia in Europe and North America but not so in Japan where multi-infarct dementia is more common. Up to half of people with AD may have a family history of the disease but only a small percentage have autosomal dominant AD. From diagnosis, life expectancy is usually seven to 10 years. No positive test exists for AD and diagnosis is by exclusion criteria and examination of behavioural, cognitive and language data, the most widely used criteria for diagnosis in research being the DSM-III-R (American Psychiatric Association, 1987). The following criteria are commonly used:

- impairment in two or more of areas of cognition, e.g. memory, language, abstract thinking and judgement;
- no clouding of consciousness;
- exclusion of non-organic psychiatric disorders;
- absence of systemic disorders.

In addition, the diagnosis of AD is unlikely if the disease is of sudden onset, has focal neurological signs or has seizure or gait disturbance presenting early in the disease.

For the speech and language therapist, Maxim and Bryan (1994) suggest that, when looking at the research on AD or when testing patients with possible AD, the following questions need to be considered:

- Are language and cognition equally disordered or is there an imbalance between these two systems?
- Which language processes are disordered, which are spared and how are they disordered?
- What level of severity is present and does this knowledge help to illuminate the current processing deficits, i.e. are these deficits severity dependent or do they contribute to the severity?

In addition, another set of questions also need to be asked which reflect functional disability:

- What communication disability is present?
- If cognitive deficits are present, what is their contribution to the communication disability?
- What is the relationship between the communication disability and other behaviours?
- If there are behaviours which are distressing to the individual or his or her carer, can a change in communication make any difference?

It is now widely recognised that there is variation within the disease entity of AD but there is considerable debate as to why this variation occurs and its relationship to the neuropathology affecting brain structures. Schwartz and Chawluk (1990, p.143) describe this heterogeneity as follows:

> Each patient presents a landscape of eroding cognitive and functional capacities, but the landscape contains peaks and valleys. One patient may be seen with particularly severe visuospatial confusion and little language disturbance; another patient may show the reverse. Patients may be 'frontal' to a greater or lesser extent.They may have marked extrapyramidal motor signs....More typically most patients show simultaneous dissolution across several domains.

AD may represent a single pathological entity which presents in different forms (Hardy, 1992) although recent genetic studies point to a number of aetiologies that eventually lead to AD. Examples of different forms of AD are:

- familial Alzheimer's (Rossor, Kennedy and Newman, 1992);
- early onset (Faber-Langendoen et al., 1988);
- late onset (Bondareff, 1994);
- Alzheimer's disease associated with Downs Syndrome (Johannsen et al., 1991).

Specific symptoms may be associated with faster rates of decline (Chui et al., 1992) but whether these symptoms reflect a different biological basis to the disease is not known. Mayeux, Stern and Sano (1992) suggest that symptoms such as extrapyramidal and psychotic disorder in AD do not define different clinical entities but are manifestations of different stages of disease progression. Joanette et al. (1992) suggest that different profiles of deficits and preserved abilities between individuals may be due to individual differences in brain organisation for cognition and normal age-related changes in this organisation.

Language deficits in AD can be significant in both diagnosis and prognosis. Chui et al. (1985) found that prevalence and severity of aphasia correlate with duration of illness and that early-onset AD predicts the early development of language problems. Early-onset AD (before age 65) is associated with greater language deficit than late onset (Faber-Langendoen et al., 1988; Seltzer and Sherwin, 1983). In contrast with this finding, Bayles (1991) did not find greater language impairment in her early onset group. Filley, Kelly and Heaton (1986) also found greater disruption in language processing in early onset AD but interpreted this disruption as being due to variation in disease progression. Boller et al. (1991) suggest that poor performance on language tests, in particular naming tests, may be a good predictor of rapid decline in AD on initial diagnosis rather than age or severity of dementia.

For some time, the most prevalent view of language in AD has been of a homogenous progressive course of semantic deficit, syntactic deficit and finally phonological deficit. As a snapshot of AD, this picture has some merits but it is not the only picture and we need to remind ourselves that patients with AD are almost as likely to be atypical as typical in their presentation and in the course of the disease. Ska et al. (1990), for example, found that only just over half of their AD group conformed to the standard account of disease progression. Whilst it is possible to describe general characteristics of the disorder in AD, the underlying processes and the nature of the disruption to these processes is still not clearly understood.

It is common to present checklists of functions showing deficits and spared areas at different stages of the disease but such lists need to be used with caution. Language is compromised in all stages of AD but there is an enormous variation in deficits amongst individuals. As a guide, we have constructed a list which is more applicable to late onset Alzheimer's disease than other subtypes.

Late-onset disease
Early stage:
Language   Low-frequency word finding impairment
                  Circumlocution in conversation
                  Word fluency impaired
                  Composite picture description incomplete

	Poor repetition of BDAE low-frequency sentences
	Utterance completion poor in conversation
	Auditory and written complex sentence comprehension impaired
	Single-word recognition maintained
Cognition	Episodic memory impaired
	Specific autobiographical memory impaired
	Time orientation impaired
	Impaired famous faces naming
	Attention impaired
	Time orientation impaired
Personality	Change of affect
	Avoidance/denial strategies
	Increased anxiety
	Depression

Mid-stage:

Language	Naming deficits on high frequency items
	Semantic paraphasias
	Reference deficit in pronoun use
	Errors in complex sentence production
	Occasional phonemic paraphasias
	Decrease in semantic cuing response
	Sentence reading aloud poor
	Single regular word reading aloud retained
	Decreased use of gesture
	Poor repetition of BDAE high-frequency sentences
	Single word recognition impairment
	Simple sentence comprehension impairments
Cognition	Impaired working memory
	Decreased knowledge of current events
	Ideational perseveration
	Time and place orientation impaired
	Calculation deficits
	Visuo-spatial and perceptual deficits
Other	Wandering and exit-seeking behaviour
	Increasing apathy
	Sleep disturbance
	Assistance needed in activities of daily living

Late-stage:

Language	Language initiation decreased/ceases
	Noun use non-specific/non-existent
	Phonemic paraphasias on repetition
	Stereotypical utterances
	Verbal perseverations
	Echolalia possible
	No use of gesture
Cognition	Time, place and person disorientation
	Face recognition poor
Other	Dependent for activities of daily living
	Poor eye contact
	Inappropriate social behaviour
	Poor mobility

Purposeless motor movements
Incontinence
Feeding and swallowing disorder.

A comparison of early versus late onset types below shows the major differences between the types.

	Early onset	*Late onset*
Language deficit	Likely	Less likely
Progression	Faster	Slower
Myoclonus	More likely	Less likely

For clinicians who wish to use such information in a clinical context, the most informed and accessible research on language function is Bayles, Tomoeda and Trosset (1992) who provide extensive information on language functions linked to stages of the disease measured on the Global Deterioration Rating Scale (Reisburg et al., 1982) and compared with normal age- and education-matched controls. More important, though, is the knowledge that we now have concerning the variation in presentation of AD and the need to test for a range of deficits.

Research methodology in Alzheimer's disease

Maxim and Bryan (1994) suggest that research into language disturbance in AD had been influenced by four separate research trends :

* group studies of the language characteristics in AD, which describe symptom clusters and severity;
* studies which have compared the language disturbance in dementia with that of aphasia, using the syndrome-based classification in the Wernicke-Lichtheim tradition;
* single-case studies which have looked closely at the underlying language deficits, sometimes longitudinally;
* small-group studies which have looked at patients who present with distinct subtypes of AD.

There is now a consensus that the language symptomatology in AD is heterogenous and that, although it is possible to describe language and cognitive functions at different stages in the disease progression, it is more useful to investigate and compare the deterioration of specific processes. One of the main problems in group studies which use a profile approach is that very little can be said about what the individual patient can and cannot do. Single case studies of AD have, to some extent, helped, particularly because they often point to specific deficits and dissociations between deficits which are unlikely to be found in group studies. Unless single case studies are longitudinal, however, only one moment in the disease process is described. Systematic research of how specific processes deteriorate in AD is still needed.

Language function in Alzheimer's disease

Language changes are most apparent at the semantic level in AD but what happens to the semantic system is complex. Most studies of AD have concentrated on investigating the reduction in naming ability and the breakdown of logical associations which are common in language produced by people with AD. Discourse analysis has also been used to describe changes in conversational interactions (Hutchinson and Jenson, 1980, Ripich and Terrell, 1988; Ulatowska, North and Macaluso-Haynes, 1981). Most studies of language in AD look at different levels of breakdown as language deteriorates (Appell, Kertesz and Fisman, 1982; Bayles et al., 1992). These studies give a valuable overall view of the range of language behaviour which can be found among people with dementing illnesses. They do not usually look at language as the reflection of a linguistic system undergoing change but see language changes as a reflection of cognitive or neurological processes in decline. More recent single-case and small-group studies have discussed the dissociations of impairment which can be found in AD and longitudinal aspects of language processing deficits (Chertkow and Bub, 1990; Funnell and Hodges, 1990; Joanette et al., 1992).

Naming and lexical semantics in Alzheimer's disease

Difficulty in finding words that are appropriate and specific to the context in which they are needed is one of the most noticeable features of AD but is not always an early feature of the disease process (Bayles and Tomoeda, 1983, Huff et al., 1986). Other aspects of lexical semantics, on the other hand, such as word fluency (the ability to generate as many exemplars of a given category in a given time) are often a presenting feature. The exploration of this system entails some of the following range of tests:

- Object naming
- Picture naming
- Word fluency/word generation
- Word definitions
- Word-to-picture matching
- Picture-to-picture matching
- Superordinate category tasks
- Probe questions on semantic features

The central question in this area of language processing concerns the nature of the deficit: is the deficit due to a problem accessing semantic information or is semantic information lost? This question is not only of theoretical interest but has very practical implications for people with AD and their carers. If words and their meanings are difficult to access but are still present somewhere, then it should be possible to find strategies which will help access in conversation. If, on the other hand, semantic information is lost altogether, then such strategies will not help and may even be distressing.

The nature of the breakdown at the level of lexical semantics is not a clear picture but there is now some evidence that, in the early stages of the disease, access to the semantic lexicon is the main problem (Bayles et al., 1992; Funnell and Hodges, 1990) but, as the disease progresses, specific items in the lexicon are lost (Funnell and Hodges, 1990; Hodges, Salmon and Butters, 1992). Despite this loss, the semantic system at a single-word level may remain partially intact in AD up to a relatively late stage in the disease process (Bayles et al.,1992; Nebes, Boller and Holland, 1986; Schwartz, Marin and Saffron, 1979). The semantic feature system may be susceptible to breakdown with more specific features being lost first. There is difficulty in correctly selecting an item from others at the same semantic level and items sharing several of the same semantic features may be confused. Semantic priming effects but not semantic cuing have been observed in AD (Chertkow and Bub, 1990; Chertkow, Bub and Seidenberg, 1989; Nebes, Boller and Holland, 1986) but the effectiveness of semantic cueing appears weak.

In an early single-case study, Schwartz, Marin and Saffran (1979) found evidence of an often inaccessible semantic system. Their patient was only able to name one out of 70 items although the patient demonstrated by gesture that some of the items were recognised. Asked to select the correct name from five written words, the percentage of correctly recognised objects went up to more than 50%. Of the errors, over one-third were choice of the semantic distracter item (item = cat/semantic distracter = dog). Schwartz et al. say that this is caused by the gradual loss of semantic features for each item with more specific semantic features lost before more general semantic features.

Schwartz, Saffran and Williamson (1981), working with a group of AD patients, found that underselection of the semantic lexical item was a cause of naming problems in AD. Given a series of four pictures and asked to identify one item, there was much greater difficulty in selecting the correct item from four items of the same class than in identifying one item from four different semantic classes. Whilst the group had difficulty selecting the correct written word when given the word verbally, they could match the spoken word more easily to conceptually related items.

Whitaker (1976) provided further evidence that the semantic system in dementia can remain partially intact and accessible under certain conditions. Her patient had no useful social language but could repeat. Given a noun phrase which contained a phonemic error, the patient would correct the phrase when shown the actual object. Some phonemic substitutions created a semantically meaningful word, e.g. *pork* for *fork*, *wooden stable* for *wooden table* but the patient still corrected the items, showing that the word had been successfully related to the object. Only when she was shown no object did she repeat exactly what the examiner had said, even when the phonemic error created a non-word, e.g. a *yellow tencil*.

Whilst there is evidence for access difficulty in AD, there is now increasingly convincing evidence that specific items from the lexicon may be systematically lost. Chertkow and Bub (1990) Hodges, Salmon and Butters (1992) and both used similar methodology of the same target items in all tests. Hodges et al. found a significant relationship between the inability to name specific items and the inability to match the same item in a spoken word-to-picture matching task. There was evidence of preserved superordinate knowledge on definitions and on category sorting when the categories were grossly different (living versus manmade) but deficits emerged as the distinctions to be made required more semantic processing. The AD group also showed a significant frequency effect when naming.

Chertkow and Bub (1990) found that semantic cuing was not effective. A semantic priming effect, however, was greater for the AD group than age-matched controls. In addition, the AD group showed enhanced priming effects on those items that were semantically degraded compared with those that were not. Chertkow and Bub point out that semantic cuing is an off-line process whereas semantic priming is an on-line phenomenon. If we characterise, albeit extremely crudely, on-line processing as effortful and non-automatic and off-line processing as automatic and not under conscious control, then there are functional implications. We might hypothesise that people with AD will be able to respond better to contexts that do not require effortful processing and interventions might be best targeted at on-line processes.

Another issue within semantic processing theory is whether the semantic system is unitary or whether semantic representations might be divided into verbal versus non-verbal systems. Chertkow and Bub (1990) found that their AD group showed a loss of conceptual knowledge for both verbal and picture-based tests and that, again, this loss was item specific. However, a subgroup within their study performed better on picture tests than on word tests for pictures that they could classify. Some people with AD may therefore be aided by pictorial material rather than verbal material.

Dick, Kean and Sands (1989) illustrate the interaction of naming skills with aspects of semantic memory. They investigated recall of self-generated words in AD patients and the normal elderly and found that

AD patients did not show increased recall with self-generated words as the normal elderly did. They suggested that this was due to a breakdown in semantic encoding as well as a deficit in semantic memory.

Phonological cueing has been used in a longitudinal study by Funnell and Hodges (1990) of a single AD patient. They suggest that access from semantics to the phonological output lexicon, in which spoken word forms are stored, may be another area of deficit. The patient, Mary, was followed over two years and initially spoke fluently although word-finding difficulties and circumlocutions were present. She had similar performance and verbal IQ, with a much higher predicted premorbid IQ. Despite a decline in single-word comprehension over two years, her comprehension scores remained much better than her naming scores. On picture-naming tests, her performance declined in line with word frequency and she could not name better when given semantic cues. She could, however, repeat the picture names accurately and read them aloud well but she had greater difficulty in repetition and reading of nonsense syllables. This discrepancy between word and non-word repetition suggests that the store of word forms (phonological output lexicon) is intact.

On the picture naming task, Mary could sometimes name when given a phonemic cue, having failed to name spontaneously. Phonemic cueing became less effective as overall naming scores decreased. Despite general word-frequency effects, specific items were consistently named or not, suggesting that the problem was not one of access to the semantic system. If items had been named spontaneously on recent testing, then phonemic cueing sometimes produced the target name. Diesfeldt (1991) describes a similar patient with primary degenerative dementia who had some preserved semantic abilities with retained ability to name and read irregular words but difficulty reading non-words and function words. Obler (1980) reported that word frequencies and the probability of co-occurrence between words-affected subjects' ability to repeat sentences. Word frequency has consistently been found to have a significant impact on naming performance (Hodges, Salmon and Butters, 1992; Howes, 1964; Obler, 1980; Skelton-Robinson and Jones, 1984).

In moderate to severe AD patients, superordinate identification (a stimulus item has to be matched to an appropriate category) is harder than a spoken-word to picture-matching task, suggesting loss or inaccessibility of semantic categories (Bayles et al., 1992). The same study suggests that confrontation naming is an easier task than superordinate naming. Sorting objects by category was found to be an easier task than recognising the function or specific features of an object (Martin et al., 1985). But AD patients have been widely reported to have difficulty on word-fluency tasks and to generate fewer exemplars of a category than controls (Kontiola et al., 1990; Troster et al., 1989).

The changing semantic system in AD produces specific naming behaviour. Descriptive phrases such as *cutting blade, hand bell, ink pen, drinking cup* will be added onto the object name or they will replace it by a descriptive phrase. Bayles and Tomoeda (1983) found that over a quarter of incorrect naming responses were correct contexts or functions. Such behaviour suggests that these patients have some ability to monitor and change their language behaviour. The concepts of underselection and specific semantic feature loss, both postulated as reasons for incorrect recognition, are not necessarily synonymous and may point to different types or even stages of lexical-semantic breakdown. Although naming errors are more likely to be semantically associated with the target, AD patients do produce phonemic paraphasias and even neologisms in the later stages of the disease process, particularly in conversational language. They may also use words, phrases or even short sentences repeatedly in their conversational language, sometimes as perseverations and sometimes as markers when other lexical items are not available. People with AD also produce intrusions or confabulations where correct information is inaccessible (Dalla Barba and Wong, 1992; Dalla Barba et al., 1992). McNamara et al. (1992) found that their AD group repaired 24% of their speech errors compared with between 72% and 92% for a healthy elderly control group. The AD group used very few single-word repairs but relied on adding new syntactic information.

Most research on large groups of AD patients has found that single-word comprehension scores are better than naming scores (Bayles, Tomoeda and Trosset, 1992). However, when the same items are used both in naming and comprehension tasks, small-group studies have found item consistency across both tasks and similar patterns of impairment (Chertkow and Bub, 1990; Hodges, Salmon and Butters, 1992; Schwartz, Saffran and Williamson, 1981). Funnell and Hodges's (1990) single-case study shows clearly that there can be a dissociation between input and output tasks.

Deficits in the use of the semantic lexicon, then, are one of the most common features of language in AD. Indeed, severity of object naming and overall dementia are highly correlated (Skelton-Robinson and Jones, 1984). These deficits also affect language used in conversation and the semantic relationships between words, although there is evidence that semantic priming and, less effectively, semantic cueing are possible (Herlitz et al., 1991).

Visual and auditory perception in Alzheimer's disease

Some researchers have argued that anomia in AD is due to an agnosic component; that is, AD patients have difficulty perceiving the nature of the object they are required to label.

People with aphasia due to focal lesions, by contrast, have difficulty finding the label. Stevens (1985) has noted the tendency of AD patients to misinterpret visual information in picture-description tasks. Similarly, Rochford (1971) argues that semantic errors in dementia have an agnosic component and Martin (1987) found that a specific subgroup of AD patients showed visuo-spatial deficits. When writing to dictation errors are often misperceptions of the stimulus.

AD patients may also auditorily misperceive and therefore guess responses. Confirmed visual or auditory agnosia appears to be rare in anything but profound AD. Usually AD patients are able to match objects and shapes without error in the earlier stages of the disease. Auditory comprehension is frequently impaired in mild and moderate AD and language-processing deficits are well documented but auditory agnosia has not been described as a feature of AD. The ability to repeat single words and short sentences accurately would suggest that auditory agnosia is not a significant component.

Visual processing problems, on the other hand, are often cited as a possible cause of naming difficulty in AD but careful analysis of the errors made when naming have concluded that the errors are far more likely to be due to semantic processing deficits (Hodges; Salmon and Butters, 1991, Smith, Murdoch and Chenery, 1989). However, AD patients do have far greater difficulty recognising degraded letters or object pictures than the normal elderly, suggesting that their visual processing can be disrupted more easily or perhaps requires more complete information to facilitate processing (Corkin, 1982; Grist and Maxim, 1992; Heindel, Salmon and Butters, 1990). Dissociations between semantic naming and visual perceptual impairment is now well documented. Schwartz, Saffran and Williamson (1981) found no relationship between naming and conceptual ability. Individuals who were able to name well might show gross conceptual problems when tested on other tasks such as figure copying, in the absence of other visual problems.

Shuttleworth and Huber (1989) found that one group of AD patients made more semantic errors on naming whereas another group made perceptual errors. Saffran, Fitzpatric-DeSalme and Coslett (1990) discuss the dissociations within the visual perceptual system of two patients and demonstrate that only careful testing can differentiate between visual, language and other cognitive deficits.

There is now clear evidence for visual perceptual difficulties in subgroups of patients, particularly as the disease progresses (Martin, 1990; Shuttleworth and Huber, 1989; Taylor and Warrington, 1971). Evidence points away from visual and auditory agnosia being part of the general picture of early deficits in AD but these deficits are sometimes present and need careful testing.

Written language skills in Alzheimer's disease

The ability to read regularly spelled single words aloud is particularly well preserved in AD (Bayles, Tomoeda and Trosset, 1992; Nebes, Martin and Horn, 1984). Reading and spelling are, however, all part of language processing and therefore likely to be impaired at some stage in the disease process. The ability to read single words aloud even in severe AD has been used by Nelson and O'Connell (1978) in the National Adult Reading Test which gives a measure of premorbid IQ. It is useful in mild and moderate AD and where patients have at least 12 years of education (Stebbins et al., 1990). Patients are asked to read a list of irregularly spelled words.

Schwartz Marin and Saffran, (1980) have noted that AD patients are able to use regular spelling rules to assist reading but they are less able to read irregular and nonsense words. Fromm et al. (1991), in a group longitudinal study of AD and age- and education-matched normal controls, found that oral word reading is sensitive to AD and that this ability does decline with time. Both AD and control groups attempted to read the NART irregular words using regular grapheme to phoneme conversion rules but the AD group produced more phonetically impossible errors, suggesting that even regularisation rules may break down. Reading sentences aloud, however, is often impaired and may, in part, be due to scanning difficulties (Hart, Smith and Swash, 1986; Stevens, 1985).

In contrast with reading aloud, reading single words and sentences for comprehension does not show the same sparing (Appell et al., 1982; Cummings, Houlihan and Hill, 1986; Schwartz et al., 1979). Bayles et al. (1992) report that their mild AD patients scored between 60% and 90% of the normal mean for reading comprehension. Their most severe AD patients scored very poorly, if at all, on reading comprehension.

Patterson, Graham and Hodges (1994) found that their AD patients had most difficulty on low-frequency words with irregular spelling. Such a pattern is not surprising but they argue that this difficulty is caused largely by the breakdown in the semantic system:

> This link from a word's meaning to the set of phonological elements comprising its pronunciation serves a prominent role in binding those elements into a unitized whole... if representations of meaning deteriorate... a major source of coherence for individual phonological representations will gradually be lost...part of what makes a phonological (and orthographic) word whole is its link to semantic memory (pp. 404–405).

They also found that there was a significant reading impairment for non-words which they hypothesise is due to an impairment in the ability to segment and blend.

Alzheimer described both dyslexia and dysgraphia in his original patients and recent reports have correlated impairment of writing to the severity of the disease (Bayles et al., 1992) and to writing deficits being characteristic of familial Alzheimer's disease. Rapcsak et al. (1989) studied spelling of regular and irregular words in AD and normal elderly subjects. They found that spelling of irregular words was significantly worse in the AD patients and suggested that this was due to a loss or impaired access of word representations from the orthographic lexicon.

Horner et al. (1988) used a writing proficiency score to rate written narrative description in AD patients and found a significant correlation between writing ability and dementia severity. Writing and spelling are both vulnerable in AD because of language disturbances but disturbances of praxis and visuo-spatial processes may contribute in the later stages of the disease (Martin, 1987). Writing in AD may therefore show spelling and language impairment but may also show difficulties in motor coordination, praxis and visuo-spatial orientation. Writing errors may be incomplete words, missed inflections, substituted letters and incomplete spelling. The ability to copy is better preserved than the ability to write spontaneously or to dictation but it also shows degradation.

Sentence processing in Alzheimer's disease

One of the first dissociations reported in AD was that of an impaired semantic system in contrast with spared grammatical structure in language output (Appell et al., 1982). Whilst language output in AD may appear well structured, sentence comprehension and more complex grammatical relations in output may be disturbed (Troster et al., 1989). Auditory comprehension of sentences and paragraphs does show deficits in AD but a close correlation between access to the semantic system and the ability to understand sentences has been suggested. Another aspect of sentence comprehension and production which requires consideration is that of working memory which may show deficits although Hart (1988) argues that increased length of sentence, for example, is less a factor in comprehension than semantic complexity.

Kempler, Curtis and Jackson (1987) found that AD subjects produced a normal range and frequency of structures, using age-matched normal controls, but Troster et al. (1989) suggest that AD patients have particular difficulty both understanding and constructing complex grammatical structures. The correction of semantic anomalies, on the other hand, can also be difficult for the person with AD (Whitaker, 1976). Kopelman (1986), however, looking at recall of anomalous sentences, found that his early-stage AD subjects did sometimes correct semantic anomalies. The process of reduction to more simple semantic and grammatical forms is a commonly reported finding although in the early stages complex sentence structure may be retained (Blanken et al., 1987; Iles, 1989).

Schwartz, Marin and Saffran (1979) looked at the relative sensitivity to semantic and syntactic context in a single case study. They devised three contextual conditions which required a written response to disambiguate.

The semantic context was most difficult for the patient, who had to listen to three words, all in the same grammatical category and all semantically related, and then write the last word, e.g. *under: on: in*, tavern: hotel: inn. The first two words were meant to act as a cue into the semantic context. Disambiguation of phrases and sentences was more difficult but the written responses that the patient gave were more than 50% correct e.g. *a nose* versus *he knows; she blew out the candles* versus *she wore a blue suit*. The grammatical framework in which a word appears may act as a better entry to that lexical item than semantic cueing (Kempler et al., 1987) although the process described in the study is closer to priming than cueing.

Williamson and Schwartz (1981) followed an AD patient over four years and, using conversational samples, charted language undergoing change. As the patient's language deteriorated, fragments of simple sentences, in the form of isolated noun and verb phrases, appeared more frequently. The number of complete, simple sentences declined as the number of fragmentary phrases went up. False starts to sentences and fillers decreased over the sampling period, thought to be due to an increasing inability to self-correct. Verbs of quotation, e.g. *think, feel*, increased at the same rate as sentence fragments because, it was suggested, they commonly appear in sentences with an embedded clause which are difficult to construct. The number of grammatically complete sentences containing a subordinate clause remained small but constant.

Obler (1980) points out that the language of Alzheimer patients contains a large range of subordinating conjunctions but they are used inappropriately, and the grammatical function of these words, which is to signal the relationship between clauses, is not fulfilled. Tissot, Duval and de Ajuriaguerra (1967), too, found that their patients who could correct morpheme agreement errors in simple sentences could not correct errors of subordinating conjunctions. Some grammatical processes continue to work, even in the very late stages of AD, and are evidence that this system has some functional independence but to say that the grammatical level is intact is ignoring the complexity of language processing.

Frequency of word co-occurrence is an important variable in sentence repetition and construction. Obler (1980) looked at the effect of word frequency on the ability to repeat sentences from the BDAE. Her AD group could repeat long sentences in which the words were both of high frequency in the general vocabulary and had a high ratio of co-occurrence, but both grammatical and semantic relationships were lost in much shorter sentences where the words were of low frequency and low co-occurrence. For example, the sentence *the spy fled to Greece* was repeated as *the fly fed to geese*. Obler's research on frequency and co-occurrence reveals another aspect of the deteriorating linguistic system which leads to simplification in both grammatical form and semantic content.

The on-line processing of sentences is dependent on spared aspects of the linguistic system which appear to operate with such variables as word frequency and canonical structures. As the disease progresses, structures become more simple but are also likely to be unfinished. Whitaker (1976) characterised the language used by the severely deteriorated AD patient as automatic and non-volitional linguistic behaviour. Phonological and syntactic systems are functioning with little back-up from the semantic system or cognition and therefore communication is severely curtailed.

Whitaker (1976) and many other researchers have characterised spoken language in later stages of AD as automatic, redundant and also elliptical (Critchley, 1964; de Ajuriaguerra and Tissot, 1975), with fluently produced language and sentence fragments. Certain features may predominate at one particular stage in the disease process (Bayles et al., 1992). Utterances tend to become shorter as the degree of dementia becomes very severe and the initiative to use language is lost (Stengel, 1964). Using the term *elliptical* is probably not accurate as ellipsis implies a knowledge of that part of the utterance which is deleted and there is little evidence that the person with AD has such knowledge. It also implies an integrated semantic and grammatical framework for the utterance on which the process of ellipsis is to occur. As some facets of both grammatical and semantic levels of language are not available in AD, then the extent to which ellipsis can take place is limited. Fragments of uncompleted utterances are a feature of fluently produced AD language and may look like ellipsis (Maxim, 1991; de Ajuriaguerra and Tissot, 1975; Ripich and Terrell, 1988) but the mechanisms by which these fragments are produced are not clear. Some of the fragments may be the unfinished and abandoned attempts at constructing an utterance, but equally some may be examples of successful and unsuccessful elliptical processes. Bayles (1981) tested the ability to correct auxiliaries and modals, using tag questions which require a knowledge that the tag is related to the main clause and that part of the process involves ellipsis. Bayles found a hierarchy of difficulty with *BE* verb tags at the top but could find no explanation for this. The ability to correct some tag question errors does show that relationships between clauses not connected by overt conjunctions may remain partially intact in AD and suggests that other processes such as the production of elliptical utterances may also be possible at some stages of the disease process.

Fluent language in AD is often due at least partly to the redundancies which it contains (Obler, 1980), as well as phonological and suprasegmental fluency. The use of adjectives and adjective strings which reduplicate aspects of each other or of the noun to which they are attached may also be a common feature (Obler, 1980; Sinclair, 1967). Exclamations also increase as the number of propositions decreases, showing a greater reliance on fixed form or stereotyped utterances, and may be inserted into declarative utterances, either appropriately or not, giving the language used the illusion of fluency. Blanken et al. (1987) compared the spontaneous speech of AD subjects with that of Wernicke-type aphasics and found no evidence of systematic syntactic disturbance in the AD subjects. They suggest that fluent empty speech in AD is due to a failure to form prelinguistic conceptual structures of speech act-like representations. These representations are assumed to control the content-related decisions of sentence production.

A study by Kern et al. (1992) found that AD and normal elderly subjects produced verbal intrusions during a series of language and cognitive tests but the normal elderly control group produced more recall inaccuracies whereas the AD subjects produced novel intrusions. The recall inaccuracies involved information within the correct semantic category which enabled the elderly person to reach the required information and was therefore said to be a compensatory strategy but the novel intrusions of the AD subjects did not contribute to coherence of the language and were therefore considered pathological.

Sentence production shows some retained features in mid-to-late stage AD. Sentence comprehension research has been hampered, to some extent, by this finding. Whilst it appears that certain grammatical processes are possibly more resistant to the disease process than the lexical-semantic system, there is ample evidence that grammatical structure processing does show deterioration.

Whilst the ability to correct sentence errors or anomalies and to match sentences to pictures suggests some processing abilities (Schwartz et al., 1979; Smith, 1989), other researchers have consistently shown deficits in sentence comprehension. AD groups have been found to perform poorly on the Token Test (Emery, 1985), sentence tasks adapted from an adaptation of, Luria's test battery (Kontiola et al., 1990) and on subtests of the ABCD (Bayles, 1992). Unless all aspects of the sentence comprehension task are controlled, results are difficult to interpret. For example, it is important to check recognition of the vocabulary used in the sentences and to control for sentence structure and complexity. Using early stage AD subjects, Rochon and Waters (1994) tested them on nine different sentence types, using a target picture and a syntactic distractor picture. The vocabulary items were chosen from a pilot test, all sentences were reversible and sentence length was controlled. Their AD subjects showed only a mild syntactic impairment even on sentences with a complex structure such as passives. Their performance was significantly poorer than a control group on all three sentences with two propositions, two of which had an embedded clause. Length was not a significant factor. They suggest that 'a separate match is required for each proposition and thus sentences with two propositions require more postinterpretive processing' (p. 346).

Clearly more carefully controlled studies of sentence processing in

AD subjects at different stages of the disease process are needed. Research above single-word level points to the need to consider how linguistic processes interact and how the disease progression in turn impinges upon these processes.

Discourse, cohesion and repair in Alzheimer's disease

The ability to use language appropriately in context becomes more severely impaired as the disease progresses and overall cognitive function deteriorates. Yet clinicians working with this population report some meta-awareness of appropriate communication. Ripich and Terrell (1988) found that their group of AD subjects used more words to discuss a topic but the conversational turns were shorter than in the normal elderly. Further research by Ripich et al. (1991) on turn-taking and speech act patterns in AD subjects showed that the AD subjects used shorter turns, fewer assertive acts but more requests and increased non-verbal information. Conversational partners also modified their discourse by using shorter turns. Ripich et al. conclude that the basic structure of the discourse is preserved and that the differences observed are compensatory. For example, shorter turns decrease the memory load in conversation, making it more likely that the conversation will continue. Ripich and Terrell (1988) found that their AD group used more words to discuss topics than the normal elderly but cohesion was disrupted twice as often. Cohesion also shows changes in AD which may be of diagnostic significance. Gloser and Deser (1990) found that measures of cohesion can discriminate between AD and aphasia.

An early study in this area by Hutchinson and Jenson (1980), comparing normal, institutionalised elderly with an institutionalised dementia group, found that the dementia group initiated topics more frequently than the normal group and also violated topic initiation rules more frequently by not signalling or explaining the change of conversational topic. The dementia group also used twice as many commands, requests and questions as the normal group. Nearly 30% of dementia group utterances were classed as inappropriate to the conversational context in which they were spoken compared with under 2% in the normal group.

The ability to use cohesion in discourse is another area of impairment in AD. When we listen to spoken language, we can normally tell easily if the utterances are related to each other. Cohesion is the linguistic relationship between utterances. The research findings in this area suggest that both structural and semantic aspects of cohesion are disrupted. AD patients have difficulty maintaining simple grammatical agreement across clauses within the same sentence. It is therefore perhaps not surprising that cohesion impairment occurs.

Lahey and Feier (1982) found that lexical cohesion was the most stable form of cohesion in their single case study of Mrs W but Mrs W reiterated the same words across sentences rather than using related words. In particular, the ability to use pronouns as reference decreased across samples, as did both intra- and inter-sentence ellipsis. Absence of a clear referent has been reported as occurring far more frequently in the language of AD patients than in the normal elderly (Ripich and Terrell 1988; Ska and Guenard, 1993). Similarly, absence of an appropriate topic is far more frequent in dementia groups than in the normal elderly (Hutchinson and Jenson, 1980). The ability to use cohesive devices is likely to be dependent on the functioning of a number of linguistic processes, as well as working and other memory components and its impairment will reflect the decline of these processes. Another pointer to the level of meta-awareness of language function is the ability to repair, either to correct errors or to change the emphasis of what is being said. Repair ability is impaired in AD in comparison with the normal elderly and with other diagnostic groups with dementia (McNamara et al., 1992; Maxim, 1991).

Shadden (1995) suggests that the following set of tasks can be used to elicit discourse samples which will be helpful in management of communication:

- narrative discourse task based on a series of pictures;
- procedural discourse task, e.g. how to make scrambled eggs;
- conversation about key topics, e.g. family, current environment and events.

She describes intervention with two clients in residential care in which discourse-defined goals were set and outcomes measured and specifically comments that discourse procedures can be integrated into other intervention procedures such as Validation Therapy.

Movement disorder and the dypraxias in Alzheimer's disease

Although movement disorders are not typical of AD, myoclonus may be present at some stage in the disease process. People with AD become less mobile as the disease progresses and a gait disorder may be present. In the last stages of AD, primitive reflexes such as the sucking and grasp reflexes may reappear. The presence of other movement disorders may be due to additional pathologies.

Far more common, particularly in the middle stages of AD, is dyspraxia: the inability to perform certain purposive movements and movement complexes, with the conservation of mobility, sensation and coordination. Ideomotor, ideational and constructional dyspraxia may coordination. Ideomotor, ideational and constructional dyspraxia may all appear in AD and these disorders will affect everyday demands of daily living. Such deficits may be discrete or part of larger decrements (Foster et al., 1986; Miller, 1986; Kempler, 1988).

Oral and verbal apraxia are both rare in early AD, unlike Pick's disease where they may be a presenting feature. Reduced praxis suggests the most likely area of cortical damage in each disease. Oral and verbal apraxia appears more frequently with lesions of the anterior cortex, as in Pick's disease, whilst other dyspraxias are a more common sequel to diseases of the posterior cortex, as in AD. Findings from a PET scan study suggest that dyspraxia for oral commands and dyspraxia for imitation show different loci of cortical deficit (Foster et al., 1986).

People with AD invariably have constructional difficulties on drawing tasks. Reichman et al. (1991) used a drawing test of increasing complexity to identify visuo-constructive deficits in AD subjects and found that such deficits were highly correlated with severity of dementia, memory and language deficits in AD.

Activities of daily living such as dressing, swallowing and feeding are compromised by the dyspraxias. In particular, the interaction between frontal lobe initiation deficits, other cognitive and language disturbance, motoric function and dyspraxia may require careful assessment and intervention in feeding and swallowing.

The progressive aphasias

There is now a considerable literature on patients whose language impairment progresses slowly over a number of years without significant cognitive impairment (Chawluk et al., 1986; Mesulam, 1982; Poeck and Luzzatti, 1988; Tyrrell et al., 1990). This progressive language impairment may be a prolonged initial phase of Alzheimer's or other dementias. Poeck and Luzzatti (1988) concluded that only a few out of over 30 patients described in the literature maintained an isolated language impairment.

The majority of patients with a progressive aphasia have a fluent form of language deficit and have been classified as anomic, transcortical sensory or Wernicke's type aphasia, although Tyrrell et al. (1990) describe one patient whose language impairment was non-fluent with good auditory comprehension and who had a number of apraxias. Weintraub, Rubin and Marsel-Mesulam (1990) describe the longitudinal course of four other non-fluent patients. There is usually left hemisphere focal atrophy and PET studies now suggest that, in some patients, there may be little or no functional disturbance in the right hemisphere (Chawluk et al., 1986; Tyrrell et al., 1990).

Poeck and Luzzatti (1988) describe a businesswoman who presented with severe word-finding problems. Medical investigations for hypertension or cerebrovascular disease were negative. Her language was fluent but showed severe word-finding problems, empty phrases and semantic paraphasias. She attempted to repair her output errors but was not always successful. She was, at that time, still able to communicate adequately with little help from her conversational partner. IQ tests showed her to be within the average range for the normal population. Over the next three years her language deteriorated to the extent that she had to stop work but she still had an active social life. Subsequent assessment showed few attempts to self-correct and increased use of stereotypes. Conversation needed support from the examiner. Her IQ was lower but still within the average range.

Mesulam and Weintraub (1992) distinguished primary progressive aphasia from Alzheimer-type dementia and suggested the following criteria for diagnosis:

- progressive decline in language;
- absence of deficits in other domains for at least two years;
- no disturbance of consciousness;
- no signs of a more generalised dementia syndrome;
- no systemic disorder or other brain disease that could account for the progressive deficits in language.

Current descriptions of people with progressive aphasia suggest that they are younger than the AD population and often develop signs of language difficulty in their mid-60s. The disease progression is slow. Cognitive impairment appears late on in the disease process or is a minor component of the disorder and cognitive deterioration is slower than language loss. The retained functional language and daily living abilities suggest that this group may benefit from different management and advice from those patients with more general cognitive decline.

Semantic dementia

Snowden, Goulding and Neary (1989) first used this term to describe a dementia in which specific aspects of the semantic system become degraded in the disease progression. Hodges et al. (1992) have described a group of five fluent patients with severe anomia, reduced vocabulary and difficulty in understanding single words, using the following criteria for diagnosis:

- selective impairment of semantic memory with severe anomia, impaired spoken and written word comprehension;
- relative sparing of other components of language output and comprehension;

- normal perceptual skills and non-verbal problem-solving abilities;
- relatively preserved autobiographical and episodic memory;
- a surface dyslexia.

This study gives detailed information on neurological, cognitive and language testing which is useful in further defining the characteristics and, in particular, the specific processing impairments which may be found.

A single case by Hodges, Patterson and Tyler (1994) looked at the longitudinal perspective of this dementia and found that cognitive functions such as non-verbal problem solving remained relatively intact but that phonological representations and structural descriptions used to recognise familiar objects deteriorated. They suggest that these language functions are ultimately dependent on the semantic system.

In a study which has important clinical implications, Snowden, Griffiths and Neary (1994) comment on the poor naming and word comprehension on testing of this group compared with the range of nominal expressions used in everyday conversation. They found that their group of five people with semantic dementia had much better single-word comprehension for items such as names of people and places which were personally relevant to them than items which were not. In contrast, their control group of Alzheimer's subjects did not show this same ability. One person in their study showed better object recognition for her own versus other items. The preservation of an autobiographical lexicon and autobiographical knowledge about this specific lexicon may be an important factor when planning management for these patients. Snowden et al. mention also that one patient showed evidence of new learning. Given a toaster to use at home where previously she had not used one, she was able to identify the specific toaster and demonstrate its function within one week.

Pick's disease

Pick's disease often presents with a specific language impairment and relatively spared cognitive function (Hodges, 1994). Pick's disease may be the cause of some cases of progressive aphasia. There are a number of reports in the literature of patients whose language impairment deteriorates only slowly over many years, who are not reported as having gross behaviourial changes and who are diagnosed as having Pick's disease on post mortem (Graff-Radford et al., 1990; Scheltens et al., 1990). Poeck and Luzzatti (1988) make the point that Pick's disease is now used to describe a condition in which altered behaviour is a prominent symptom and which has a distinct pathological picture whereas Pick's original patient had a severe progressive language disorder and a different pattern of cortical damage.

The disease is said to have three stages (Cummings and Benson, 1992):

- initially patients present with personality changes such as lack of spontaneity and inactivity and emotional changes such as inappropriate laughter. Impaired insight and judgement are also a feature, but language abnormalities are among the earliest intellectual deficits;
- as the disease progresses, language impairment increases, often with relative sparing of cognitive functions such as mathematical skills, memory and visuo-spatial skills;
- in the final stage of the disease, patients develop extrapyramidal disorders, intellectual decline in all areas, mutism and incontinence.

The disease process is commonly seven to 10 years between diagnosis and death.

Pick's disease begins at an earlier age than Alzheimer's disease, often in the 50s (Lishman, 1987). Diagnostic criteria on post mortem include the presence of Pick bodies and Pick cells in the brain matter. Cortical atrophy is most likely to be significant in the frontal and temporal lobes where one or both hemispheres may be affected. There are also rare reports of parietal, occipital and subcortical changes (Holland et al., 1985; Munoz-Garcia and Ludwin, 1984; Wechsler et al., 1982).

Mutism is often reported although this is not usually a presenting symptom, tending to appear in the middle stages of the disease process, unlike Alzheimer's disease where it is common only in the final stages of the disease process. Why people with Pick's disease become silent is not clear but a specific verbal dyspraxia may be present. In the single case study by Holland et al. (1985), it is reported that Mr E was heard to make non-speech sounds for two years after he stopped talking. Early on in the disease process, his speech was described as stumbling and he produced what might have been phonemic paraphasias but there is evidence that he might have had dyspraxic difficulties too.

Progressive dissociation of the semantic system from the phonological and assembly processes needed for spoken language may also account for the increasing mutism. For Mr E, this mutism was restricted to speech output. At first, he was able to communicate well by writing and even in the later stages of the disease he could still communicate meaning through single words although he was unable to construct sentences correctly. Looking at his written language samples, he was able to produce a variety of constructions but not necessarily the appropriate structure at the right time. His problem in syntax appears to be one of access, with less structure becoming accessible as the disease progressed.

Mr E's writing showed that he initially retained good access to his semantic lexicon although low-frequency words were sometimes substituted for higher frequency ones. He was still able to understand most written material until one year before he died. The most striking feature of his progressive language disorder is his auditory agnosia. Hearing acuity was good but he had difficulty understanding spoken language. At first he could understand if the speaker slowed the rate of speech or repeated for him. He understood better, he wrote, if the conversational context was known to him. Approximately seven years after language changes were first noted, he asked his family to write when they wished to communicate with him. He had also largely stopped talking at this point. A trial training period of Amerind was begun about 18 months before he died. He learned 50 signs but could not combine or use them despite encouragement from his family. That he could learn shows some intact memory skills. Mr E showed no sign of echolalia but he did have auditory comprehension deficits. These two symptoms are signs of transcortical sensory aphasia, the aphasic syndrome Pick used to describe his patient.

Pick's disease is a rare form of dementia but should be considered if there are initial personality and/or specific language changes. The case of Mr E suggests that communication can be maintained until late on in the disease process because of specific modality sparing. Another patient EK, however, presented with significant behaviour changes but developed quite marked changes in language and cognition over a one-year period; (Maxim and Bryan, 1994; Thompson, 1986). She was a 78-year-old widow who lived alone and was diagnosed as having Pick's disease after referral to a psychogeriatric assessment team. A CT scan demonstrated frontal atrophy. EK had a history of ten years' deteriorating relations with family and neighbours. She developed suspicious thoughts about the local butcher. On assessment, she was found to have a moderate dementia, with disorientation in place and a poor knowledge of current events. She was able to identify objects by name and function without difficulty but her auditory comprehension was reduced. Like Mr E, her verbal output and, in particular, her ability to initiate language deteriorated but she did not demonstrate the same depth of specific modality sparing and her behavioural symptoms were very apparent.

Diffuse Lewy body disease

Diffuse Lewy Body disease (DLBD) is a primary degenerative dementia characterised by interneuronal inclusions similar in structure to the Lewy bodies found in Parkinson's disease. These inclusions reflect neuronal loss and are found in the cortex and the subcortical nuclei in DLBD. It was considered a rare form of dementia, but now is thought to be the second most common form of dementia after Alzheimer's disease (Burns et al; 1990; Homer et al., 1988).

The clinical features of DLBD are:

- patients present with early fluctuation in cognitive state with periods of acute confusion;
- cognitive impairment is less than would be expected in Alzheimer's in the early stage;
- extrapyramidal deficits of rigidity and tremor are present;
- psychiatric symptoms, particularly visual hallucinations, are a common finding;
- the progress of the disease is variable but all patients develop dementia and have at least one extrapyramidal deficit (Byrne, 1992).

Byrne et al. (1989) describe a spectrum of symptoms ranging from a Parkinsonian syndrome with subsequent dementia to dementia with subsequent Parkinsonian syndrome in 15 DLBD patients. They specifically mention fluctuations in severity of symptoms from day to day which have clinical implications for assessment and intervention. Galloway (1992) found a specific pattern of memory deficits and motor disturbances. Fearnley et al. (1991) described a patient with features of hyperkinetic dysarthria and nominal dysphasia. Studies of speech and language functioning in patients with DLBD are needed. Some overlap with Alzheimer-type pathology has been found in some studies but a strong case is now being made for its distinction as a separate form of dementia (Dickson et al., 1992).

Huntington's disease

Huntington's disease is inherited as an autosomal dominant condition and, because of the familial nature, the diagnosis is not usually difficult. Members of those families in which it is present are often aware of the possibility that it may develop. This progressive and familial disease, affecting both sexes, usually has a mean age of onset between 30 and 45 years, beginning with either involuntary movement or personality changes. It is associated with cortical and basal ganglia degeneration.

A hyperkinetic dysarthria with sparse speech, altered prosody, decreased phrase length and lack of speech initiation is a feature (Podoll et al., 1988; Ross et al., 1990). Impairment of comprehension of prosody (Speedie et al., 1990) and language changes including simplified syntax and press of speech (Illes, 1989) have been reported. Visual processing impairments may contribute to word-finding difficulties, rather than specific semantic impairment (Bayles and Tomoeda, 1983; Hodges et al., 1991). Patients with Huntington's disease have difficulty on initial letter and semantic category fluency tasks but their performance shows the same pattern as a normal age-matched control group, suggesting that the difficulty is one of initiation and retrieval rather than lexical semantic loss (Rosser and Hodges, 1994).

Butters et al (1978) compared the neuropsychological deficits found in subjects with recently diagnosed and advanced Huntington's disease. The recently diagnosed group had specific memory disorders associated with difficulty in acquiring new information and reduced verbal fluency. This deficit was due to difficulty in retrieval from long-term memory rather than a specific language dysfunction as naming was intact on other tests. The advanced group showed generalised non-focal cognitive disturbance but picture naming was preserved, suggesting less wide-spread deterioration than in other dementia-producing disorders.

Parkinson's disease

Parkinson's disease (PD) is characterised by disturbance of motor function, in particular muscular rigidity and/or tremor. It is a common disease, with a prevalence of 108:100 000 in Britain which is comparable to the average reported prevalence across countries (Sutcliffe et al., 1985). It is most likely to begin around 60 years of age and affects men and women equally.

PD patients have consistently shown a good response to several forms of group therapy for their communication disturbance in a number of well-validated studies (Johnson and Pring, 1990; Robertson and Thomson, 1983; Scott and Caird, 1981, 1983).

The dementia associated with Parkinson's disease has been described as subcortical but there is ample evidence that both cognition and language functions show deficits. The average dementia prevalence in PD is thought to be just over 35% but, for idiopathic PD and adjusting for age-related cognitive changes, the figure is probably between 15% and 20% (Brown and Marsden, 1984). There is also co-occurrence of Alzheimer's disease and PD. Alzheimer-type cortical changes have been found in neuropathological studies of PD patients. Some studies have suggested that advancing age in a PD population may account for the Alzheimer-type changes (Heston, 1981).

PD patients show impairments on tasks which require them to use their own internal cues but perform much better when external cues are provided (Brown and Marsden, 1988). Tasks which require set shifting are more difficult for PD patients than for normal controls despite the absence of dementia (Taylor, Saint-Cyr and Lang, 1986). Tweedy, Langer and McDowell (1982) found difficulty in the ability of their PD group to utilise semantic cues as memory aids.

Several studies have investigated whether increasing cognitive loads, while keeping motoric aspects of the task constant, cause difficulties for PD patients. The majority of these studies show no evidence of processing decrements with increased cognitive load when age-matched groups of PD and normal subjects are used (Brown and Marsden, 1986; Rogers et al., 1987) although one study found a decrement in an older but not a younger group of PD patients (Wilson et al., 1980).

The features of Parkinsonian dysarthria may convey an impression of slowness of thought and cognitive dysfunction which is not necessarily confirmed on testing. Slowing of the processing of auditory, visual and tactile sensory information is called bradyphrenia. Bradykinesia (slowness of movement) may have an impact on language performance because there may be slowed initiation of motor acts, motor responses may be carried out slowly or motor planning may be slowed (Brown and Marsden, 1991).

Damage to subcortical structures may in itself affect language processing in PD but the language deficit may be caused by reduced cortical functioning as shown in more recent metabolic scanning studies (Kuhl, Metter and Reige, 1984). Language skills in PD may show deficits in complex areas of language processing. Scott, Caird and Williams (1984) found that their PD patients had difficulty in appreciating intonation and facial expression but showed no language deficits on a shortened aphasia test battery.

There is some evidence of difficulty in interpreting linguistic information in PD. Although Scott et al. (1984) found no impairment of auditory comprehension, either at single-word, sentence or paragraph level, McNamara et al. (1992) suggested that PD patients are less able to monitor their own language errors. Using language produced when describing the Boston Cookie Theft picture (Goodglass and Kaplan, 1983), they found that PD patients corrected only 25% of their own errors compared with a normal elderly group whose correction rate was over 82%. The PD group, who had an average age of 61.3 years and had been screened to exclude dementia, had a correction rate similar to an Alzheimer group but there were qualitative differences. The PD group were able to correct single words and make reformulation repairs, i.e. corrections that alter the grammatical structure of the phrase or sentence in which the error occurs, but the Alzheimer group used mainly reformulation type repairs. This evidence corresponds to other evidence on word retrieval in PD. PD patients can make single-word corrections because they have better access to their lexicon whereas naming disorder and specific word-retrieval deficits are pervasive in Alzheimer patients.

McNamara et al. (1992) suggest that the PD group have monitoring difficulties due to frontal system dysfunction. Huber, Shuttleworth and Freidenberg (1989), using a PD group with an average age of 70.4 years and matched for cognitive function on the Mini Mental State Examination, replicated the findings of many studies (see Knight, 1992 for a review) that PD patients are significantly worse at word fluency tasks than normals and, on Huber's study, worse than the Alzheimer group. Hanley, McGuire and Boyd (1981) suggest that the significant difference in word fluency disappears if age and vocabulary scores are matched. On a naming test, the PD group performed significantly better than the Alzheimer group although they were significantly worse than the normal controls. No deficits in comprehension of single words and commands was found in the PD group who were tested on the Western Aphasia Battery.

Understanding and production of sentences may show deficits, in particular syntax (Grossman et al., 1991; Lieberman, Friedman and Feldman; 1990; Obler and Albert, 1981). Both spoken and written language have been shown to be different from normal age-matched controls, having shorter phrase length in spoken language (Iles, 1989) but using more words per theme and more complex sentence structure in written language (Obler and Albert, 1981). Sentence comprehension seems to be impaired when syntax becomes more complex but increased length of sentence does not increase comprehension difficulty (Grossman et al., 1991, 1992). PD patients' ability to understand may be helped by semantic constraints such as non-reversibility of sentences (Grossman et al., 1992).

Whilst medication may alleviate some features of PD, there are highly complex patterns of drug response in PD patients. Medication may be the cause of some learning impairment in PD which is not present when medication is withdrawn (Gotham, Brown and Marsden, 1988). Improvement in general mobility with medication does not necessarily carry with it any corresponding change in speech patterns and vice versa.

Depression is common in PD with a reported incidence of up to 50% (Gotham, Brown and Marsden, 1986). Depression is obviously not necessarily an abnormal reaction to a degenerative disease but it may require treatment and needs to be taken into account in assessment and management.

Maxim and Bryan (1994) suggest that signs of dementia in PD may, for most clients, be no more than an interaction between age, motor dysfunction and drug effects. Careful investigation of drug effects, patterns of performance during the day as well as cognitive performance, need to be made before dementia is diagnosed.

Progressive supranuclear palsy

Alternatively called Steele Richardson Olszewski syndrome after the authors who first described it, progressive supranuclear palsy (PSP) typically includes:

- a gaze palsy;
- pseudobulbar palsy;
- dysarthria;
- dysphagia;
- dystonic rigidity of the neck and upper trunk.

It may be diagnosed as Parkinson's disease at first because extrapyramidal signs are prominent and the age range for presentation is similar. The dementia of PSP has been described as consisting of the following (Maher and Lees, 1986):

- forgetfulness;
- slow mentation;
- dysarthria;
- emotional or personality changes;
- impaired ability to manipulate acquired knowledge in the absence of dysphasia, agnosia and perceptual abnormalities.

The disease is progressive and usually results in death within six years, unlike Parkinson's disease which is not necessarily life-threatening. It is a subcortical dementia and most investigations of small groups of PSP patients have shown no definite signs of primary language difficulty although other deficits such as initiation problems and dysarthria may produce a communication disturbance (Lebrun et al., 1986). A study by Maher, Smith and Lees (1985) examined cognitive deficits in PSP subjects at the time of diagnosis and reported mild word-finding difficulty but no evidence of dysphasia or comprehension difficulties. Podoll, Schwarz and Noth (1991) have found evidence of language impairment secondary to other cognitive deficits which include increased rates of repair and misnamings. Other deficits in reading and writing appear to be due to visual processing changes or to the gaze palsy. Sentences are well formed but syntactically simple and memory function equals that of normal controls (Milberg and Albert, 1989). The dysarthria in PSP is characterised by a slow speech rate, low volume and restricted prosody due to both poor pitch variation and difficulty in altering loudness for stress. Palilalia is sometimes found but as the disease progresses speech is initiated less often and response latencies are great (Albert, Feldman and Willis, 1974).

Creutzfeldt-Jacob disease

Creutzfeldt-Jacob disease (CJD) has a mean age at onset of 60 years and can progress rapidly. Even in its chronic form, the average length of time from diagnosis to death is two years. A recent cause of CJD in young adults between 20 and 34 has been virus contamination of growth hormone, given to stimulate physical growth in undersized children (BMJ, 1992). It is a rare degenerative disorder caused by a slow transmissible virus which principally affects the frontal and occipital lobes of the cortex, the brain stem and cerebellum.

The initial diagnosis may be of psychiatric disorder but other symptoms such as aphasia, agnosia, apraxia, dysarthria and memory disturbance follow quickly. The dysarthria is most likely to be a combination of cerebellar and extrapyramidal types. Motor disturbances include myoclonus which may be an early feature of the disease, rigidity and tremor due to extrapyramidal involvement, cerebellar ataxia, visual disturbances and cranial nerve palsies (Bieliauska and Fox, 1987; Cummings and Benson, 1992). An isolated Wernicke's type aphasia may be a presenting feature (Mandel, Alexander and Carpenter, 1989). In later stages of the disease, patients become mute and may go into a coma for some weeks before death.

Depression, confusion and dementia

There is a complex interaction between dementia and depression which is a common symptom in elderly people (Cooper, 1987). Communication in an elderly person with endogenous (i.e. of unknown origin) depression is often impaired, with reduced intonation range and slow response latency. Language is often impoverished, the patient giving brief replies which are unlikely to lead on to further discussion. On specific tasks, however, depressed patients may do well. Descriptions of the Cookie Theft picture by depressed elderly people may be as good or better than those given by the normal healthy elderly (Maxim, 1991). On the Western Aphasia Battery, Emery (1989) reported that depressed elderly subjects performed significantly better than Alzheimer patients on all measures and were only scoring significantly lower than normal controls on measures which involved errors on the most complex items.

There is a chance of misdiagnosis of the clinically depressed elderly person who presents with a history of cognitive impairment, sleep disturbance, appetite loss, psychomotor slowing, depressed affect and poor memory (Jarvik, 1982; Cummings and Benson, 1992). Accurate diagnosis of the dementia syndrome of depression from organic causes is obviously essential because appropriate drug intervention and therapy may be successful (Grossberg and Nakra, 1988). Early on in the course of Alzheimer's disease, patients may have a co-occurring depression (Reifler, 1986) or may be referred with a diagnosis of depression which is then found to be a primary dementing illness (Feinberg and Goodman, 1984), sometimes called pseudo-depression. Depression can also be a major feature in the dementias associated with subcortical damage such as Parkinson's disease and Huntington's disease.

The AIDS dementia complex

Navia, Jordan and Price (1986) described two forms of dementia in AIDS, one being steadily progressive at times punctuated by accelerated deterioration and the other occurring in 20% of cases, having a much slower and protracted course. Van Gorp et al. (1989) found that subcortical functions were more affected in AIDS encephalopathy than those in the cortex. In the early stage there may be a dysarthria and motor problems with speech and writing. Mild word-finding problems were found in some subjects and language was affected by slowness of thought and mood changes. As the dementia progresses, verbal responses become slower and less complex with virtual mutism in the final stage of the disease. Most patients with AIDS develop dementia associated with an HIV encephalopathy but a smaller percentage develop a dementia before AIDS has been diagnosed (Cummings and Benson, 1992). The AIDS dementia complex usually includes lethargy, progressive cognitive impairment and slowing of movement and speech (Bannister, 1992).

Wernicke's encephalopathy/Korsakoff's psychosis

These conditions are amnesias rather than dementias, caused by a thiamine deficiency secondary to chronic alcohol abuse. Chronic alcohol abuse and an associated head trauma can lead to alcoholic dementia. The conditions are characterised by an isolated loss of recent memory in an otherwise alert person with little other evidence of remote memory, immediate recall or other cognitive changes. As head injury has a peak of incidence in old age, it is important for clinical management that these two conditions are understood to be linked and that an underlying or frank Korsakoff's psychosis may complicate subsequent recovery from head injury. Alcoholic dementia has been described as being more severe in the elderly and clinically the progression is slow with impairment in abstracting ability, short-term memory and verbal fluency (Cutting, 1982). If the patient ceases to consume alcohol there is usually an improvement in cognitive abilities but return to pre-alcoholic levels is unusual (Grant, Adams and Reed, 1984).

Communication ability is reduced because memory for recent events is poor but language remains intact. Murdoch (1990) describes the relationship between the two conditions as follows: 'Wernicke's encephalopathy represents the acute stage of this process and Korsakoff's syndrome the residual mental deficit that usually occurs in the late stages of Wernicke's encephalopath' (p. 172). Kopelman (1991) suggests that frontal lobe dysfunction causes a disorganisation of retrieval processes and that this in turn contributes to the retrograde amnesia.

Conclusions

Communication disability and specific language impairment are components of most dementias but do not necessarily co-occur.

Someone with Alzheimer's disease may have a communication disability but very little evidence of language deficits. Another person with a progressive aphasia may show very specific language deficit but be able to communicate effectively. Intervention and management of language and communication problems in the dementias now needs to differentiate between the needs of people with different forms of dementia.

Chapter 4:
Issues in Service Provision: a Management Perspective

SUE STEVENS

Introduction

Fifteen years ago the concept of a planned speech and language therapy service for the elderly mentally ill (EMI) was a rare, if not unknown, phenomenon (Griffiths, 1991). It is a credit to the initiative and dynamism of therapists working with the elderly that this branch of speech and language therapy services has developed, and is now regarded as an essential part of a comprehensive service.

In 1978 Marsden predicted that, by 1980, there would be seven million people in Great Britain over 65 years of age. In 1991 Griffiths stated that eight million (15%) of the population were over 65 years, then quoting Wicks and Henwood's prediction that between 2001 and 2021 there would be a further 17% increase in this age-group.

The incidence of psychiatric disorders increases with age, with possibly 40% of the age-group being affected (Kay, Beamish and Roth, 1964). The most common condition is depression, whilst dementia affects about 5%, rising to 20% in those over 80 years (Brayne and Ames, 1988).

This population growth is one factor that has precipitated the development of services to the elderly mentally infirm. It may also have been fuelled by the increase in the numbers of day hospitals, both geriatric and EMI, and memory or dementia clinics. All of these service outlets may require speech and language therapy input.

Throughout the 1980s and early 1990s several examples of excellent service practice have been written up (Baker et al., 1992; Heritage and Farrow, 1994). However, this level of service has not been universal, usually because of funding or staffing limitations, or perhaps lack of interest in this aspect of speech and language therapy on the part of managers or therapists. The quality of service to this client group has been underpinned by the publication in 1991 of the Royal College of Speech and Language Therapists' quality guidelines in *Communicating Quality*.

Changes in the way services are planned and delivered in the post-community care health service mean that discrepancies will still exist. These may relate to the differing priorities established by the service purchasers, who will be the local health authorities (commissioning agency), together with fundholding GPs and/or private organisations such as private nursing or residential homes or charities.

The control of the service will have moved therefore, in broad terms, from individual consultants and therapists to health care purchasers. Doctors and therapists retain control on a day-to-day basis, but may be constrained by restrictions placed on them by the formal contracting process, such as which and how many clients can access the service, and what is offered in terms of assessment and follow up.

This chapter sets out the main topics that need to be considered when negotiating the most appropriate and acceptable model for EMI service provision. The negotiating process is likely to be smoother and more satisfactory if an ongoing dialogue is maintained with purchasers and, ideally, if purchasers have some experience of the service through information and, preferably, observation.

Many members of purchasing authorities do not have a clinical background, so invitations to observe the service in action together with succinct reports about its form and potential can provide a meaningful basis for discussion. However, the service required by purchasers will vary from area to area because of the way they perceive local need and the make-up and priorities of their population, the size of which may vary markedly from area to area.

Service aims

The provision of a speech and language therapy service to the elderly mentally infirm (EMI) should have clear aims, concisely conveyed by an appropriate mission statement. These can be summarised as:

- enabling individuals to achieve maximum functional communication;
- assessment and management of dysphagia problems;
- appropriate advocacy for clients;
- prevention of communication breakdown between clients and carers;
- education of other professionals.

The overall aim of the service should be to allow any elderly individual with psychiatric and/or cognitive problems to function communicatively at their optimum level, whatever their surroundings. A speech and language therapist will determine the communication skills and deficits of that individual by objective assessment and will institute suitable management programmes.

Part of this aim may be achieved by enabling staff and carers to understand better the process of communication, and the possible communication problems they may encounter. It is facilitated by working together as a total care team, with the focus often on working with, and through, staff and carers, rather than directly with the client.

Any EMI service should also aim to cover the assessment and management of dysphagic problems, ensuring that any risk to individuals is minimised, and that all carers are aware of such risks and how to manage them.

In order to achieve the main aim of effective functional communication, a therapist may need to highlight a client's needs for other services such as audiology or dentistry, and will sometimes act as the client's advocate in ensuring referral to such services. Such intended action will need to be discussed with the original referrer, probably the general practitioner or consultant psychogeriatrician. All such recommendations should be recorded in patient notes, and a written request made. The therapist may subsequently need to check with client and/or carer that the appropriate action has been taken. As some clients' insight into, and awareness of, the effect of their communication deficits may be limited, the therapist needs to ensure that problems are addressed in an ethical manner, taking into account the legality of consent. Any coercion to comply with therapy is unacceptable. This is discussed in more detail in the section on 'legal considerations' (p.96).

It is also in keeping with the UK Government's 'Health of the Nation' policy to focus on the benefits of preventive care, with education of other professionals and carers being essential in this context. Explanations about the actual or likely communication problems faced by patients and their carers, and subsequent discussion and support, may help to relieve carer stress, anger and possibly depression.

Contracting

The basis upon which any service is now provided is the contract. Three main types of contract are negotiated at present in the NHS:

1. *Block*: an agreed sum of money over an agreed period of time covering all aspects of the service, with no limit on client numbers.
2. *Cost and volume*: an agreed sum of money over an agreed period of time with agreed client numbers and service commitments.
3. *Extra-contractual referral* (ECR): a one-off agreement for provision for an individual for an agreed sum of money, of a specialist or out-of-area service.

The block contract leaves the provider open to lack of workload control, whilst the purchasers may get very poor or very good value for money depending on client throughput. The cost-and-volume contract ensures both purchaser and provider have greater control over their commitments, whilst ECRs tend to be used in exceptional circumstances only. An example of an ECR, in the context of an EMI service, might be the referral of an individual to a out of area memory/dementia clinic, as these are not run by all trusts or health districts.

A problem in some areas is that separate contracts may have to be negotiated for 'acute' and 'community' provision, if the purchasers and/or the providers are different, i.e. acute and/or primary care commissioning. Acute (or secondary) care is provided in an acute hospital. The EMI service will probably be under the direction of a consultant in old age psychiatry and administratively placed in a directorate/division of medicine. Any contract will be negotiated between an acute commissioning unit for the area or fundholding general practitioners and the directorate concerned.

Community (or primary) care is provided in the community, i.e. domiciliary, health/day centres, residential/nursing homes. The service may again be under the direction of a consultant in old age psychiatry. Any contract will be made between the primary care commissioning unit for the area or fundholders and the community healthcare or mental health trust.

In some circumstances these different contracts may relate to the *same* patients using different parts of the system at different times according to the needs of their disease. The best option is a cost-and-volume contract which covers the provision of a speech and language therapy service to all service provision locations in any geographical area, in order to simplify management and facilitate seamless care.

Any contract will need to cover the following areas of provision:

- quantity;
- quality;
- price;
- skill mix;
- monitoring systems;
- service cover;
- sanctions.

Quantity, quality and price are known as the contract triangle (Ovretveit, 1994), and negotiation may centre around those three headings.

Sites of provision

Currently there is frequent talk of services being moved from 'hospital' to 'community'. However, there is a need for any service to the elderly mentally infirm to be provided in both, although the greater part of any such service in the future may be community provision. A good service is a comprehensive one without arbitrary geographical or administrative boundaries, i.e. seamless.

There are several possible sites for the provision of all or part of an EMI service:

1. acute geriatric/psychogeriatric ward;
2. slow-stream rehabilitation ward;
3. long-stay geriatric rehabilitation/psychogeriatric ward;
4. geriatric/EMI day hospital;
5. memory clinic/dementia clinic;
6. day centre (Social Services: voluntary sector);
7. residential/nursing homes (Social Services, charity and private);
8. domiciliary.

Locations 1 to 5 will come under the heading of acute care provision, i.e hospital, whilst locations 6 to 8 are 'community' provision. The situation may slightly vary from area to area, with, for example, NHS nursing homes being something of an anomaly. The site of service provision will influence the composition of the team with whom the speech and language therapist works. Examples of possible multidisciplinary teams are given below:

Acute hospital ward for the elderly

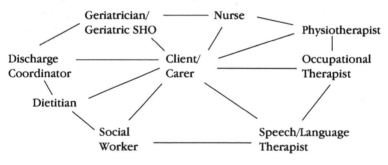

Domiciliary

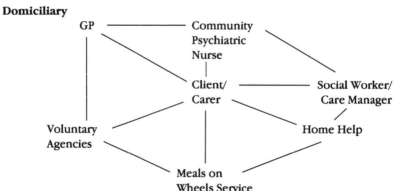

It also may affect the ease and manner which a multidisciplinary team can work. It is probable that an acute unit will have a regular ward meeting or case conference at which care needs and objectives are discussed. These meetings ensure team members meet at least weekly, but because members are likely to be based on the same site, chance meetings may occur frequently, providing opportunities for informal discussion and exchange of information.

Face-to-face contact with other team members may be a greater problem if the service is community based, with less likelihood of chance meetings with other team members, and case conferences perhaps being related to a particular issue for an individual client, rather than being a regular occurrence. The speech and language therapist's skills at, and appreciation of, the importance of liaison may then be invaluable in the formation and maintenance of a cohesive team approach.

Referral

The site of provision will also inevitably have an effect on who is referred to the service, from whom and how.

Although the greatest proportion of people referred to such a service are likely to be suffering from a variety of different types of dementia, it may also be appropriate for people with the following diagnoses to be referred:

- depression;
- paranoia;
- schizophrenia;
- acute confusion;
- alcohol abuse.

No one over the agreed age with communication or swallowing problems should be excluded from assessment, although the extent of therapeutic management for some cases may be limited.

In an acute unit, still probably based on a medical model, referrals will tend to come from the consultant or one of his or her team. Nurses, who often know patients better than anyone else, may also refer, as will social workers, who nowadays frequently require information for Complex Needs Assessments. Self- and carer-referrals are extremely uncommon, so a service contract may not need to take account of that possibility. However, all managers and therapists should be aware of their employer's policy with regard to self-referrals as attitudes are variable.

In a community setting, such as a Social Services day centre, referrals may come from centre staff, such as the client's keyworker. Other referrals, perhaps for domiciliary consultations, may come from a GP.

Although self-referrals are again uncommon, carer-referrals are sometimes made, so unless it has been agreed in a contract that 'non-agency' referrals are accepted, any self- or carer-referral may have to be referred back to, and agreed with, the individual's general practitioner before being acted upon. This process also enables the therapist to acquire the appropriate medical information.

The method of referral, i.e. verbal and/or written, should be identified in the contract. Any referrals for assessment and management of *dysphagia* must be written (RCSLT, 1991), although it varies from place to place, at the time of writing, as to whether a written referral is necessary for communication problems.

Just as hospital referrals are made on a specified form, it may be more efficient for an agreed form to be used by staff working in the community. This eases the referrer's task by avoiding the need to write letters, and should, if appropriately formatted, give the speech and language therapist the background information she or he might need.

Monitoring of referrals

Regular monitoring of the number and type of referrals is essential throughout any contract period. If the contract is of a cost-and-volume type, any +/- 5% deviance from the agreed referral numbers, perhaps over a quarterly period, needs to be brought to the purchaser's notice and discussed.

If there are noticeable changes in the types of referrals, e.g. a greater number of depressed clients, the reason for such a change should be established and the contract amended if appropriate. This could be caused by changes in a unit's medical staffing, with a resulting alteration in the type of client care.

In order to carry out appropriate monitoring, accurate statistics need to be kept and to be available. Many services or units will be keeping statistics in computerised form, but discussion with computer staff may be necessary about what data are required, how they are recorded and the format in which they are printed out. A suggested format for a 'paper' record of such data is given in Appendix 1.

Intervention

It is rare that intervention for this client group takes the form of 'conventional regular individual therapy'. It is more likely to be facilitated intervention, which will largely be concerned with creating the right environment, both physical and psychological, for the client to communicate as effectively as possible.

Clear and realistic therapeutic goals should be set and regularly monitored, with agreed written standards establishing how this monitoring may take place. Reassessment to confirm or re-evaluate the original diagnosis is often necessary, and should be regular practice in dementia, as with other progressive conditions.

If any intervention required relates to dysphagia or feeding problems, the speechl/language therapy service manager needs to be aware of the possible practical, ethical and legal considerations (Grimley Evans, 1989). The management of a client may be contentious in situations where he or she is deemed unable to give consent owing to cognitive impairment.

Comprehensive assessment of swallowing/feeding problems may be difficult because of the patient's lack of insight, and, at times, inability to cooperate fully. Videofluoroscopy examination may not be available due to cost, lack of access for older clients, physical difficulties and/or clients' lack of ability to cooperate adequately.

At all times the therapist needs to record fully and clearly in his or her own service records, as well as client notes, any assessment findings and management recommendations. These notes should always be signed. Although decisions about whether to use joint case notes will be made by consultants or unit managers, the speech and language therapy service may be well served by a joint case note system, such as that used with clients in the community serviced by Optimum Health Service Trust in south London, or the Problem Orientated Multidisciplinary Records (MUDI PORS) used in the Regional Rehabilitation Unit at Northwick Park Hospital, London. Such record keeping may increase the likelihood of others being exposed to information about speech and language therapy diagnoses and management recommendations.

Discharge

Although discharge completes the process of intervention, discharge planning should start from the time of initial assessment.
Planning should include:

- discussion of client's and carer's needs and wishes;
- liaison with the multidisciplinary team;
- referral to appropriate agencies/organisations;
- appropriate type of ongoing support.

Because of the progressive nature of some pathologies, discharge may only take place if:

- client/carer no longer requires intervention;
- client transfers out of area;
- client's health deteriorates;
- client dies.

Discharge standards agreed with purchasers should include the necessity for appropriate information to be given to the client, although, for many clients with impaired cognition, it is often carers and other multi-disciplinary team members who need to be informed.

Because EMI clients are often unable to act as their own advocates, agreed standards of service are one way of ensuring that a quality service is provided and maintained. They should be regarded as a useful set of checks and balances, rather than a hindrance to professional judgement. EMI service managers need to set up audit systems which can highlight any loss of service quality or abuse of this client group.

Service components

The form of any service will depend on what purchasers are prepared to pay for, or possibly what the providers can supply. During the contract negotiation process agreement will have been reached which takes account of:

- purchaser's priorities;
- provider's staffing/facilities;
- client/carer needs;
- local population information, e.g. age, epidemiology;
- practicalities of provision, e.g. site, transport;
- money available.

Contracting should not be seen as restricting a service. A good contract may provide opportunities for expanding a field of care that has historically tended to be neglected in the past. It should allow for speech and language therapy clinical provision, together with teaching and clinical research, and should also take account of the need for staff training and support, in what is often a stressful area of work. Purchasers will be looking for quality, flexibility and value for money, whilst the clients and their carers want a friendly and responsive service providing the information and support they feel they need. There are times when a 'Rolls Royce' service may have to be traded in for a Ford Mondeo or even a Mini, but regular communication with purchasers may prevent it happening too frequently.

Listed below are factors that need to be considered as part of any service provision:

1. *Assessment*:
(i) communication and/or swallowing problems;
(ii) differential diagnosis;
(iii) baseline for therapy/management;
(iv) provision of complex needs assessment information.

2. *Therapy/Management*:
(i) communication and/or swallowing problems;
(ii) individual/group – if groups, are they for therapy/communication/ reality orientation?;
(iii) length/frequency;
(iv) direct/indirect;
(v) advice/support to other team members;
(vi) carer support – individual/group;
(vii) reassessment over time (possibly years);
(viii) reasons for, and timing of, discharge.

3. *Teaching*:
(i) to whom, and by whom;
(ii) lectures/workshops/observation;
(iii) subject;
(iv) frequency;
(v) uni-professional or part of multidisciplinary programme;
(vi) part of recognised qualification programme.

4. *Research*:
(i) clinical or pure;
(ii) funding;
(iii) assessment for inclusion in projects;
(iv) staff requirements.

5. *Outcomes/audit*:
(i) who monitors?;
(ii) how is monitoring carried out?;
(iii) when?;
(iv) to whom are results given?;
(v) how are subsequent changes implemented?

6. *Quality standards/protocol*:
(i) common protocols/standards;
(ii) agreed between purchasers/providers;
(iii) monitored by whom, how and when?

Staffing

Speech and language therapists who have worked in this field will appreciate some of the difficulties and challenges of providing a service. It therefore is implicit that any service manager should have some experience and specialised knowledge of the work. However, there are probably not enough such therapists around to fill managerial posts. Also the increasing, often financially-based, trend of employing therapists of lesser experience in managerial roles may mean that the service manager's experience is limited. Managers and therapists in such situations can use the Royal College of Speech and Language Therapists' advisory network to good advantage.

If the service is an assessment-only one, it is essential to have therapists of some experience, whereas if therapy/management components are included, skill-mix analysis indicates some scope for less experienced therapists, assistants, students or even volunteers to carry out some tasks. The more experienced therapists in a comprehensive service would appraise and support other staff. Table 4.1 shows a skill-mix analysis of various tasks.

Table 4.1

Type of Work	Staff	SLT Grade
Service Management	SLT	3
Assessment		
i) Communication	SLT	2
ii) Swallowing	SLT	2
Therapy/Management		
a) individual:		
i) communication	SLT	2 (1/2 under supervision)
ii) swallowing	SLT	2
b) group:		
i) therapy	SLT, assistant with volunteers, students	2
ii) communication	SLT, assistant with volunteers, students	2/1/2
iii) reality orientation	SLT, assistant with volunteers	2/1/2
Teaching		
i) Other staff	SLT	2
ii) Patients/Carers	SLT	2
Research		
Administration		
i) Secretarial	Secretary	–
ii) Other clerical	Secretary/ Assistant	–

Key: Grade 1 – a clinical post suitable for a new or recently qualified therapist where support from specialists or managers is available.

Grade 2 – a post with more responsibility where experience, special skills or managerial skills are required.

Grade 3 – a top-level practitioner's post which may be generalist, specialist or managerial.

Whilst the service workload dictates staffing levels and skill mix, the broader management structure, within which a department is working, will be influential.

Three management structures found at present are delineated below:

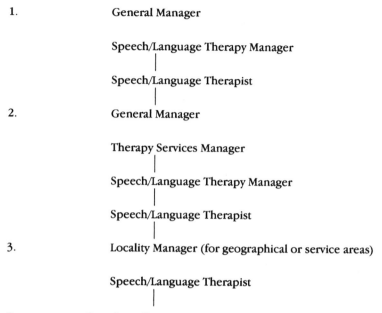

1.   General Manager

            Speech/Language Therapy Manager
                        |
            Speech/Language Therapist
                        |
2.   General Manager

            Therapy Services Manager
                        |
            Speech/Language Therapy Manager
                        |
            Speech/Language Therapist
                        |
3.   Locality Manager (for geographical or service areas)

            Speech/Language Therapist
                        |

Supporters of each will present it in the most favourable light, e.g. cost-effective, available professional and peer support, but in reality all have plus and minus points. Whether any particular structure works depends on

(i)   the way individuals communicate;
(ii) the flexibility within the structure;
(iii) whether it is adequately funded;
(iv) the numbers and grading of staff which may relate to:
   • numbers of clients;
   • complexity of service;
   • range of service;
   • amount of face-to-face contact time;
   • amount of other patient-related activity;
   • multidisciplinary team commitments;
   • teaching;
   • research;
   • amount of management time required;
   • other team tasks, i.e. audit, standards, outcomes.

Recruitment of staff can be difficult in some parts of the UK, but if therapists work in a dynamic team atmosphere, with good managerial support and opportunities for career development, recruitment and retention problems may be averted. A recent survey by speech and language therapy managers in what was the North West Thames Region found that job design, management attitudes, resources and funding were more important to recruitment and retention than other factors such as pay (Edelman and Hughes, 1994).

Links with voluntary agencies

In recent years voluntary agencies have been increasingly involved in service provision. Those organisations with whom the speech and language therapist working in this area may have contact are:

- Alzheimer's Disease Society;
- Parkinson's Disease Society;
- Age Concern;
- Help the Aged;
- MIND;
- Crossroads Care Scheme;
- Hospital League of Friends;
- Local Volunteer Bureau.

It would once have been exclusively other professionals on whom the speech and language therapist relied for information, support and implementation of therapy or environmental changes. Now, it is frequently likely to be volunteers from some of the above organisations who may have more to do with clients on a day-to-day basis, especially those in the community. This change raises questions about the type and extent of training individuals working for these organisations may have had, or may need. When working with other disciplines, e.g. nurses, occupational therapists, a certain level of knowledge and experience is assumed. It is likely that volunteers will have a more disparate knowledge base and varying levels of experience.

In order for speech and language therapy management to be implemented, support may need to be sought from individuals working for these agencies, as well as the client's family or friends. It may therefore be appropriate to suggest that some form of training related to communication and swallowing problems should be provided for volunteers and other care workers. Observation of a therapist at work can be helpful, but it can be better to suggest input into an existing training programme run by the organisation concerned.

If there are problems in funding such teaching activities, interested volunteers may be able to participate in teaching or workshop sessions run locally for professional staff, although any therapist running such sessions will need to be aware of these participants' needs. Some pre-

prepared but flexible training packages are available, such as Working with Elderly People (Stevens et al., 1992), Dysphagia Training for Nursing Staff (Heritage and Knapp, 1994) and Action for Dysphasic Adults Communicate Scheme (ADA, 1995), which reduce the amount of time needed for preparation of workshops and talks.

Literature and handouts should be available as an accompaniment to any session whether run for professionals or volunteers. Some specifically relating to communication, notably in dementia, have been produced by speech and language therapists (Tanton, 1993). The Alzheimer's Disease Society and the Parkinson's Disease Society also produce useful booklets.

It is possible that, in the foreseeable future, links with voluntary agencies will be formalised by contracts. If so, that could clarify issues related to training, as the commitment to give and receive such training programmes might be part of any contract.

Private patient provision

Earlier in the chapter mention was made of provision to private residential and/or nursing homes. The 1980s saw an enormous expansion in the provision of residential care by the private sector, due to a number of factors:

- closure of NHS long-stay units;
- increase in the 'old-old' population;
- enhanced financial status of the elderly:
- increased involvement of charities;
- potential for financial gain in residential home ownership.

Most speech and language therapists working in this area have had some referrals from these homes for assessment and/or therapy. Although not all of these will be appropriate to the present discussion, many will have come under the umbrella of elderly mentally infirm provision.

Owing to the recent recession, a number of these homes and the residents therein may have found themselves financially stretched, and so the perceived luxury of (a) a speech/language therapy assessment and (b) staff training may not be a high priority. However, that does not mean that any speech/language therapy service should exclude these clients from provision, although any financial implications of service provision must be fully discussed at a managerial level before a therapist becomes involved.

If residents are registered with an NHS general practitioner, they may be able to receive care without a financial outlay to home or individual. The Royal College of Speech Therapists offers guidance with regard to private patient charges, and speech and language therapy managers should agree charges with their employer's financial or costing department.

Costing

The cost of all areas of service must be agreed with the finance managers of the service provider. Any cost calculation needs to take into account:

- staff time (including preparation, travelling and administration);
- grading of staff;
- costs and overheads;
- consumables.

Costs should be established before any contracting negotiations are entered into.

Income generation

Although not the most likely clinical area to produce ideas of income generation, with the potential for private patients being limited, other possibilities need to be considered. Some suggestions are:

(i)   staff teaching, e.g. private residential/nursing homes;
(ii   publication of literature (e.g. Tanton, 1993);
(iii) direct access contracts with GPs;
(iv) development and publication of assessment tools, i.e. for differential diagnostic assessment procedures;
(v) lecturing;
(vi) provision of courses and conferences.

Although each of these may in itself be able to generate only relatively small sums, the total may not be negligible. Some of these possibilities would not be regularly available so any income thereby generated should be regarded as a bonus rather than part of a planned cost improvement programme.

Service standards

It is now common practice when any contract is negotiated that standards of service should be agreed. These may relate to areas of:

- service access;
- referral;
- assessment;
- treatment/management;

- discharge;
- outcomes;
- communication;
- audit.

Although local variations in standards should always be considered, speech and language therapy managers should base standards on *Communicating Quality* (RCSLT, 1991), with core standards being met at least 80% of the time.

For this client group standards will, broadly speaking, be no different than for any other group, but some possible differences are worth highlighting:

Referral:

(i)   If referrals from all disciplines are accepted, accurate background medical information should always be sought before the individual is seen. This may sometimes prove difficult in community settings, but is essential to good practice.

(ii) A simple re-referral practice should be considered because of the progressive nature of many pathologies found in this group.

(iii) Access to the service should be by community and/or hospital routes as clients may frequently cross boundaries and need to access provision through either.

Assessment:

(i)   Assessment may need to be carried out over a period of time in short sessions perhaps in a variety of settings and at a number of different times of day. Assessment may include:
- observation;
- discussion with other relevant staff/carers;
- evaluation of the environment;
- informal/formal assessment.

(ii) Standards should allow for the fact that it may not be possible to discuss assessment results meaningfully with the client, and that carer involvement is crucial.

Management:

(i)   Ongoing reassessment and carer support are part of a quality service as the communication situation will change over time.

(ii) The patient's previous level of function must be taken into account.

The procedure for the regular monitoring of standards should be agreed by purchaser and provider, together with the action to be taken if standards are not being met. Some purchasers in the UK are levying financial penalties if standards are failed consistently. If this is a possibility, due, for example, to recruitment problems, purchasers should be alerted as early as possible before the situation affects the service.

Legal considerations

As stated in *Communicating Quality* (RCSLT, 1991, p. 198), 'a client has the right under common law to give or withdraw consent prior to examination or treatment'. In the case of some of the patients seen as part of an EMI service the ability of the patient to give reasoned consent may be in doubt.

For any assessment or therapy intervention, oral consent is always solicited, but with some clients incapable of giving informed consent, appropriate mechanisms for carer consent should be established. Difficulties are most likely to arise when the problem is one of swallowing/feeding. Information obtained from, or advice given to, the carer should be clearly and accurately recorded in patient and speech and language therapy notes.

If there is any doubt, the service managers should consult their employer's legal adviser. If it appears that the disregard of speech and language therapy advice will lead to increased risk for the client, lack-of-consent forms such as those shown in Appendices 2 and 3 may be of use.

Although most work in this field relates to communication problems, an increasing number of referrals are being made for people with feeding and/or swallowing difficulties. Ethical problems arise if the client is unable, or refuses, to carry out speech and language therapy management recommendations, thereby putting him or herself at risk. In such situations the legal status of the client is important. If a carer has legal responsibility for the client's affairs, i.e. Enduring Power of Attorney has been activated, the legal responsibility for care will have shifted, and the therapist needs to ensure the carer has been asked for consent to treatment, and made aware of any risks involved.

Appendix 2 relates to a legal guardian of a client and Appendix 3 to the representative of a cognitively impaired client. The latter should be signed by the client and representative together.

There should be no coercion in the process of gaining a client's consent and, above all, the therapist must record, clearly and factually, activity related to all contacts. Any entries in the client's notes should be signed.

Speech and language therapy training

In order to ensure the future of the speech and language profession, student observation and clinical experience are essential. Students need to have the opportunity to view and treat as wide a range of clients as possible, of whom EMI patients will be one group.

As EMI clients present complex clinical problems, some ethical and legal considerations may arise with regard to student involvement, which may not be present for those in whom cognition remains unimpaired.

Since the 1991 UK regrading of therapists, when the student allowance was subsumed in Grade 2 salaries, managers have had an obligation to provide facilities for student training. Such facilities need to be acknowledged in any contracting arrangements.

Considerations concerning teaching practice should be made explicit in any service standards. As stated on p.222 in *Communicating Quality* (RCSLT, 1991), it is 'clinicians who should request and obtain permission of the client or relevant Unit Head before observation or treatment'.

Some students may find work in this field depressing or pointless, as few patients are 'treatable' in the conventional sense of the word. Good student placement planning should therefore include adequate time for discussion of the aims and practice of the service, and the student should be placed with a therapist with some experience of this type of work. The importance of multidisciplinary team working needs constantly to be emphasised.

Any written reports by students should be checked and counter-signed by the therapist with responsibility for the student placement before being filed or written in patient notes.

It is possible that future changes in clinical training programmes, such as the increased use of teaching videos, will overcome some of these difficulties. However, nothing can entirely replace the benefits of good 'hands-on' experience, under the supervision of an experienced and enthusiastic therapist.

Research

The need for research in all areas of speech and language therapy clinical practice is widely acknowledged. It is even more important in some respects in a relatively new area of practice such as this when new assessment techniques and therapeutic approaches are being developed.

A number of different approaches may be viable:

- validation of a particular therapeutic approach;
- measurement of treatment/management outcomes;
- development and standardisation of appropriate assessments;
- effect of communication problems on carers (both professional and non-professional);
- single-case studies;
- case/service audit, unit or multidisciplinary.

Research is time consuming and demanding. Any therapist undertaking research needs to be enthusiastic about the project, and well supported clinically and administratively. Research must be carefully planned. Although small-scale research may be done as part of a therapist's clinical remit, more comprehensive work will need specifically allocated time, and therefore funding. Quite commonly it will be undertaken as part of a postgraduate qualification, e.g. MSc, MPhil or PhD.

In the UK all research should follow the Royal College of Speech and Language Therapists' ethical guidelines for research, and must fulfil an employer's ethics committee requirements. This also applies to students, undergraduate and postgraduate, doing any original research work in a particular unit or department. In these instances any time schedule needs to allow for submission to the appropriate research ethics committee.

If research is undertaken, clients, carers, unit managers and purchasers all need to be kept informed of plans and progress. The latter will be primarily interested in the potential benefits of research to them, i.e. income generation potential, improved quality of care, more cost-effective care, and better use of resources, so results need to be presented with those factors in mind.

Because this is such a new area of care it is essential for the development of the profession's knowledge base that any research findings, positive or negative, are made known. Special interest group meetings, refereed journals, conferences and publications such as *Therapy Weekly* are four possible channels of communication. However, for the quality of the profession's work in this field to be acknowledged all effort should be made to get papers published in refereed journals of national and international repute.

Summary

This chapter has looked at management of an EMI speech and language therapy service under the following headings:

- Service aims;
- Contracts;
- Sites of provision;
- Referral;
- Intervention;
- Discharge;
- Service components;
- Links with voluntary agencies;
- Private patient provision;
- Costing;
- Income generation;

- Service standards;
- Legal considerations;
- Speech/language therapy training;
- Research.

It is not intended to be prescriptive, but rather to raise awareness of certain issues in those who are new to this area of service management.

It is a service area which is likely to change in the reorganised health service, and speech and language therapy managers will need to ensure that clients or potential clients are not disadvantaged as a result of that change.

Chapter 5:
The Team Approach to Working with the Elderly Mentally Ill

KIM ZABIHI AND KAREN BRYAN

Introduction

This chapter will consider the various disciplines and agencies that are likely to become involved in providing care those elderly people who are suffering from psychiatric disorders associated with old age. Psychiatric illnesses, with their concomitant social, medical and emotional problems, are an important cause of loss of functional independence by elderly people.

Although they are not exceptional in terms of proportions, the numbers of elderly people who are suffering from mental illness do pose a profound challenge for all those who become involved in caring for them: from their families, friends and neighbours, through to workers in the health and social services, residential care facilities and the voluntary sector. Two examples of elderly people with psychiatric disorder are given below. Their management is seen to be complex and requires a range of professional inputs including speech and language therapy, but the role of community and family agents is also vitally important.

Case example 1

An 85-year-old widow was referred by her GP to the day hospital, after what appeared to be a small stroke at home. She had had an initial stroke two years previously, but made a complete recovery. Her daughter told day hospital staff that her mother's memory had begun to fail over the last two years, although she had been able to communicate well and manage at home without help from social services.

The speech and language therapist found this client's communication to be severely impaired by a fluent dysphasia and accompanying press for speech; the occupational therapist confirmed that this lady appeared bewildered and unable to carry out simple sequential tasks in the kitchen. On her next attendance, day hospital staff noted that she appeared unwell; her speech was copious, incoherent and rambling; she could not settle and appeared generally confused by her surroundings. Her daughter felt she had deteriorated over the weekend and might have had another stroke.

Admission to the hospital ward was therefore arranged as it was felt that she was at risk if she returned home. The team felt that further investigations, including a brain scan, should be carried out to identify the cause of her progressive memory loss and other difficulties. During her admission, further assessments were carried out by the team, and a joint care planning meeting was organised with the family in order to discuss the patient's future support needs.

Case Example 2

An 84-year-old married woman attended the day hospital for assessment of her mobility and communication skills following a recent stroke. She was known to have suffered two previous strokes. She was pleasant and talkative, but rather reluctant to cooperate in assessment procedures. She presented with:

- a slight weakness to her right arm and leg ;
- associated difficulties with fine motor movements;
- slight slurring of speech;
- occasional dribbling.

She denied any other difficulties and maintained that she was managing to look after herself and her husband at home. However, she was experiencing word-finding difficulties during speech, and appeared unable to retain information given to her about the day hospital routine. Discussion with her husband revealed that she had been experiencing a progressive forgetfulness for about two years. She was becoming increasingly reluctant to socialise except with her family, and became anxious whenever her husband went out of the house, for example to go shopping. She was unable to walk long distances and was apprehensive about 'going out', except to go in the car to visit her daughter.

She tended to repeat the same questions to staff at the day hospital. The team assessment indicated that this woman appeared to be in the early stages of dementia due to multiple infarct episodes. The occupational therapist carried out a home visit in order to assess whether the couple would benefit from the provision of any aids or adaptations in the home, for example to assist with bathing or in the kitchen. A referral was made to the social worker to arrange for a day centre place, which would also give her husband time during the week to do the shopping and other necessary jobs. It was also decided to review this client on an outpatient basis in order to monitor her progress and provide further help at home for the couple should this become necessary.

This chapter will consider the implications for multi-agency involvement in meeting the support needs of the mentally ill elderly and those of their carers.

Why the team approach?

The elderly person with a mental illness is likely to experience a variety of problems which can reduce independence in life skills and require the intervention of care-giving personnel representing various disciplines and agencies. The major mental disorders which are encountered in clinical practice with the elderly are:

• confusional states;
• the dementias;
• depression;
• paranoid conditions or 'paraphrenia'.

In practice, however, the elderly are frequently found to present with a combination of interrelated mental and physical symptoms. In addition, psychiatric disorders may coexist in the elderly and each of the four conditions named above could in practice mistakenly be diagnosed for any of the others.

In many cases, there may be no clear psychiatric disorder but a combination of handicaps and home circumstances which can act as the trigger for the onset of mental health problems. For example: an elderly woman in her 80s living alone in an upstairs flat was unable to move around or get out easily owing to severe arthritis. A severe hearing loss made social interaction difficult and her anxiety about burglars encouraged feelings of suspicion so that she became increasingly isolated and lonely.

The diagnostic process is therefore complex and requires careful multidimensional, multidisciplinary analysis. It is because of the multiplicity of problems that are usually presented that services for the elderly are commonly provided by a team rather than by an individual.

Such a team typically comprises medical staff, psychologist, social workers and physio-, occupational and speech/language therapists. This enables the skills and specialisations of workers from the various disciplines to be utilised in formulating an overall care plan.

The following sections will describe the typical multidisciplinary team which is likely to become involved in service provision for an elderly mentally infirm person in the UK, the role of individual members within that team, and the implementation of multi-agency care in hospital and community settings.

Networks of care

Within the literature, the terms formal and informal networks have been used to describe the services which are available to help elderly people and their carers (Gilleard, 1992).

Formal services are provided mainly by statutory organisations such as the health authority (hospitals and primary health care teams) and the local authority (social services and housing agencies), and involve paid workers. Some private services (residential homes, nursing homes, housing schemes and respite care schemes) and the larger voluntary organisations can also be included under the heading of formal networks.

Informal care networks involve the elderly person's family, friends, and neighbours – all those individuals who are involved in providing flexible help on a day-to-day basis in the home setting. Some locally organised volunteer schemes in the community may also be included as informal networks.

The help provided by family and friends can cover anything from weekly help with the shopping to providing care on a 24-hour basis for a frail and profoundly disabled elderly person. Thus the role of family and friends remains crucial in supporting the elderly person and in complementing the formal care provided by the statutory services. *The Rising Tide* (Health Advisory Service, 1982) describes the commonest pattern of care for the elderly as consisting of support from within the person's family and social networks, with help when needed from social services and primary health care teams, backed by specialist hospital services.

In the case of a progressive disease such as Alzheimer's disease, the global cognitive impairment and progressive deterioration mean that help from both formal and informal sources is likely to be required. The amount and type of input will vary depending upon the degree of impairment being experienced by the elderly person.

Formal networks of care: the multidisciplinary team

The speciality of psychogeriatrics was developed as a branch of psychiatry to provide expertise in the total management of mental illness in old age. Pitt (1982) states that the efficient running of a psychogeriatric service begins with a team which has a special interest in the psychiatry of old age, provides a full range of psychiatric skills, and has good knowledge of general medicine and social interventions.

Most psychiatric services for the elderly are based on a team of workers from different disciplines who, as well as providing services directly, also liaise with people outside the 'core' team (Wattis and Martin, 1994).

Multidisciplinary input to the team ideally enables the physical, psychological and social needs of the elderly patient with psychiatric illness to be addressed concurrently. The core team providing a specialist service for the elderly mentally ill normally includes representatives from each of the following disciplines:

- medicine;
- psychiatry;
- nursing;
- social work;
- physiotherapy;
- occupational therapy.

The following professionals are also likely to have an input to the core team:

- clinical psychologist;
- speech and language therapist;
- dietician;
- audiologist;
- dentist;
- chiropodist.

The core team should aim to involve principal carers such as relatives, neighbours and home helps, who are likely to be most familiar with the elderly person and the daily problems which are being experienced in the home setting.

The role of the speech and language therapist

Speech and language therapists have specialist skills and knowledge for the evaluation and treatment of communication disorders. The speech and language therapist is concerned with the person's total ability to communicate. Speech and language assessment can help to identify communication abilities that are still working well and those that are impaired as a result of the underlying disorder.

Speech and language therapists working with the elderly are usually based within hospitals, and offer services on both an inpatient and outpatient basis. Some districts offer a domiciliary service to elderly people at home, or in residential institutions.

Speech and language therapy assessment is an important component of the multidisciplinary assessment and diagnostic process. For example, the specific pattern of language deterioration in Alzheimer-type dementia is recognised as distinct from the linguistic deficits consequent upon focal neurological lesions such as stroke. The assessment of the pattern of communicative breakdown can contribute to the differential diagnostic process.

The most frequent differential diagnosis that the speech and language therapist will be asked to make is that between a dementia and aphasia (Gravell, 1988). Where a dementia is suspected, the assessment must include measures of cognition as well as language because evidence of more general cognitive decline is essential to the diagnosis of dementia. According to Gravell, the separation of language assessment from cognition will be of little clinical value.

A comprehensive test battery should include assessment of cognitive functions such as orientation, memory and learning as well as expressive and receptive language skills and communication ability. Such assessment necessitates a multidisciplinary approach.

Periodic reassessment of communication skills can provide information for the rest of the team about whether the causative disorder appears to be stable or progressive in its pattern of linguistic deficits. For example, if a dementia of the Alzheimer type is present, a deterioration will usually be evident on reassessment after a time delay of six months.

Griffiths and Baldwin (1989) point out some benefits arising from the speech and language therapist working as a recognised member of the core team. Attendance at weekly team meetings results in on-the-spot referrals of cases for assessment; another benefit is the raised consciousness of the rest of the team towards communication problems, as a result of exposure to the speech and language therapist's skills and clinical procedures.

The speech and language therapist's role as a member of the multidisciplinary team involves providing information relevant to the management of individual patients, and also being a source of advice and expertise on the nature and management of communication problems in the elderly population.

Heritage and Farrow (1994) found that the work of the speech and language therapist was best understood and appreciated, most effective, and most rewarding, when the therapist was a specialist and permanent member of the multidisciplinary team.

Several specific areas can be identified where the skills of the speech and language therapist can make a significant contribution to the overall care of mentally impaired elderly people. However, work with this client group is very different from the speech and language therapist's traditional role involving individual face-to-face therapy (Tanner and Daniels, 1990).

Gravell (1988) points out that the speech and language therapist working with the elderly must be 'convinced' of his or her own role in order to ensure that others understand it; this may present problems for speech and language therapists beginning to take on more 'indirect' functions such as training, as contrasted with 'direct' treatment work with communication-impaired patients.

However, as the numbers of elderly people in our community continue to increase into the next century, so have there been accompanying changes in the overall philosophy of care applied to this population, with greater emphasis on informing people about the ageing process and the communication disorders which can accompany it.

The current management emphasis is on detailed assessment of the elderly person's communication breakdown, as a basis for advising relatives and care workers on strategies which they can use to facilitate their own communication with the elderly person. The ultimate aim of teaching must be to inform staff about how elderly people communicate and the specific comunication disorders which can be experienced by elderly people. Heritage and Farrow (1994) found training to be a significant role for speech and language therapists providing a service to the elderly mentally ill. In their survey, therapists were providing teaching input to staff and also to local relatives' support schemes. Nursing staff were found to perceive training through demonstration, i.e. the opportunity to observe the therapist communicating in informal settings, as the best way to teach basic communication skills.

The speech and language therapist has an important role to play in identifying environmental and other factors which may be limiting the mentally impaired person's communication attempts and skills (Lubinski, 1995).

Gravell (1988) emphasises the importance of setting up training programmes for staff working in residential homes and other institutional settings. Such training programmes must promote the principles of a 'quality communication environment' which encourages communicative interchange by its elderly residents. The therapist can advise on alterations to the physical environment which may be necessary to encourage communication attempts by the elderly person. Physical changes could include rearranging furniture in communal rooms to a layout which promotes social interaction; reducing intrusive background noise from radios and televisions; ensuring suitable lighting to compensate for auditory impairment, and providing memory aids such as name labels.

The speech and language therapist may be involved in planning and running groups to stimulate communication skills. Such groups may be organised in day hospital or residential care settings and can involve other members of staff. Different types of groups can be set up depending on the needs and abilities of the elderly people invited to participate; some groups may use specific treatment techniques such as reality orientation and reminiscence therapy, whereas other groups are less formal and focus on encouraging conversation and open discussions relevant to current events.

Speech and language therapists can be involved in devising training and support programmes for the families and carers of elderly mentally infirm people. Tanner and Daniels (1990) set up a project in which they observed the behaviour of carers (husbands or wives) while communicating with their dementing elderly relative. The researchers were able to identify carer behaviours which facilitated communication and behaviours which were unhelpful. They subsequently used their findings to run a series of practical communication workshops for carers. Projects such as this help to reinforce the role of the speech and language therapist in providing training for all those involved in communicative interactions with elderly mentally ill people.

Health care teams: hospital and community

In the UK, health care workers may approach the elderly mentally frail person from either hospital or community-based services. The hospital team normally operates under the leadership of the consultant in that particular medical discipline. The specialist hospital team for old-age psychiatry is normally headed by the the psychogeriatrician, a consultant psychiatrist who holds special responsibility for the psychiatry of old age. A psychogeriatrician will normally work with a team of staff who also have a special responsibility for the elderly (Fraser, 1987). Typical team members are:

- the community psychiatric nurse;
- social worker;
- occupational therapist;
- physiotherapist;
- psychologist.

Most referrals to the psychogeriatrician are through the general practitioner, and diagnosis in the first instance is usually the premise of the consultant (Fraser, 1987). There is normally close collaboration between the psychogeriatricians and the geriatricians (physicians specialising in the medicine of old age). Substantial overlap has been noted between the elderly who are physically ill and those with dementia (Copeland et al., 1975).

Hospital facilities for the elderly mentally infirm may be sited in local community hospitals or at the district general hospital, and include:

- acute admission beds;
- continuing care or long-stay beds;
- holiday relief and respite beds;
- day hospital places;
- outpatient clinics;
- specialised assessment facilities such as memory clinics.

Access to the hospital is usually via the general practitioner, although in urgent cases following a crisis situation the admission may be via the accident and emergency department.

It is important that the nuclear health care team in one facility – for example the hospital-based consultant and specialist team – should work in close collaboration with the primary health care team and support networks which are based in the community. The primary health care services provide health and supportive care to sick or disabled elderly people in the community. Old-age psychiatry is an area where a more integrated model of care often exists between hospital and community-based health care services (Wattis and Martin, 1994), with the same core team involved in assessment and management of the patient in the community and within the hospital.

The family doctor or general practitioner (GP) is usually the focal point of the community-based primary health care team (Bennett, 1989). GPs are moving increasingly towards work in group practices, which involve a number of doctors based at a health centre together with other primary health care workers such as the district nurses and specialist nurses attached to each GP practice. Community physiotherapists and speech and language therapists are also part of the primary health care service.

The GP is frequently the first point of contact for a confused or depressed elderly person and his or her anxious family. The GP may be regarded by many elderly people and their families as the gatekeeper to services which they feel they may need, and an advocate in ensuring that their needs are met expeditiously (Williamson, Smith and Burley, 1987).

The GP therefore is, or should be, the key figure in the management of the elderly mentally ill at home. Being locally placed, the GP should be familiar with local support services, and with how to obtain specialist help for the elderly mentally ill person.

It is, however, necessary that elderly people with mental illness are known to their GP. The implementation of an age/sex register, as recommended by The Royal College of Physicians' report (1981) enables the GP to be aware of the elderly population in the practice and to develop specific services for this group.

The report also recommended (Royal College of Physicians, 1981) that the population especially at risk for dementia (i.e. those aged over 65) should be involved in regular screening programmes. The revised (1990) GP contract includes an offer of an annual check-up and home visit for over 75s (O'Neill, 1991). Screening programmes for the elderly, often utilising health visitors or district nurses in implementing the programmes, are being developed (Bennett, 1989; O'Connor et al., 1993). However, there is some doubt as to whether the elderly will benefit unless such a service is followed up by accessible management and support (Mcintosh and Power, 1993).

The district nursing service provides nursing care to elderly people in the community. District nurses are qualified nurses who have undergone specialist community nurse training. District nurses are traditionally attached to GP practices and work closely with the GP. Access to the service is usually through the GP.

The work of the district nurse covers various aspects of nursing care such as wound care, supervising medication and giving injections. Home nursing of frail and dependent elderly people can also involve help with washing, dressing/undressing and getting in and out of bed.

Specialist nurses have expertise in the management of particular problems such as diabetes and incontinence. For example, continence advisers are nurses who have a special interest and expertise in helping with mainly urinary, but also faecal incontinence. They assess continence problems and advise on available aids and services. They may be based in the hospital or community. Help with managing incontinence may be required by those caring for elderly relatives with dementia.

District nurses may require advice from speech and language therapists on how best to communicate with elderly clients who have dementia. In particular, advice on how much the client can understand in relation to instructions for taking medication, etc. District nurses may refer clients directly to speech and language therapy as they may be in regular contact with an elderly person and may be first to notice difficulties with communication.

Community psychiatric nurses (CPNs) are nurses with specialist training in psychiatry. They offer help and support in the community to people who are affected by mental illnesses, including dementia, and to their carers. Their role includes advising on medication, supporting relatives and monitoring patients living at home who are already known to the service. The majority of well-established psychogeriatric services have CPNs attached (Health Advisory Service, 1982). CPNs are employed by the health authority; their work involves close liaison with both health and social services.

The CPN may work from a local hospital, where he or she liaises closely with the psychogeriatrician; many are based at local health centres and therefore work in close collaboration with the GP and other members of the primary health care team.

The CPNs play an essential role in maintaining elderly people with dementia at home. Much of their work involves intervening in crisis situations and monitoring the situation afterwards.

Whatever services visit the elderly person at home, they and the carer should keep a record of the worker's name, contact number and date of the visit. Such information can be especially important when care is being provided in the home for elderly people who are confused and unable to remember which services (a hot meal, help with medication, bathing) they have received that day.

Therapy services: hospital and community

Occupational therapists (OTs) have specialist training in assessing the problems a person may have in managing daily life activities. They advise the person and their carers on practical ways of coping with the disability. Some occupational therapists work in hospitals, whilst others are employed by the local authority and work in the community.

The occupational therapist can advise on adaptations to the home and provide aids and specialised equipment (safety rails, commodes, bath boards, modified kitchen utensils) which improve safety and functional performance especially in the areas of personal care (washing, dressing, toileting) and domestic tasks (safety in the kitchen, ability to prepare meals). The mentally impaired elderly experience difficulties with routine skills. Self-care may be neglected because of grief, depression or delusions; confusion and forgetfulness present safety hazards in the home. Signs of such difficulties can be picked up during home visits, and are manifest as burnt pans or items put away in the wrong place, for example clothes in the refrigerator.

Assessments of domestic functioning are usually carried out by the occupational therapist in the person's own home, but may also take place at the day hospital or during admission to a hospital ward. The information from the OT assessment is taken into consideration by social services when planning support services provision at home, or when a move into residential care may be be necessary.

The occupational therapist can also be involved in providing therapeutic activities on an individual or group basis for confused or depressed elderly patients in the hospital or day hospital settings (Bach et al., 1995). Group activities may be run jointly with other staff such as speech and language therapists and thus promote joint working (Bryan and Drew, 1987).

Again, occupational therapists may need to refer clients to speech and language therapy if they detect communication difficulties during everyday activities. Speech and language therapists and occupational therapists may also liaise in the assessment of functioning at home and the provision of practical aids such as louder telephone bells for the hard of hearing and the format and siting of memory aids such as lists of telephone numbers.

Physiotherapists have expertise in maintaining and, wherever possible, improving all aspects of mobility. They can be based either in hospitals or in the community. Physiotherapy is part of the care of the elderly mentally ill because such clients commonly experience mobility and balance problems which may be associated with specific disease processes (e.g. cerebral infarctions), fractures following falls or injury, or age-related deterioration in sensory abilities (vision and hearing) (Pickles, 1995).

Physiotherapy treatment techniques for the frail and mentally ill elderly can involve individual or group exercise programmes, which can be implemented in partnership with nursing staff and other members of the team in the hospital or residential environment, in order to maximise functional mobility skill.

The physiotherapist is also involved in the selection, provision and supervision of mobility aids (e.g. walking sticks, frames) and adapted furniture (e.g. chairs, cushions and back rests), tailored to meet individual needs (Smythe, 1990).

Physiotherapists may also require advice from the speech and language therapist on how best to give instructions to a client who is undergoing therapy for example to improve walking. Physiotherapists and speech and language therapists may also be involved in joint programmes, for example to improve sequencing skills in everyday activities in a client with dementia.

Principles of effective teamwork

The involvement of a diversity of disciplines and organisations in services for elderly people with mental illness provides opportunities for creative and effective cooperation between the workers and their respective organisations. But, equally, a special effort is required to ensure that the team works towards the greatest benefit for the elderly person.

There are a number of factors which can influence the overall effectiveness of multi-agency teamwork, including:

* quality and style of leadership;
* personality and attitudes of individual team members and their previous experience of teamwork;
* frequency and organisation of team meetings;
* accommodation or location of the workplace.

Leadership is a vital function within the multidisciplinary team (Wattis and Martin, 1994). An effective team leader seeks to create a climate in which the skills and knowledge of team members can be fully utilised in the provision of effective services.

Hierarchichal structures differ within different disciplines, and may be a potential source of conflict in the context of multidisciplinary working. Close collaboration is needed to prevent conflict, and to facilitate the blurring of role demarcations and status hierarchies. There must be a mutual recognition of, and respect for, each other's skills and professionalism.

The multidisciplinary team will consist of a mixture of unique and shared skills. The extent of overlap and skill sharing in any team will be determined by the training, experience and special interests of individual team members. Each discipline represented on the team has its own area of expertise and responsibility. For example, the doctor has the responsibility for prescribing medication; the home-care manager is responsible for allocating support services to elderly people in their homes.

There will be some aspects of care, for example counselling skills, in which many members of the team have relevant experience and training. Team members must therefore be flexible with respect to overlap of roles and responsibilities. A successful multidisciplinary team makes full use of the expertise of each of its members, pooling skills and effort to achieve a coordinated plan of care which will be of maximum benefit to the elderly person and his or her caregivers. Each professional involved with the elderly person must also recognise the limitations of their own expertise and responsiblity and be prepared to refer on to other disciplines for further assessment or intervention.

The diversity of personnel and working styles requires good communication between all concerned. It is vitally important that each member of the team is aware of what other members are doing; in the absence of interagency communication, there is the risk of duplicated effort, or some aspects of care being left uncovered.

Regular contact with colleagues from other disciplines can take place through informal on-the-spot discussions or at organised team meetings and is important on several counts: to improve communication, maintain continuity of care, and ensure a consistency of approach in care provision. This gives the opportunity to pool skills and efforts for the most effective use of resources. This is particularly important as a continuously ageing population means that the demand for resources is always likely to exceed the available supply. Where weekly team meetings are part of the care planning process, there should be an atmosphere which encourages each team member to share relevant information and participate in the care-planning process. Successful teamwork promotes honest discussion between disciplines, such that individual points of view are acknowledged and incorporated into improved total care for the patient (Gray, 1982).

Joint working and liaison can be made easier where all members of the team share the same premises or work in close geographical proximity. This makes weekly team meetings and case conferences easier to organise and easier for team members to attend. In the hospital setting, for example, the multidisciplinary team has the advantage of being based at a single geographical location (Brocklehurst,1995).

In the community setting, workers from different disciplines may operate from different locations which are widely dispersed. Regular face-to-face meetings may prove costly in terms of travelling time. However, effective team working and liaison can be achieved in the context of collaborative ventures such as joint assessment visits to the elderly person's home (Arie, 1991; Neill and Williams, 1992).

The success of the multidisciplinary team ultimately depends upon each individual recognising and acknowledging the contribution of each fellow worker on the team. Membership of the team is not confined to the health and social service professionals; recognition should also be given to the role played by workers from organisations such as the home care service and voluntary agencies, and the contribution of the elderly person's family or other caregivers.

Those involved in caring for the elderly mentally ill, many of whom are dependent and in need of long-term care, need to share a common philosophy with respect to caring for the aged and the quality of that care. This is best achieved within the context of collaborative and harmonious teamwork, which in turn depends largely upon effort and goodwill from each member of the team.

Joint working to plan coordinated care

The vast majority of mentally ill elderly people in the UK live at home (Wattis and Martin, 1994), either alone or with family or friends. These people have the right of access to help and care when needed.

The overall philosophy underlying intervention with the mentally ill elderly should be to provide a supporting structure to enable each person to maintain a satisfactory quality of life either in their own home, or in an alternative residential environment should such a move become inevitable.

Wattis and Martin (1994) view a comprehensive psychiatric service for old people as providing the following compartments of care:

- treatment and support in the community;
- acute inpatient treatment;
- long-stay residential or nursing care.

The effective functioning of such a service depends upon a comprehensive assessment process, which is implemented at the point of entry to the service and whenever needs change, or a move from one compartment of care to another may be necessary (Grimley Evans, 1993; Utting 1993). Assessment must go hand-in-hand with good communication between all those involved in providing care for the elderly person. It is also important to ensure that information is passed appropriately between the various care agencies as an elderly person's needs and resulting care change.

Assessment is the essential preliminary task which forms the basis for any intervention process. The aim of assessment is to provide a diagnosis of the underlying illness, together with an evaluation of the elderly person's social, medical and psychiatric needs.

The assessment process may be seen as a collaboration between the elderly person, his or her main carers, and the multi-agency team, with the end goal of pooling and coordinating resources to agree and implement a programme of care for each individual. In line with recent government 'care in the community' initiatives, providers of both health and social services in the UK are now required to institute what is referred to as a 'care-planning' procedure (Jolley and Arie, 1992) (previously referred to as 'case' management). Social services authorities have a lead role in this process, and are required to:

- carry out an appropriate assessment of an individual's social needs (including residential and home care and involving medical, nursing and other care agencies;
- design packages of services tailored to meet the assessed needs of individuals and their carers, with appointment of care managers where necessary;
- secure the delivery of services by purchasing and contracting as well as by directly providing services (Department of Health/Social Services Inspectorate, 1991).

This enables joint care plans to be designed in cases where people are likely to require help from more than one agency.

Workers from all agencies concerned, together with the elderly person and his or her relatives or caregivers, are involved in the process of producing an individually tailored 'package of care' which meets the person's perceived need. This usually involves joint case conferences to which relevant members of the health care, social services and home care teams are invited, together with the elderly person's main caregivers (Coles, von Aberdorff and Herzberg, 1991).

Each member of the team undertakes his or her own assessment of the elderly person's abilities and difficulties, the findings of which contribute to the overall picture. The overall care plan or long-term goal will be designed on the basis of the collated assessment findings. It will be concerned with the level of care and support that the elderly person is likely to need, and consideration of where the person is likely to reside in the future, be it remaining in their own home with a supporting package of care services, or perhaps an inevitable move into residential or nursing home care. (Working in the community and care management are discussed further in Chapter 8.)

For the team seeing an elderly person for the first time, it is the caregivers such as relatives who are able to provide vital information about recent events at home and any difficulties which they have been facing in caring for their dementing relative. The assessment process must take into account not only the availability of care provision in the community, but the needs and limitations of carers and the wishes of the elderly person him or herself. Skilled assessment also includes a weighing up of any risks or potential dangers in the existing situation for the elderly sufferer and those who are likely to be directly affected – the carers and neighbours.

Elderly clients change relatively quickly in terms of functional ability and needs; constant review is therefore essential (Gravell, 1988). Members of the multidisciplinary team must be prepared to reassess the elderly individual on a regular basis in order to evaluate progress or deterioration in relation to set management goals. Effective follow-up can ascertain whether the services offered are sufficient to deal with the problem, and the care plan should be modified as circumstances change. Carers at home should also be given a key person or service to contact should the situation deteriorate and more or different types of help be required.

The holding of regular team meetings or case conferences, for example in the hospital setting, enables the group to share information, discuss setbacks or difficulties and reach agreed criteria of success in relation to each person's care plan. Good communication strategies ensure that each team member is informed about decisions relating to the overall care plan, and that information is not misunderstood or omitted.

As far as is practicable, the elderly person and his or her caregivers must be consulted about what is happening and his or her opinions and preferences taken into consideration in the decision-making process. It is important that each member of the team retains sight of the elderly person as a whole individual and not as a series of functions or disabilities. Elderly people who are unable to decide for themselves, as a result of physical or mental incapacity, will need others to do this on their behalf. In most cases, it is the elderly mentally infirm person's next of kin who takes on this responsibility.

Leng (1990) emphasises that caring means doing only what is necessary, and not too much, to help the older person care for him or herself. The overall aim of caregiving should therefore be to encourage independence while maintaining the elderly person's dignity, self-esteem and psychological well-being, all of which are just as important as any aspect of physical care.

Teamwork in practice: the day hospital

Day hospitals form part of the treatment resource to the community. They are run by the health authority and are usually situated on hospital premises. Referral to the day hospital for patients from the community is usually through the general practitioner. The purpose of day hospitals is to bridge the gap between staying at home and admission to hospital; they provide medical, nursing and therapeutic input on a 'day' basis and so avoid the need for admission in many cases.

Jolley and Jolley (1991) describe day hospitals as holding a dynamic balance between care in the community and care on an inpatient basis for those with persistent or progressive disorders. Day hospitals can have a medical or psychiatric basis, providing treatment facilities for the elderly physically frail or elderly mentally frail, respectively.

The day hospital incorporates the multidisciplinary team and has the benefit of one or more workers from each of a number of disciplines working together within the same premises. The team typically includes the consultant psychiatrist or consultant physician and one or more doctors on their team; nursing staff; occupational therapists, physiotherapists and their assistants; and a social worker. There is also likely to be input to the day hospital from other disciplines including speech and language therapy, psychology, dietetics, pharmacy, chiropody and dentistry.

Other staff who are involved in the day-to-day functioning of the day hospital service include secretaries and reception staff; the drivers who provide transport to and from the day hospital; the domestic staff who prepare hot drinks and meals; portering staff who take patients to other departments in the hospital for investigations such as X-rays, hearing and eye tests; and any volunteers, for example volunteer drivers, who may provide an input to the day hospital service.

In some areas where the population is relatively scattered, the 'mobile day hospital' facility has been developed, whereby a team of staff travel from the base hospital to different locations in the community (Wattis and Martin, 1994).

Most patients will be attending the day hospital for a course of treatment of finite duration; the progress of individual patients is reviewed at multidisciplinary team meetings which are usually held on a weekly basis. Some day hospitals accept elderly patients on a long-term basis (Fraser, 1987). This will especially apply in the case of patients with dementia, for whom discharge rates are noted to be very low (Arie, 1979).

Patients usually attend the day hospital on a twice or three times weekly basis, and stay for a full day of treatment from morning until mid-afternoon. In some cases the help of relatives, home carers or other community agencies may need to be enlisted to ensure that the elderly person is able to get ready in time for the transport and does attend the day hospital on scheduled days.

The typical day hospital will include a communal lounge and dining area, separate rooms for individual or group treatment and easily accessible bathroom facilities. The day hospital usually incorporates an occupational therapy 'flatlet' with kitchen, bedroom and bathroom furniture and equipment to enable the occupational therapist to assess performance in daily living skills.

Day hospitals may serve several different functions for elderly people with mental health problems. In addition to providing assessment, diagnostic advice and specialised therapeutic activities for people with functional illness and the dementias, the day hospital can also offer support and counselling services to carers, for example by the setting up of support groups for relatives. By liaising with local voluntary services it may be possible to organise 'sitter' services to enable carers to attend such meetings while their elderly dependent relative is at home. The day hospital provides opportunities for social contact and friendship with others who may be attending for treatment at the same time, which can be of particular benefit to elderly people who live alone and/or suffer from mood disorders such as depression.

Attendance at a day hospital perhaps most importantly also allows respite for the carers, for example a spouse or other family member looking after an elderly person at home. The setting provides opportunities for specialist and innovative therapeutic work with the elderly mentally ill. Techniques such as reality orientation or reminiscence therapy can be implemented on a routine basis by members of staff as well as carers. Reality orientation aims to orientate the elderly confused or dementing person to their environment by constant repetition of information: the date, place, time of day, peoples' names and what is happening that day. Reality orientation acts as an informal or '24 hour' philosophy of care (Holden and Woods, 1988) although it may be presented in the context of organised group sessions.

Reminiscence therapy uses the recall of past experiences to help the older person adjust to the present and to cope with the problems of old age. Reminiscence therapy can be carried out with groups, and requires 'aids' such as old objects or photographs; a collection of such objects in the day hospital can be used in therapeutic tasks with individual patients, or may be displayed to form a 'talking point'.

The effective functioning of day hospitals may depend to a large extent upon the availability of facilities for day care provided by social services or voluntary agencies, to which patients who need ongoing social support and maintenance can be discharged. This involves close liaison with the social worker, who usually organises day centre attendance. In the absence of such day care provision, the balance of places at the day hospital can be disrupted.

Gilleard (1992) suggests that in order for psychogeriatric day hospitals to fulfil their central role within a community, they should expand their role as a resource and training centre and work in conjunction with existing statutory and voluntary services in the community. This may include setting up 'open days' to demonstrate the available service facility to family doctors and other members of the primary health care and domiciliary care teams. Workshops and seminars could also be held for home helps and other groups to enable discussion of issues surrounding care of the elderly mentally ill at home.

Support in the community

It is the case that the majority of those with dementia, even severe dementia, live at home and are cared for by their relatives (Fraser, 1987). Because of their dementia, all are to some degree handicapped and require certain supports in order to enable them to continue living satisfying lives at home. Services provided on a domiciliary basis may be able to maintain people at home despite extreme levels of disability (Bebbington and Charnley, 1990; Henwood, 1992).

The elderly are the greatest consumers of local authority welfare services in Britain (Jolley and Jolley, 1991); in addition, families who care for an elderly person with mental illness are likely to require support from services such as carer support groups, respite care and sitting services. The majority of services which enable elderly people to be supported at home are provided by the social services department of the local authority. Such services include:

- day centres;
- the provision of home care;
- meals on wheels and aids ;
- adaptations to property.

Other schemes such as social clubs, support groups and sitting services are often provided on a smaller scale by voluntary organisations.

The general practitioner and area social workers act as the first line of contact for services in the community. The *social worker* provides a link between the elderly person and his or her family, and the available services. Social workers have the lead-agency role in assessing the elderly person's need for community services (such as home care, meals on wheels or day centres) and in coordinating the necessary services (see previous section on joint working to plan coordinated care). They also give advice on available benefits and how to obtain them.

Social workers can also be involved in helping elderly individuals and their families cope with crises such as bereavement, the effects of serious illness, or the dilemma which often surrounds the elderly person needing to move from his or her ownr home into residential care. In this area of work there is likely to be overlap with the work of the community psychiatric nurse. Social workers operate from an area or neighbourhood base in the community, or they can be based in hospitals where they are attached to the specialist team.

There are several forms of community support that may be offered to elderly mentaly ill people.

Day centres

Day centres for the elderly and elderly mentally ill are run by the social services department. Some social clubs and centres are set up in the local community by voluntary agencies. The function of a day centre is to provide opportunities for companionship and social stimulation.

Day centres operate on a weekday basis and normally provide care between the hours of 10.00 a.m. and 3.00 p.m. They usually have a programme of activities (for example Bingo, artwork) and many arrange outings. Transport to and from the day centre is provided if necessary, and the elderly person is given a midday meal and hot drinks. Unfortunately, day centres frequently have a waiting list, mainly as a result of limited transport spaces and high demand for places. In addition, they are not normally able to provide care over weekends or in the evenings, when an elderly housebound person is most likely to be isolated and vulnerable.

Some local authorities provide specialised day care facilities which cater specifically for the elderly mentally ill with dementia. Such centres are often the key element in maintaining at home the frail, confused or dementing elderly person who is dependent upon daily care (Fraser, 1987). Day care can help to prevent or defer admission to long-term care. As well as providing stimulation and social contact for the elderly person, day centres provide relief for caregivers. For those caring for an elderly relative, a little time to themselves during the week, made possible by their dependant attending the day centre, may be invaluable. The day care facility can also provide daytime supervision for an elderly person whose carers are at work during the day.

Help in the home

Williamson, Smith and Burley (1987) state that a well-run home help service is the 'linchpin' of community care for the elderly. Traditionally home help services have concentrated on domestic tasks, whilst the community nursing services have incorporated help with daily living activities relating to personal care.

However, in recent attempts to remove artificially created divisions between domestic service provision and health care provision, and to acknowledge the wider needs of elderly housebound people, some local authorities have redesignated the home help services 'home care' services.

The input of a *home carer* is another vital component in supporting a mentally confused elderly person at home. The home carer, who is usually a female worker, helps the elderly person with everyday necessities such as shopping, making hot drinks and light snacks, collecting pensions or prescriptions, paying bills and light housework. The amount of home care input required is usually based on the assessment of the elderly person's ability to cope at home. This enables close collaboration and liaison with the occupational therapy service.

Home care managers are responsible for recruiting members of their staff to provide the care necessary for each individual case. The home care manager liaises with the multidisciplinary team, for example through care planning meetings, when a package of care is being organised for an elderly person going home from hospital. The home carer input is monitored so that the service can be tailored to individual need, or ceased as needs change.

Home care staff, not surprisingly, are in a position to establish close relationships with the elderly people they visit. They may often be the only point of social contact for a housebound frail person, and their visits offer the opportunity for companionship.

The *meals-on-wheels* service aims to deliver a hot midday meal, on a daily basis if necessary, to elderly people at home who are unable to prepare their own food. Meals on wheels is usually run as a joint enterprise between the social services and a voluntary organisation such as the Women's Royal Voluntary Service or Age Concern. The meals are delivered in heated containers with the help of volunteers, and recipients make a small contribution to the cost of the service.

The meals-on-wheels service probably works best for those elderly people who are mentally alert but unable to prepare a hot meal for themselves due to illness or physical disability. The effectiveness of the service may be compromised in the case of elderly people who are confused, forgetful or depressed and therefore unlikely to eat unless there is somebody available at home to supervise the meal.

Voluntary organisations

Voluntary organisations are non-profit-making bodies which are usually funded by donations and may receive some central or local government top-up. Voluntary bodies have been formed all over the country in response to perceived local needs which are not being met by the statutory services.

There are a large number of voluntary organisations concerned with elderly people and their carers. Many of these organisations exist at a national level, for example Age Concern, Help the Aged and the Alzheimer's Disease Society. Voluntary organisations can provide practical help for elderly mentally ill people in many ways. They may run day care facilities or 'lunch clubs'. In some areas, care schemes such as 'Crossroads' provide volunteer visitors who will 'sit in' with the elderly at home to allow carers a break during the day.

Many organisations provide emotional support, advice and counselling through setting up self-help and carers' groups. Such groups also offer support and social contact to those who have become isolated in their caring role. Many carers and sufferers find great strength in meeting others who have experienced the same problems. (A list of addresses of voluntary organisations is given in Appendix 4.)

Conclusion

The increasing number of very old people in our society means that all carers, both family and professional, will be faced with enormous challenges which can only be successfully met by multidisciplinary teams. Such teams should provide a close degree of partnership, collaboration and understanding between all involved. The need to develop and establish key workers and/or case manager schemes is apparent so that multidisciplinary teams are appropriately 'led' and are able to function as real 'teams' which can provide the type of highly integrated, multifaceted care which many older people with psychiatric illness require.

Bennett (1989) emphasises that maintaining the quality of life should remain the overriding principle in providing a service of care to the aged in our society. In other words, we should aim to 'add life to years'. We must ensure that the care we are instrumental in providing enables each elderly person to maintain independence and physical and psychological well-being for as long as possible given their particular life circumstances. Workers must also strive to ensure that their practices reflect a service of care which is innovative as well as effective in its provision for the elderly who are incapacitated by psychiatric illness.

Chapter 6:
A Survey of Service Provision to the Cognitively Impaired Elderly in the USA

DANIELLE RIPICH AND ELAINE ZIOL

Introduction

For four intensive days in May 1995, Washington, DC was the venue of the Fourth White House Conference on Aging at which delegates from across the United States met to discuss a variety of issues that will affect the ageing policies of the USA over the next ten years. Key topics focused on the future of funding for medical and ageing services, issues of universal health care, and health problems of later life such as dementia. Alzheimer's disease (AD) research was fifth on the list of the 75 resolutions that the delegates voted to adopt as documented priorities.

The first conference on ageing was held in 1961 and resulted in the passage of the Older Americans Act and the creation of Medicare, medical insurance coverage for eligible elderly. Although the second and third conferences had less effect on the country's ageing policies, the impact of the most recent conference is yet to be seen. There is little doubt, however, that radical reform by policy makers and legislators and a shift in concentration of services by health professionals will be required to meet the rapidly growing population of older Americans.

Demographics of dementia in the USA

The United States Congress Office of Technology Assessment (1987) has estimated that there were 1.4 million persons with severe dementia in the USA in 1980. This number is expected to increase to 2.4 million in 2020 and 7.3 million in 2040. However, these estimates may significantly under-represent the prevalence of persons with dementia according to a report (Evans, 1990) that applied the results of a community study in East Boston to the US population with consideration for age, sex and education strata. Evans indicated that the number of persons over age 65 with Alzheimer's disease in 1980 was 2.88 million which is 11.3 % of persons in this age-group. This estimate is in close agreement with the 11.2% reported by Pfeffer, Afifi and Chance (1987). Evans's projection for the year 2050 of the number of persons in the USA over age 65 with AD ranges from a low projection of 7.5 million to a high range of 14.3 million. A sevenfold increase in the oldest age-group over 85 years of age compared with 1980 will account for most of the projected increase. This estimate is substantially higher than previous studies because it includes:

- a full range of cognitive impairment from mild to severe;
- persons who may have passed screening tests who actually are afflicted with dementia;
- persons whose dementia is not formally recognised and documented in the medical chart;
- persons with dementia from causes other than probable AD alone.

This projected increase in the number of persons with dementia is also a result of the demographic phenomena of this century. First, the number of older persons in the USA has risen from 4% of the population in 1900 (3 million persons) to 11.9% in 1984 (about 28.5 million persons). Second, the oldest segment is the most rapidly increasing group; so that by the year 2000, the number of people aged 65 to 74 will have increased by 23%, those 75 to 84 by 57%, and those 85 and over by almost 100% (Lawton, Brody and Saperstein, 1991). Because severe dementia increases with age, implications for the future clearly include a vast increase in the number of persons with dementia in the USA.

The Hoover Institute of Stanford University estimated the costs of medical care, long-term care and loss of income due to brain failure at US$28–31 billion per year in the mid-1980s (Hay and Ernst, 1987). The Office of Technology Assessment estimated the cost in 1985 at $24–48 billion (Batelle Memorial Institute, 1984) with an additional $10–20 billion of indirect costs taken up by caregivers.

Despite limitations of prevalence studies, these estimates have significant implications for service provision as a public health issue. The increase in prevalence of persons with dementia will place demands on extended care facilities in the USA and other developed countries with a growing ageing population. Although the goal is prevention of the dementing condition, the need for services to this group will continue to increase in magnitude unless there should be a major biomedical breakthrough that prevents or ameliorates the disease.

The purpose of this chapter is to provide an overview of services provided to the cognitively impaired elderly in the USA. It will discuss the types of service provision available in the health care system and current federal legislation influencing assessment and intervention for the cognitively impaired elderly. It will also address federally funded programmes for treatment, research and education in this area, professional education for speech–language pathologists who serve the cognitively impaired, and interventions to maintain and enhance communication for persons with dementia. In this discussion of services to the cognitively impaired elderly in the USA, AD and other dementing conditions will be considered. The terms dementia and cognitive impairment will be used throughout this chapter to describe the irreversible condition most commonly manifest as AD or multi-infarct dementia. The communicative needs and practical problems are similar in these conditions. (The issue of differentiation between the different types of dementia is discussed in detail in Chapter 3.)

Types of service provision in the USA to the cognitively impaired elderly

Extended care facilities

Extended care facilities (also called long-term care facilities or nursing homes) provide medical, residential, custodial, social and rehabilitation services to persons who cannot perform activities of daily living independently or with community-based support. In 1985 about 1.5 million persons lived in extended care facilities compared with 1.7 million persons in 1990 in over 16 000 facilities throughout the USA (US Department of Commerce, 1992). The majority of residents in extended care facilities are white (92%), women (72%), and 35% are over 85 years old. Chronic conditions of these residents include mental disorders (79.1%), cerebrovascular disease (26.2%), chronic obstructive pulmonary disease (24%), heart disease (21%) and diabetes (19.5%) (National Center for Health Statistics, 1985). The 1985 National Nursing Home Survey (Hing, 1987) reported that 63% of all residents in extended care facilities were disorientated or memory impaired. Other studies suggest that the percentage may be even higher (Kay and Bergmann, 1980; Sloane and Pickard, 1985). The frequently quoted statistic that 4% of elderly reside in an extended care facility may indeed be an underestimate of both present, and certainly future, extended care needs given the exponential increase in the number of very old elderly and the increase in two-career households.

As a response to the increasing numbers of cognitively impaired elderly, many extended care facilities have developed specialised units for persons with AD with separate living quarters, special physical design and the provision of activities tailored to persons with dementia (Sloane and Mathew, 1991). Of approximately 22 000 extended-care facilities in the USA in 1987, 150 to 200 had dementia units (US Congress, Office of Technology Assessment, 1987). Opinions of professionals regarding the effectiveness of such units remain divided. Maas (1988) and Rabins (1986) have identified the following advantages of specialised units:

- specially designed environments;
- specialised staff;
- ability to develop formal behaviour programmes;
- reduced family anxiety;
- separation of cognitively impaired elderly from intact in the facility.

The authors cite disadvantages as:

- higher financial costs;
- difficulty in admission criteria;
- resistance to placement by the person with dementia or his or her family;
- difficulty recruiting staff;
- negative labelling of the unit;
- higher staff turnover;
- lower staff expectations of residents.

Although the question of whether to segregate residents remains unanswered, specialised units continue to increase in the USA. Proponents of the traditional model, in which persons with dementia are integrated with other residents, suggest that residents can receive behavioural management as part of the extended care mainstream. Much literature has been published about numerous innovative programmes and their worth (Peppard, 1985; Coons and Weaverdych, 1986; Johnson, 1986; Millard, 1989). It is now widely recognised that the person with dementia needs a different approach from that offered for other residents of extended care facilities (Sloane and Mathew, 1991). However, more data are needed on dementia units to justify costs, determine effective therapies, develop standards and assist families in seeking out the best care possible.

Respite services

The US Department of Health and Human Services describes respite as 'short term inpatient or outpatient care delivered to an elderly person in lieu of his or her regular support' (US Department of Health and Human Services, 1981). Although a fairly new option in the USA, respite services for caregivers have gained widespread interest in community care for the cognitively impaired elderly. Respite has the potential to reduce strains on family caregivers and to prevent or delay admission to extended care facilities. Caregivers consistently rate respite as their top priority unmet need (Danis 1978; Crossman, London and Barry, 1981; Horowitz and Dobrof, 1982).

Originally developed in the 1960s to serve families of the developmentally disabled, respite services for caregivers of the elderly have similar goals of reducing caregiver strain and postponing institutionalisation. These programmes have been common in Europe over the past 25 years. In the USA, respite services are sometimes available through programmes primarily designed for other purposes. For example, hospice services for the dying often include a component of some institutional care for the dying patient. Some hospitals offer day care or 'vacation stays' for persons with dementia when caregivers need time away. However, there is no regular public or private funding for consistent respite in the USA (Lawton, Brody and Saperstein, 1991).

The types and availability of respite vary. These include *in-home respite* where companions, homemakers, volunteers and home-health-care aids come to the home or occasionally take the person with dementia to the home of the worker. *Overnight respite* refers to short-term stays in extended care facilities, hospitals, group homes or foster homes. Maximum hours or days of respite vary from programme to programme. *Day care* services range from small programmes for socialisation to large, multiple service settings (Lawton et al., 1991).

Only inconsistent efforts to provide funding for respite services through privately financed demonstration grants and other funding mechanisms have been noted. In addition, there has been little research and practical knowledge to guide programme development (Meltzer, 1982). Despite availability of education and counselling, reports of under-utilisation of respite services by caregivers persist (George, 1988; Brody, Saperstein and Lawton 1989). Although part of the problem may be a lack of information to the caregiver, many overburdened caregivers view respite as an end-of-the-road option to be used only when absolutely necessary (Montgomery, 1986). Another major barrier may be the physician's lack of awareness of services (Cohen, Hegarty and Eisdorfor, 1983).

Adult day care

Adult day care is increasingly acknowledged as a key component of community-based care by providing the support required by persons with dementia so that they can remain in their own homes. Caregivers use the service for blocks of six to eight hours allowing them to rest or do home chores. Other advantages include lower costs than home care and an opportunity for socialisation and stimulation for the person with dementia (Lawton et al., 1991). Although initially slow in development, adult day care is becoming increasingly available as community-based care for the elderly. Approximately 64 000 community-dwelling elderly used adult day care in 1989, compared with 1.5 million persons in extended care facilities in 1985 and 2.3 million elderly using some type of home care in 1987. Of all adult day care centres, 40% were established after 1984 (Wallace et al., 1991). Nearly 3000 centres are currently located throughout all 50 states (National Institute on Adult Day Care, 1992).

Surveys consistently report a wide range of services offered by adult day care centres (Zawadski, Von Behren and Stuart, 1992; Hedrick et al., 1993). The majority offer medical services which include nursing management, health assessment, restorative therapies including physical, occupational and speech–language therapy, pharmacology assistance, podiatry services, respite care and phone reassurance systems, health monitoring and nutrition counselling. The centres surveyed frequently offer additional services including formal exercise, movement therapy, individual/group psychotherapy, pastoral/peer/social service counselling, weight control and opportunities for social/personal interaction.

Weissert et al. (1990) reported that the average age of day care participants was 78 years with just under 20% older than 84 years. Most were unmarried women who lived with a family caregiver. More than half were functionally impaired with almost 40% diagnosed with a mental disorder. Average cost per day was $31 with a median cost of $20 (Von Behren, 1986). Payment for adult day care services comes from a variety of sources including self-payment, Medicaid, Title III-B of the Older Americans Act and local funding programmes (Weaver, 1994). In the study by Weissert et al. (1990), approximately 45% of participants paid for some part of their care charge.

In-home respite care

In-home respite care is the most common type of programme in the USA (George, 1986; US Congress, Office of Technology Assessment, 1987) Home health care is becoming more available and can reduce the use of extended care facilities. Traditional home health care may include nursing services, home health aide visits, physical therapy, speech therapy and social and homemaker services. Home health aides can assist with personal care and help with exercise. Other community services, either paid or volunteer, provide the elderly with assistance with chores, home delivery of meals, mental health services, transportation, escort services and housing assistance (Cohen, Hegaty and Eisdorfer 1983).

Federal legislation affecting services to the cognitively impaired elderly

The federal government provides numerous programmes that directly or indirectly support the care of persons with dementia. Many of these services are available through local or state agencies or private providers. Several federal programmes have an impact on support care. The Social Security Amendment of 1965 established Medicare with Title XVIII and Medicaid with Title XIX. Medicare and Medicaid are the primary health care programmes in the USA.

Medicare

Those 65 and over, the disabled and those with kidney disease receive funding for acute medical care through Medicare, a federally sponsored health insurance programme. The programme is divided into Part A and Part B. Part A covers primarily hospital services and is supported by payroll taxes on those who are working. Part B covers physician charges and is funded by premiums and from general revenues. For elderly persons with dementia, Medicare covers a fraction of the costs of diagnosis and medical treatment. Because the programme excludes custodial care, the person with dementia qualifies for coverage only if he or she requires skilled care on the basis of another condition. Medicare does not cover the cost of his or her extended care or services needed on a continuing basis (Cook-Deegan, 1990).

Medicare coverage may also be denied for home health and therapy services because the care is often for maintenance and to prevent deterioration rather than to actively treat persons with dementia. With physician services, Medicare pays 80% of the physician's approved fee, which may be below the physician's actual fee. Families may be required to pay the 20% difference along with any difference between approved and actual fees. Fortunately, some physicians will agree to accept the Medicare-allowable fee in full (Chavkin, 1990). With the growing numbers of persons with dementia requiring services on a long-term basis, it is anticipated that service coverage will be modified by Congress.

Medicaid

Medicaid is a programme with two foci:

- a health programme for the indigent;
- an extended-care programme for the indigent.

The programme is funded both by the federal government and by the individual states, with the federal government paying over half the costs. States with more resources pay a larger proportion. Although the federal government mandates a minimal set of services, states differ widely in services covered, eligibility of participants and amount of funding.

Medicaid covers acute medical care and extended care for the impoverished. Elderly persons paying out-of-pocket fees for extended care for any length of time may become impoverished and eligible for Medicaid. The new Catastrophic Health Act of 1988 prevents spouses from losing all assets in paying for their partners' extended care by allowing them to split assets up to a limit. Medicaid, historically, is a programme difficult to control and has tried to shift costs from one funding source to the other or to the users of the programme (Cook-Deegan, 1990). Furthermore, the administration of the programme is complex with no uniformity in any aspect – eligibility, organisation, administration, reimbursement, extent of coverage and type of coverage (Cook-Deegan, 1990). It continues to be, however, the largest extended-care programme in the USA with approximately two-thirds of persons in extended-care facilities receiving Medicaid coverage for at least part of their care costs (Chavkin, 1990).

Title XX

This is a federal block grant which transfers funds from the federal government to the local county and state governments. These funds often support services for persons with dementia.

The Older Americans Act

Title III of the Older Americans Act of 1965 supports senior services and distributes funds to area or state agencies to develop systems to help older people remain in their homes in the community (US Department of Health and Human Services, 1993). Although the act aims to serve elderly persons who need transportation, delivery of meals, senior recreation centres and other programmes, the recent focus has been on persons with dementia to include more attention for day care, care coordination and dissemination of information for persons with dementia (Cook-Deegan, 1990).

Federal programmes for treatment, research and education for the cognitively impaired elderly

The Veterans Administration (VA)

The VA has a variety of services for those who have been in military service with its own set of hospitals, clinics and extended-care facilities throughout the nation. To be eligible for services a person must be a veteran or a dependant of a veteran. VA centres have been innovators of care for persons with dementia. AD and related disorders are a significant concern for VA as the number of veterans with severe dementia is expected to increase from an estimated 400 000 in 1990 to 600 000 in the year 2000 (Office of Geriatrics and Extended Care, 1994.) The VA Alzheimer's/Dementia Program includes both inpatient units and outpatient clinics which serve veterans with AD or other dementias. Three types of units provide specialised services:

- diagnostic units (up to 30-day stay) which focus on the differential diagnosis of dementia, a plan of care, short-term behavioural stabilisation, and discharge placement;
- behavioural units (30- to 90-day stay) which focus on significant behavioural and physical problems of persons with dementia;
- long-term care units (greater than 90-day stay) which focus on the needs of persons in the later stages of dementia.

The programme includes dementia consultation teams, outpatient dementia programmes and dementia registries. A VA survey in 1988–89 indicated that 56 (or 33%) of VA facilities had one or more types of dementia units.

As of 1992, there are 16 VA Geriatric Research, Education and Clinical Centres (GRECCs) which are designed for the advancement and integration of research, education and clinical achievements in geriatrics and gerontology for the total VA health system. Four of the GRECCs (Boston, MA, Minneapolis, MN, Palo Alto, CA and Seattle, WA) have a major focus on AD and related dementias. In 1993 there were approximately 300 active research projects with nearly 200 investigators addressing a wide number of topics related to dementia. These projects were funded by $4.7 million of VA funds, as well as $14.6 million of non-VA monies. The VA provides educational materials including guidelines for the diagnosis and treatment of dementia, a series of caregiver education pamphlets, and videotapes to assist caregivers in the home and health care setting (Office of Geriatrics and Extended Care, 1994).

A survey (Ripich and Ziol, 1995b) that studied the therapeutic approaches for educational activities related to the cognitively impaired elderly showed that 100% of GRECC respondents provided education about the disorder to professionals, 80% provided education about treatment in groups to the cognitively impaired elderly, 40% provided education about treatment to individuals and 60% provided information about communication strategies. All respondents provided programmes for families, individual support and family education about dementia; 60% included information to families about communication and dementia. Respondents indicated that interest levels in programmes were high to moderately high. Although respondents suggested that education about communication disorders was addressed 'frequently' or 'often', none responded that the topic was 'always' adequately addressed in their GRECC.

Geriatric Education Centres (GECs)

Since 1983, the Bureau of Health Professions has supported a nation-wide network of Geriatric Education Centres. The 20 centres that are currently funded maintain resource clearing houses and develop and disseminate curriculum and teaching materials. Participants include health and allied health professionals who are faculty, practitioners, students and informal caregivers. Purposes of GECs include the improvement of training for health professionals in geriatrics through development and dissemination of curricula related to geriatrics, support and retraining of faculty who teach geriatrics and establishment of new affiliations with health care facilities which treat the cognitively impaired elderly.

Ripich and Ziol (1995a) conducted a survey of GEC activity on issues related to the cognitively impaired elderly. Results showed that 92% of those who responded provide education to professionals on the disorder, 5% provide education on group treatment, 79% provide education on individual treatment and 75% provide information on communication strategies for interacting with persons with dementia. GECs reported that for family caregivers, 75% of respondents provide information about dementia, 66% have group programmes for family members, 50% provide individual support and 66% provide family members with education about communication and dementia. Responders reported high to moderate interest in the programmes. Although 17% of responders indicated that they felt education about communication disorders was always adequately addressed in their GEC, 83% stated they felt it was 'rarely' to 'occasionally' addressed.

National Institute on Aging (NIA)

NIA is the lead agency in the federal government supporting efforts in research and AD-related issues. Since 1985, the Alzheimer's Disease Research Centers (ADRC) programme has supported research on AD along with providing clinical service, disseminating information to professionals and the public, and sponsoring educational activities. There are currently 28 centres at major medical institutions and 27 satellite facilities in the USA doing collaborative studies from a variety of disciplines in basic clinical and behavioural research (US Department of Health and Human Services, 1993).

The Consortium to Establish a Registry for Alzheimer's Disease (CERAD), funded by NIA, was developed to standardise the assessment of AD using reliable clinical measures. Thirty-two participating US centres have enrolled 958 persons with AD and 457 controls for longitudinal study as of 1 July 1992 (Morris et al., 1993). Five CERAD task forces are dedicated to the following:

1. developing uniform assessments for AD;
2. standardising methods for neuropsychological measurements;
3. using magnetic resonance imaging to develop rating scales for AD;
4. standardising autopsies;
5. establishing data management centres (US Department of Health and Human Services 1993).

Education of speech–language pathologists in the treatment of dementia

Due to the increasing need for communication services to the cognitively impaired elderly, whether with traditional assessment and treatment or through programmes that create positive environments by the training of professional or family caregivers, communication disorders training programmes for speech–language pathologists should incorporate the topic of normal and pathological aspects of ageing into the curriculum and practicum experience (Lubinski, 1995). Two studies in the early to mid-1980s on the inclusion of geriatrics in graduate programmes in communication disorders revealed limited coursework in gerontology (Nerbonne, Schow and Hutchinson, 1980; Raiford and Shadden, 1985). More recently, Clark, Ripich and Weinstein (1994) surveyed graduate programmes in the USA and reported that 81% of the responding programmes included geriatric content in their curricula, and 91% of those responding offered at least some limited clinical training with older adults. The authors caution, however, that only about half of the responding programmes provide coursework focusing on normal ageing and communication. As clinical practicum experiences are limited in number of hours and practicum sites, geriatric coursework continues to be a necessity in the field of communication disorders (Lubinski, 1995).

There is a continuing need for speech–language pathologists, as communication specialists, to convey information about interacting with the cognitively impaired elderly to others in extended-care facilities and to family caregivers, in order to facilitate meaningful contact between persons with dementia and their caregivers. As communication specialists, speech–language pathologists should attempt to prioritise inservice training to meet the needs of changing staff and to educate caregivers of those newly diagnosed with dementia.

Treatment and intervention for persons with dementia

Speech-language pathologists and other health care professionals need to shift from a more traditional medical model, based on assessing pathology and restoring function, to a more holistic model, based on maintaining function and preventing excessive response to disability (Clark, 1995). The American Speech–Language and Hearing Association (ASHA) has two position statements (ASHA Committee on the Communication Problems of Aging, 1988a, 1988b) on the general role of speech–language pathologists and audiologists in the extended care setting. The papers stress increasing involvement in the assessment and management of persons with AD and related disorders, providing programmes to maintain functional communication for as long as possible, and improving the quality of life/quality of care. The speech–language pathologist should provide effective communication interventions both to persons with dementia and to those who care for persons with dementia, including family members, nursing assistants and nursing staff.

Direct intervention for persons with dementia

Using a direct approach, the communication specialist works with persons with dementia in groups or individual sessions to train persons with dementia in compensatory strategies such as:

* use of memory aids such as notebooks, memory wallets, or written signs;
* asking for repetition or review of the topic;
* circumlocution for word-retrieval deficits.

Group treatment often consists of simple, informative reminiscence sessions that review previous life experience. This treatment has been successful for persons in the moderate stages of AD (Hughston and Merriam, 1982).

Indirect intervention for caregivers of persons with dementia

Communication breakdown is consistently listed among the top stressors in family caregiver surveys of stress, strain and burden. That communication problems of persons with dementia contribute to caregiver stress is well documented (Rabins, 1982; Zarit, 1982; Kinney and Stephens, 1989). The exact nature of the communication problems and their impact on caregivers is less well established. Previous investigations have generally grouped communication problems with other stressors to derive burden measures, and therefore obscured the specific effects of the communication breakdown on the caregiver. In a pilot survey completed by 53 caregivers (two African-American and 51 white), the top two hassles reported from 42 possible items on the Caregivers Hassles Scale (Kinney and Stephens, 1989) were communication based. The mean score for the seven items related to communication was significantly higher than the mean of the other 35 items. This suggests that communication problems contribute disproportionately to stress and burden.

Many stressful communication difficulties may result from the caregivers' failure to understand the nature of the communication problems associated with AD (Clark and Witte, 1990) or a lack of appropriate communication strategies to keep communication from breaking down. This lack of knowledge and skills means caregivers may:

(a)   develop misconceptions about communication changes,
(b)   develop unrealistic expectations of the person with AD (either too high or too low), or
(c)   develop non-productive patterns of communication.

Ripich and Wykle (1990a) reported that communication training for caregivers has a broad impact. Their study of communication training for nursing assistants demonstrated that educating these caregivers in communication skills enhanced their control over the social interaction and increased their satisfaction with communicating with persons with AD (Ripich, Wykle and Niles, 1991). Primary caregivers of persons with AD reported a gradual erosion of sociability, and maintained that communication was the single most distressing problem they faced (Poulshock and Deimling, 1984; Carroll, 1989). Zarit, Anthony and Boutselis (1987) advocated an educational management approach to stress reduction. The goal of quality caregiving should clearly be to prolong and promote communication between persons with AD and primary caregivers for as long as possible and at the most interactive level (Clark, Witte and Macchia, 1989).

Although there is an emerging acknowledgment of the problems in communication of persons with AD (Shadden, 1988), the literature fails to delineate the problems that are particularly acute for persons with AD and their care providers. Caregivers have direct daily contact with persons with AD and are often frustrated in their attempts to establish a mutually satisfying rapport. Clinical experience has demonstrated improvement in interpersonal relations between the caregiver and person with AD when the caregiver understands the nature of the linguistic and intellectual problems experienced by the person with AD (Bayles and Kaszniak, 1987).

A caregiver communication training programme: the FOCUSED programme (Ripich, 1996)

Santo Pietro et al. (1990) examined conversations between speech–language pathologists and persons with AD and found that certain communication strategies were effective in facilitating conversation whereas others were detrimental. Researchers report that family caregivers are sensitive to their relatives' communication problems and can identify the progression of the symptoms (Bayles and Tomoeda, 1991; Orange, 1991). It would appear that caregiver training in facilitating strategies could provide useful tools to the caregiver communication partner.

'Front line' care of persons with AD could be improved significantly by enhancing the communication skills of caregivers. The ability of caregivers to draw on strategies and techniques for dealing with communication problems in these persons would reduce their own stress and frustration, and improve their competence in delivering quality care. In addition, caregivers would be better able to promote the use of residual functional communication abilities and provide appropriate social communication opportunities.

Improved communication could benefit family caregivers by reducing stress and burden and possibly allowing persons with AD to remain at home longer. Nurses and nursing assistants could also benefit from improved communication with persons with AD. In all cases, quality of life for persons with AD would be improved through better communication. The quality of interpersonal interactions is thought to be inextricably bound to quality of care provided (Adelson et al., 1982; Elliot and Hyberston, 1982; Shadden, 1988), and, subsequently, the quality of life of persons with AD. To improve communication with persons with dementia, caregivers require some instruction regarding the sufferer's communication problems (Bayles and Kazniak, 1987).

The use of the FOCUSED programme of communication training (Ripich and Wykle, 1990a, 1990b) allows for assessment of the caregivers' current level of knowledge and presents training modules designed to:

- provide information;
- correct misconceptions;
- offer techniques to maximise communication potential;
- assist caregivers in developing appropriate expectations of persons with AD.

Instruction in developing communication skills in group settings is most effective because the caregivers accept suggestions from one another (Clark and Witte, 1990); it provides an opportunity for role play (Hayter, 1982); and it allows participants to share information and build self-esteem (Aronson, Levine and Lipkowitz, 1984). Videotapes demonstrating different communication strategies have proved to be a helpful teaching tool for caregivers (Witte, 1986).

This seven-step programme uses the acronym FOCUSED to identify the major elements for communication maintenance and to help the caregivers recall the strategies. This programme was based on an interactive discourse model of conversational exchanges (Terrell and Ripich, 1989).

The following is a summary of the seven points:

- F   Face-to-face and functional
- O   Orient to topic
- C   Continuity of topic-concrete topics
- U   Unstick any communication blocks
- S   Structure with yes/no and choice questions
- E   Exchange conversation – encourage interaction
- D   Direct, short simple sentences

The FOCUSED programme, which addresses the day-to-day functional communication problems faced by caregivers of persons with AD, was designed to improve the quality of interactions between the caregiver and the person with AD. This programme was designed to develop and test didactic materials that would better prepare family and professional caregivers to communicate with persons with AD. The specific aims of the programme were to educate caregivers regarding:

- AD and the associated communication and language decline;
- the differences among memory changes in the normal ageing process, depression and AD;
- communication skills and the value of such skills in the care of persons with AD;
- the seven specific communication strategies to enhance and maintain communication with persons with AD;
- the stages of AD and concurrent communication characteristics, including how to assess and recognise the person with AD at each stage and maximise their communication through the use of the specific strategies;
- an optional section for professional caregivers on cultural differences and how these may affect the communication process with persons with AD.

Materials

A set of materials was designed to assess learning needs, educate and assist in the carryover of training programme content. The following items are included:

1. *Trainer's Manual*: This manual contains a word-for-word text of the programme information provided to the caregivers and also includes:
  (a) questions throughout the text of the programme to stimulate discussion and test understanding during training;
  (b) role-play activities designed to simulate common patient communication problems;

(c) practice assignments for use in the work or home setting to carry over what had been learned in each session.
2. *Caregiver's Guide*: The guide contains outlines of topics and key information in an easy-to-read format. Participants can keep the guides to review material and share the information with others. The materials included are outlines and text covering the six information content areas:
(i) AD and language decline;
(ii) depression and normal memory problems in ageing;
(iii) importance of communication skills;
(iv) strategies to enhance communication;
(v) stages of AD and communication;
(vi) cultural differences in communication (optional).
3. *Transparencies*: These are key points to present on an overhead.
4. *Pre- and Post-assessments*: These assessments of knowledge of AD and communication satisfaction attitudes are used to compare incoming levels of information and new information acquired from this training. They are completed by participants before and after training.
5. *FOCUSED Cards*: These 2 × 3 inch cards contain the acronym FOCUSED and serve as a reminder of the communication principles taught in the programme. The cards are given to participants upon completion of the programme to be placed in strategic places.
6. *Videotape Vignettes*: An instructional videotape was developed containing illustrations of various communication problems caregivers encounter with persons with AD and demonstrations of appropriate use of techniques.
7. *Programme Evaluation Forms*: These forms are completed at the end of training by participants to provide feedback to the trainer.

Training content

The training programme is divided into five two-hour modules for family or professional caregivers with a section on cultural differences as an option for professional caregivers. The modules address the following:

Module 1. Alzheimer's disease and the associated communication and language decline. This module discusses characteristics, pathology and incidence of AD. The components and processes of language are discussed. Participants learn how physicians make a diagnosis of probable AD and how language in aphasia and AD differ.

Module 2. The differences between memory decline in normal ageing and AD and the effects of depression on the person with AD. In this module the caregiver is taught to understand changes in memory in the normal elderly, to recognise symptoms of depression and to differentiate these symptoms from those of dementia. Discussion of the effects of depression on the person with AD's already decreasing ability to communicate with others is included.

Module 3. Interpersonal skills and the value of effective communication skills in the care of persons with AD. The critical importance of social communication to keep the person with AD engaged in communication to prevent excessive functional decline and to maintain abilities is discussed. Participants learn verbal and non-verbal approaches to good communication. A discussion of empathetic sensitivity (Egan, 1986) provides a foundation for promoting sensitive interpersonal exchanges that demonstrate respect for the demented patient and support the self-esteem of both the caregiver and the person with AD.

Module 4. The FOCUSED strategies to promote effective communication with persons with A. This critical module outlines the seven-point programme. The programme incorporates numerous strategies into a framework that is easy to recall and apply. A series of role-play exercises and videotaped vignettes is used to demonstrate the seven points of this communication enhancement programme. Table 1 shows specific examples of how to use the seven points.

Table 1: FOCUSED communication strategies

F = Face	1. Face the person with AD directly
	2. Call his or her name
	3. Touch the person
	4. Gain and maintain eye contact
O = Orient	1. Orient the person with AD to the topic by repeating key words several times
	2. Repeat sentences exactly
	3. Use nouns and specific names
C = Continue	1. Continue the same topic of conversation for as long as possible
	2. Restate the topic throughout the conversation
	3. Indicate to the person with AD that you are introducing a new topic
U = Unstick	1. Help the person with AD become 'unstuck' when he or she uses a word incorrectly by suggesting the word he or she is looking for
	2. Repeat the person with AD's sentence using the correct word
	3. Ask, 'Do you mean...?'
S = Structure	1. Structure your questions to give the person with AD a simple choice to respond with
	2. Provide two simple options at a time
	3. Use yes/no questions
E = Exchange	1. Keep up the normal exchange of ideas we find in conversation
	2. Keep conversations going with comments such as 'Oh, how nice, or 'That's great'
	3. **Do not ask test questions**
	4. Give the person with AD clues as to how to answer
D = Direct	1. Keep sentences short, simple and direct
	2. Use subject–verb-object sentence structure
	3. Use and repeat nouns rather than pronouns
	4. Use hand signals, pictures and facial expressions

Module 5. The stages of AD and concurrent communication charac-teristics including how to assess and recognise the person with AD at each stage and maximise his or her communication. Though fully aware of the heterogeneity of the progress of AD and the fact that dividing the progression into stages is an arbitrary device, the literature repeatedly reports three main levels of language deterioration designated as mild, moderate and severe. These stages have transitional phases between them that mark the specific changes in person with AD's capacity to communi-cate. In Module 5 these stages are described and guidelines given for:

- assessment and recognition of stages;
- communication strategies to maximise rapport at each stage;
- methods of non-verbal and verbal interaction that enhance feelings of successful contact for both the person with AD and the caregiver.

Table 2 summarises language at each stage of AD.

Table 2: Language stages in AD

Early Stage (Stage I)	
Pragmatics	Able to maintain conversations. Some difficulty with giving instruc-tions and storytelling. Some breakdown in pronominal referencing. Frequent requests for clarification and confirmation
Semantics	Word fluency and word finding compromised. Difficulty with comprehension of abstract and/or complex concepts
Syntax	No errors generally
Phonology	No errors
Middle Stage (Stage II)	
Pragmatics	Poor topic maintenance, poor use of pronominal reference and other cohesion devices
Semantics	Poor word fluency, confrontation naming, diminished vocabulary, circumlocutions and empty speech frequently use
Syntax	Occasional grammatical errors. Some difficulty with comprehension of complex structures
Phonology	No errors
Late Stage (Stage III)	
Pragmatics	Lack of coherence, mutism in final stage, prosody intact
Semantics	Paraphasia, echolalia, palilalia, comprehension poor
Syntax	Grammar generally preserved with some use of elliptical clauses. Poor comprehension of grammatical structures
Phonology	May have occasional errors, but no non-native language sound combinations

After a review of the seven points in the FOCUSED programme, a discussion of how its implementation would differ for persons in each of the three stages of AD is presented:

Stage I. Communication Goal: Maintain normal communicative interaction as far as possible. Even persons with AD at Stage I can benefit from all seven points in the FOCUSED programme. The use of these strategies to keep persons engaged and in contact with others can have the added benefit of improved morale and overall mental status at this stage of the disease.

Stage II. Communication Goal: Maintain turn-taking exchanges and the form of conversations even if communication content is confused. Some persons with AD will be seriously compromised by this stage. Whereas all seven points of the FOCUSED programme are still relevant, the concept of maintaining an exchange pattern of shared interaction is critical. Although often the topic is not followed by persons with AD or their speech and language is confused and fragmented, it is important that the form of human communication, i.e., turn-taking patterns, be continued. Turn taking requires the cooperation of both conversational participants. Even if the person with AD's turn merely consists of a head nod or making eye contact, it signals engagement in a two-way, turn-taking interaction.

Stage III. Communication Goal: Maintain communication through residual channels such as non-verbal gestures, key written words and pictures. Even when the person with AD no longer speaks, the caregiver should continue to use the FOCUSED principles when communicating. In addition, particular attention should be given to alternative forms of communication. For example, using cards with single words ('bathroom', 'ice cream'), pantomime (hands under head to show sleep) and pictures of family members can sometimes stimulate a person with AD to interact. The person's communication may only be a nod or a smile, but contact is made that is successful communication.

Optional Module for Professional Caregivers: Cultural considerations in communicating with persons with AD. Cultural considerations are extremely important issues in helping the professional caregiver care for the person with AD. The conflicts that arise in a caregiving situation may be further complicated by the differences in cultural and socioeconomic backgrounds of extended care residents and nursing assistant staff. The resultant disparity in values and interpersonal dynamics accentuates the communication difficulties that are characteristic of persons with AD. Therefore, didactic and experiential content that enhances the caregivers' understanding of cultural considerations affecting interpersonal communication processes is presented.

Studies of the FOCUSED caregiver training programme

Seventeen nursing assistants (16 women, 1 man) participated in a pilot project using the FOCUSED training programme. The mean age was

48.5 years, education mean = 11 years and experience mean = 14.25 years. Results of comparisons of pre- and post-test knowledge measures demonstrated increased knowledge across all areas with significant ($p < 0.001$) gains in Modules 4 and 5 which present the FOCUSED programme. This is somewhat predictable, given the specific nature of the FOCUSED training information. Nevertheless, results suggested marked gains in information regarding communication strategies. Results of the attitude survey generally indicated improvement in attitudes of nursing assistants toward persons with AD. Significant changes ($p < 0.001$) occurred on the question regarding communication satisfaction with persons with AD. There was a doubling in the percentage of nursing assistants reporting that they found communicating with persons with AD more satisfying compared with other patients. Anecdotal comments from participants suggested this training provided them with new insight into the problems persons with AD experience. They reported a greater 'feeling of control' during conversations with persons with AD, contrasting greatly with the frustration and inability to make contact with the persons prior to the training. Their newly acquired skills, reportedly, made it more likely that they would attempt to communicate with persons with AD instead of ignoring or patronising them. The new enthusiasm of the nursing assistants regarding the importance of good communication was noted by a number of their supervisors.

A FOCUSED training project for African-American and white family caregivers of persons with AD (supported by National Institute on Aging grant No. AG-08012-06) is being conducted to study the effects of communication skills training on communication patterns and stress and burden of these family caregivers. Preliminary results show similar positive effects for family caregivers in increasing knowledge about communication and AD and in reducing the hassles related to communication. In this study, 19 caregivers (13 women, 6 men) completed questionnaires to assess knowledge, attitude and stress and burden before and after completion of the FOCUSED communication training programme. Table 3 shows significance ($p < 0.001$) for responses on the Knowledge Questionnaire and for the seven hassles related to communication from the larger, 42-item *Caregiver Hassles Scale* ($p < 0.046$) (Kinney and Stephens, 1989).

Family caregivers have commented that 'strategies were helpful in everything' and that 'role-playing was very helpful in carrying out the strategies'.

Persons with dementia experience communication changes in both expressive and receptive communication, especially pragmatic and semantic functioning (see Chapter 3). The communication breakdown that occurs is a major source of stress and burden to professional and family caregivers. Communication training for caregivers can improve interactions, knowledge of AD and attitudes of caregivers. Specifically, the FOCUSED communication skills programme can increase knowledge, improve communication satisfaction and decrease hassles related to communication breakdown for caregivers of persons with AD. Education in specific communication strategies can alter attitudes towards persons with AD. Providing caregivers with adequate training is essential to quality of life issues. Additional benefits may be caregivers' greater satisfaction and sense of accomplishment in their critical day-to-day activities. Caregivers can benefit from training in communication strategies and this training may improve the quality of life for persons with AD. (Working with carers is discussed further in Chapter 11).

Table 3: Comparison of family caregivers' self-reported measures pre- and post-FOCUSED training

	n	Pre (% possible)	Post (% possible)	% change
Knowledge Assessment (Ripich, 1996)	13	55	83	+28*
Caregiver Hassles Scale (Kinney and Stephens, 1989)	15	25	24	-1
Communication items	19	28	23	-5*
PANAS (10 item) (Watson, Clark and Tellegren, 1988)	19	70	72	+2
CES-D (12 item) depression scale (Radloff, 1977)	19	43	43	0
Subjective Health (3 item)	19	79	79	0
Communication Attitude (Ripich, 1996)	19	70	72	+2

Notes: Sample size differs on two of seven measures due to missing data on questionnaires.
* <0.05.

Conclusion

This chapter has provided an overview of services available to the cognitively impaired elderly in the USA, describing the types of service provision available in the health care system and current federal legislation regarding support for these services. Federal programmes for treatment, research and education have also been discussed, as well as the educational needs of speech–language pathologists in the treatment of dementia. Finally, some intervention techniques for persons with dementia have been presented, including a discussion of the importance of training and education of caregivers of cognitively impaired elderly. The FOCUSED Communication Strategies for Caregivers of Persons with AD (Ripich, 1996), a communication skills training programme, and its effectiveness have been discussed as an option for intervention. Targeting an increase in knowledge of AD and effective communication strategies throughout the course of the disease, the programme may be used with both family and professional caregivers of persons with dementia.

The need for communication services for the cognitively impaired elderly will continue to increase with the inevitable growth of this population. Speech–language pathologists and others who work with persons with dementia should be prepared to work efficiently to meet the communication needs of both cognitively impaired persons and their care providers.

Chapter 7:
Service Delivery
in the UK

BARBARA TANNER AND KAREN BRYAN

Introduction

In this chapter we will attempt to focus specifically on speech and language therapy services for people with dementia and associated psychiatric problems of old age. This is not as simple as it may seem as some services are targeted exclusively at people with dementia, whilst others provide help to the elderly population as a whole.

The first part of this chapter describes the establishment and the development of the speech and language therapy service in a psychiatric hospital which focused primarily on the needs of the elderly. It is evident from the description below that the service has developed due to both the growing expertise of speech and language therapists in this field and in response to NHS changes such as community care.

An example of service delivery

The unit described here is part of a psychiatric hospital which is currently undergoing a process of retraction and relocation to smaller premises. The only part of the hospital remaining unchanged is the area being discussed here, an assessment unit for the elderly mentally ill. When the unit was opened in 1985 the hospital still had eight wards each of about 30 beds for the care of elderly, long-term psychiatric clients. With the introduction of Care in the Community (Department of Health, 1989a) the clients in these wards have been moved out of the hospital, most of them going into nursing homes either in the local area or the area they came from originally. Acute and forensic wards, plus a day hospital for functionally ill clients, are being relocated to new premises. The result of these changes is that the speech and language therapist's job has changed from being predominantly hospital and NHS based, to one in which more clients are seen in the community, and in social services and private establishments.

The unit was opened in 1985 with a full-time post for a speech and language therapist being established in 1986. For the first 18 months the speech and language therapy department was able to provide only six sessions per week, but in July 1988 the whole-time post was filled, with two therapists initially sharing the job.

When the post was being established it was recognised that the majority of speech and language therapists had only basic knowledge of dementia, and minimal information about any communication changes in dementia. There was little published information about working with these clients or how to manage their clinical needs. It was therefore recognised that the new therapist would need to spend time familiarising herself with the clients and their needs, learning as much as possible about dementia and its effect on communication, and establishing the maximal way to help these clients. From the start the post included one session each week to be spent reading or researching dementia and dementia care. As the therapists gained confidence in what they were doing these sessions were used to pursue small research projects which subsequently led to one therapist undertaking a part-time master's degree.

How the assessment unit operates

The structure and policies of the unit had a considerable bearing on how speech and language therapy input developed. The unit had already been running for a year before the SLT began working there so it was important that the new therapist fitted in with the routine already established. Because the unit was purpose built a lot of thought had gone into providing an appropriate environment for patients, and providing a base for all professionals working within the unit.

Originally the unit consisted of a 25-place assessment ward and a 30-place day hospital. In-patients came for approximately four weeks prior to being discharged to the most appropriate environment, and four beds were maintained to offer respite care. Clients attended the day hospital on a respite basis for anything from one to seven days per week. Since the introduction of care in the community the policy of the unit has changed somewhat. The assessment ward no longer offers respite except for those clients and carers who received it prior to April 1993, and the day hospital offers respite care only to those patients whose behavioural problems are such that alternative day care cannot be provided in the community. The day hospital now operates primarily as an assessment unit with patients being assessed on the days they attend. Whilst much of the work done with day hospital clients has always involved close liaison with their carers, it is only recently that we have started to carry out purely domestic assessments, i.e. with patients attending neither the day hospital nor the inpatient assessment ward.

Thus, although the amount of hospital-based work has decreased there has been an increase in purely domiciliary work for all disciplines.

Staffing

Assessment is multidisciplinary. The team is led by two consultants assisted by one clinical specialist and one house officer. As well as nursing staff there are social workers, community psychiatric nurses, occupational therapists, physiotherapists and a speech and language therapist based within the unit. There is no in-house psychologist, but the unit has access to the District Psychology Department which carries out assessments on a referral basis only.

A considerable amount of time is spent liaising, formally and informally, with other disciplines. Each consultant holds a ward round or multidisciplinary meeting once a week. These meetings are often quite lengthy but are a forum for discussing all aspects of each client's care, and for deciding what further assessments or interventions are necessary before discharge. Day hospital staff, including all therapists, meet every morning to plan activities to be carried out that day, and to share information about individual patients. In this way it is possible to plan which assessments should have priority and to avoid overloading the patient or the carer by bombarding them with too many visits or 'tests' in one day. All disciplines are welcome at the inpatient nurses' handover meeting when they change shifts after lunch.

Development of the speech and language therapist's role

During the first few weeks of working in the unit it was found to be extremely useful to shadow each discipline for at least half a day. In this way the speech and language therapist gained a clear idea about the role of each different profession and observed how they meshed with one another without any unnecessary overlapping. It also became very clear how much each nurse, therapist or social worker benefited from the information received from other disciplines. For example, during their time spent interviewing carers, the social workers obtain very detailed social histories of patients, which are very useful when trying to assess a client who has little memory about his or her past. It would clearly be inappropriate and unnecessarily obtrusive for other disciplines to go over the same information with carers, who are under a lot of stress, when a major problem is that they have too little time of their own.

The speech and language therapist also found it extremely helpful to visit other therapists working with the elderly severely mentally ill (ESMI), and subsequently a small group of speech and language therapists from neighbouring health authorities met on a regular basis to discuss their work, and to share any information or knowledge they had gained about the patient group. This group subsequently developed into a northern Special Interest Group which continues to meet twice a year and offers support to new and established speech and language therapists working with these patients.

The speech and language therapist also had responsibility for clients in the long-stay wards for people with advanced dementia, and could also be called upon to assess clients referred from any other ward or unit in the hospital. In 1988 this involved work in four elderly mentally ill long-stay wards, four wards for people who had grown old in the psychiatric hospital (graduate wards), as well as occasional referrals from the forensic ward, acute wards and rehabilitation areas. As more patients have moved out into the community, the number of long-stay wards and graduate wards has been halved and these will eventually disappear by the end of 1995, so that work in those areas has diminished. However, there has been a subsequent increase in referrals from the community. The speech and language therapist's greatest input has always been to the assessment unit, and there has been a marked difference in how work has been carried out in different parts of the hospital.

In this post the role of the speech and language therapist does not include much traditional hands-on therapy, but there is involvement with other disciplines in planning treatment, management or therapy, as any input is very dependent on the communication abilities of the patients, and their ability to respond. The SLT's roles are seen as the following:

- assessment and diagnosis;
- advice to other professions;
- maximising functional communication;
- counselling carers;
- training and education;
- research.

Within the unit the post involves all these functions, whereas in the long-stay wards training and one-off assessments and advice take place. In the acute areas, assessments, advice and, where appropriate, treatment programmes are part of the speech and language therapist's remit.

Assessment

Clients who attend the assessment unit, either as day or inpatients, are automatically referred to all disciplines. Referrals of non-attenders (i.e. community patients) come mainly from the two consultants, or from other disciplines via the consultants. Other community referrals come from GPs and other speech and language therapists. A small number of clients are referred by their carers or by social workers asking for a specialist assessment.

As with any other client group, assessment is both formal and informal; it involves standard and non-standard tests, conversation, observation, and discussion with other disciplines and carers. One of the first problems facing a speech and language therapist working with a new client group is deciding how to assess and what assessments to use. Most speech and language therapists who work with adult neurological patients will encounter cases of dementia when assessing the elderly. They will recognise that the client is not aphasic but that there is 'something else' happening. Originally speech and language therapists identified this by using the sort of assessments that were used traditionally in testing adults with neurological disorders, and by applying their knowledge of communication in general to the client's conversation.

When this post was established, information about assessment of elderly clients with psychiatric disorders was not widely available, although some authors were beginning to write about it, e.g. Obler and Albert (1981), Bayles (1982), Bayles and Boone (1982), Hier, Hagenlocker and Schindler (1985), Cummings, Houlihan and Hill (1986), Gravell (1988). Since then there has been considerable interest in ageing and dementia with the subsequent publishing of many useful articles and books. Both therapists in this unit found Bayles and Kaszniak's (1987) *Communication and Cognition in Normal Aging and Dementia* to be particularly helpful. More recently the publication of the *Arizona Battery for Communication Disorders of Dementia* (Bayles and Tomoeda, 1993) has proved a useful addition to the available assessment material.

Because Alzheimer's disease and other irreversible dementias are caused by neurological changes it was felt appropriate to begin by using assessments designed for other clients with neurological language disorders. It was found to be useful to score not only quantitatively, but also qualitatively and descriptively, and to look at *how* clients responded, whether they were right or wrong. By establishing a baseline, retests would show how much the client had deteriorated. At first the SLT was able only to describe each client's communication skills, and discuss whether and how his or her language changes compared with other language disorders. With more experience, and as confidence increased, the speech and language therapist became able to use assessments to diagnose different language disorders and to contribute towards diagnosis of different types of dementia.

There are times when a client will not cooperate with formal assessment of any kind but the speech and language therapist can gain invaluable information from observing the client interacting with other patients, with nurses and with other therapists, and often this is the only way to assess the client. However, because of the SLT's own communication skills a relationship can often be established with clients and the therapist is able informally to assess cognitive skills such as orientation and memory when others are unable to do so.

As well as continuing to use relevant literature, the speech and language therapist has found it very beneficial to attend the Special Interest Group described earlier where speech and language therapists exchange ideas about assessment, discuss recently published papers and describe their own work.

Advice to other professionals

This is a two-way process as comments and advice given by other disciplines can be very helpful in determining how the speech and language therapist approaches a client or a carer. It can be given (or received) in a variety of ways: informally in relation to a particular patient, or formally in ward rounds, when all clients are discussed.

Although all the staff on the unit are highly trained, there are times when they are unable to achieve cooperation from a client simply because of the way that they are communicating with the person. By careful observation of the client, the speech and language therapist can often give the member of staff advice on simple changes in style which make the client more likely to respond to them. The therapist can also give very specific advice about levels of comprehension, and alternative forms of communication, based on the SLT assessment. Sometimes it is simply a matter of reminding staff that the client is deaf, or is not wearing his or her glasses! To illustrate this point the speech and language therapist observed two quite experienced care assistants helping a new (and very small) patient walk to the dining room. The woman was very anxious and seeking reassurance about where she was and where she was going. The two care assistants were answering her questions but they did not gain the woman's attention or establish eye contact but spoke from alongside her and above her head, so that she did not hear them and was becoming more anxious and beginning to be verbally aggressive. By standing in front of this woman and gaining her attention, the SLT was able to give her the reassurance she needed. It was thus possible by example to demonstrate effective communication with this very worried patient who was also very deaf!

Formal feedback is given in the form of written reports, discussion at multidisciplinary meetings and participation in writing care plans for clients. Whilst these careplans are generally written by nursing staff, the assessments and observations of all professionals are discussed before writing the plans.

Day hospital clients are reviewed and reassessed by all disciplines every three months. The results of these reassessments are discussed at a multidisciplinary meeting and as a result care plans may be modified or changed. A weakness in our system is that carers do not necessarily attend these reviews, but they will be consulted by a member of staff, usually a nurse from the day hospital or a community psychiatric nurse, both before and after the review, so that they are involved in their relative's care. Day-to-day changes or observations are discussed at a brief meeting each morning. The speech and language therapist is also able to advise the occupational therapists in the unit on the communicative abilities of clients in their reality orientation, reminiscence and conversation groups.

Maximising functional communication

Because people with dementia have a progressive illness, their communication will deteriorate along with other cognitive functions. They are also unlikely to have the motivation or ability to respond to therapy so the role of the speech and language therapist must be to maximise communication by recognising the client's intact strengths and to advise carers on how to change their own communication and thus reduce the burden of communication for the carer. Carers can be informed specifically about their relatives' expressive and receptive skills, and can be advised on how to change the environment in order to put less pressure on the person. Carers can be taught strategies to use with the person, such as those described in Bayles and Kaszniak (1987), and Tanner and Daniels (1990). This might be something very simple such as reminding them to remove distractions such as loud television noise, or gaining the person's attention by calling his or her name first.

Carers may also need to be taught to be realistic, and not to expect too much from the person that they care for. For example one very caring husband, who was struggling to come to terms with the real implications of dementia, was still quite unrealistic about what his wife could and could not do. He felt she should be kept occupied, and because she had been a successful shopkeeper, was trying to teach her the value of new coins. When she made mistakes he got very frustrated and angry, and directly contradicted her, shouting 'No, no, not that one'. He frequently showed his frustration in all sorts of situations which only made his wife upset and bewildered. The speech and language therapist discussed with him (as had the community psychiatric nurse and day hospital nurses) why his wife was unable to perform such tasks requiring new learning, but was also able to discuss which strategies he could try and which behaviours to avoid with his wife. It was suggested that he avoided direct contradiction or confrontation and instead said something like 'Let's try it this way' and that it was his tone of voice and reassuring manner that were more important than the words he used. He was also advised, when he was very frustrated and angry, to walk away from the situation and try again later. He found it extremely difficult to avoid contradiction but soon recognised the value of using a warm, positive tone of voice, and walking away from confrontation. He found the latter strategy particularly useful once he realised that his wife forgot *her* confusion and anxiety very quickly and was not upset by him leaving her. In some cases the only way that the speech and language therapist can help the carer is by admitting that he or she too finds communication with the client extremely difficult. Furthermore, as a speech and language therapist, it is essential to learn that sometimes you cannot change how carers communicate. If they have talked to their husband/wife in a particular way for 50 years it is very difficult for them to change.

Counselling carers

This is a role shared by several disciplines working in the unit. The community psychiatric nurses (CPNs) tend to be the first professionals to have lengthy contact with carers, and they offer considerable support, explaining about the illness and its possible effects. They are also able to recognise the problems that other professionals are better equipped to deal with, and will pass this information on at multidisciplinary meetings. There is likely to be considerable overlap when counselling is offered, but for several reasons this is probably beneficial to the carer rather than just repetitive. First, the cognitive and behavioural changes caused by dementia do not occur on their own, rather there is usually a cluster of symptoms presenting at the same time and interacting with one other. Hence each professional is likely to be approaching the same problem but from a slightly different perspective. Second, most carers find it extremely difficult to come to terms with dementia, and need to hear about it and talk about it as much as possible. It seems that it cannot be overstated that their relative's changed behaviour is caused by an illness, and not by anything else. Further discussion of working with the carers of people with dementia is given in Chapter 11.

Training and education

A considerable amount of time is spent in training, educating and sharing information; about communication in dementia, and about the role of speech and language therapy. Information sharing and support for carers is provided in the form of relative support groups (RSGs), and in workshops specifically about communication. RSGs are run fortnightly in the unit, organised by a multidisciplinary committee. The groups are facilitated by a member of the RSG planning committee and speakers include both staff from within the unit and a wide range of contributors from outside.

The speech and language therapist also contributes to other RSGs run by social workers in the community, and by voluntary agencies such as Age Concern and the Alzheimer's Disease Society. Communication workshops are run for carers, other staff within the unit and staff on long-stay wards. The aim of these is to make people aware of normal communication, communication changes in dementia, and to help them identify strategies which help communication and behaviours which are likely to have a deleterious effect. The speech and language therapist is also involved in training home care assistants, social workers, other speech and language therapists, and speech and language therapy students from a nearby university. At present the speech and language therapist is investigating, together with colleagues working with the elderly in the community, the initiation of training for nursing home staff.

Speech and language therapy students are placed with the speech and language therapist, preferably as part of their adult clinical experience. Whilst it is extremely useful for them to be aware of communication changes in dementia, these are more easily understood when seen against a background of other neurological language disorders.

Research

Both speech and language therapists who have worked in this post have undertaken research projects. One of the first projects examined the effects of seating arrangements in the day hospital where chairs were arranged in a circle around the edges of the room. The study showed that patients communicated more often and for longer when seated in small groups, and by involving day hospital staff in the project it was possible to make them aware of the effect of changing the seating arrangement, and therefore more likely to support and implicate the change.

Other projects undertaken, with colleagues from other areas, have included producing a profile for scoring Alzheimer patients' naming abilities; examining the strategies used by carers when communicating with their relatives with dementia (Tanner and Daniels, 1990); the effect of using objects or pictures to facilitate conversation; and a study of whether people with dementia can provide linguistic reference – specifically their ability to use the given – new distinction (Tanner, 1993).

Developments

It has already been mentioned that there has been an increase in the number of clients seen solely in the community. As with all other clients, this group is discussed at multidisciplinary meetings, but not all disciplines are necessarily involved. As clients move out of hospital care and into care in the community there will be an increased need to provide training for the nursing home staff who will be providing that care. As well as the speech and language therapy training described earlier, unit staff are currently discussing how best to provide multidisciplinary training for homes which cater for elderly people with psychiatric disorders. Since being in the post, it has become clear to the SLT that many clients with dementia have eating difficulties; these may be actual swallowing problems, but very often the problems are behavioural, drug related or stem simply from the fact that the patient no longer remembers what food is, what to do with it or to swallow it once it is in the mouth. Thus the speech and language therapist's role includes assessment of feeding problems, to determine whether or not the patient is dysphagic and to manage accordingly. Even if the problem is not dysphagia, the speech and language therapist's advice on communication during feeding, posture, food taste and texture are all useful in managing the problem.

Standard assessments of dysphagia are very difficult to use with people with dementia as they are often not able to cooperate. Therefore, it is essential to use observation skills and to obtain a thorough case history from carers involved with feeding the person, as well as any information the client can provide.

There has been close liaison with the hospital dietitian which has resulted in workshops throughout the hospital, helping staff to recognise eating and swallowing problems, and to identify how they can help. We have also aimed to inform them about the role of non-nursing disciplines in the management of feeding difficulties, and the importance of a team approach to management.

This approach is also being discussed by the North West Special Interest Group in Psychiatry of the Elderly and the speech and language therapist has joined a subgroup interested in developing a supplementary assessment schedule for looking at the swallowing and feeding problems seen in these patients.

As the post has developed there has been a move away from roles directly related to speech and language therapy, but these roles are important in a multidisciplinary environment. The speech and language therapist is a member of the RSG Committee, and a member of the group which plans and organises entertainments and outings for clients. The speech and language therapist is also a member of the local editorial board of the 'Carer's Newsletter' produced by social workers for all carers in the community.

The speech and language therapist is supported both by the team within the unit and by colleagues working with other adult clients. All speech and language therapists in the adult team work according to protocols and standards which have a core structure but with slight variations depending on the exact nature of the post.

The job has evolved both because of changes within the Health Service and through the speech and language therapist's developing interest in working with elderly people who have psychiatric disorders.

Future developments are likely to include closer cooperation with social services, nursing homes and voluntary agencies, who are caring more and more for these patients, and the provision of training to help them manage people with dementia as well as possible.

Service variation

There remains tremendous variation in the service provision for elderly people with dementia in the UK (Moriarty and Levin, 1993). This is very evident in speech and language therapy with provision varying from specialised services providing a full range of assessment and treatment to areas where there is no specialist elderly or psychogeriatric service. Indeed there may be positive exclusion of clients with dementia from the therapy provision for acquired disorders. The Royal College of Speech and Language Therapists (RCSLT) published a report on speech and language therapy for the elderly with dementia in 1993 in which a survey of the provision for this client group was conducted, the findings being based on the information given by managers or their representatives from 134 districts. The survey revealed that 42 out of 134 districts had no service for clients with dementia whilst 29 offered a specialist EMI service with the majority of the therapists working in psychiatric, geriatric or psychogeriatric teams. Of the individual clinicians who took part in the survey, 97% had contact with this client group but this varied from full-time involvement to an occasional 'on-request' remit. Between one and 20 clients with possible dementia were referred each month. This large range was again said to reflect the contrast between 'on-request' services and existing specialist services.

The average referral rate for elderly mentally ill patients with dementia was 50 per annum which was at that time as frequent as other client groups such as those with dysphagia and acute medical referrals. The sources of referral were mainly geriatricians and other hospital specialists, with psychogeriatricians ranked third. The emphasis on referrals from hospital specialists may reflect their access to current speech and language therapy provision. Referrals from general practitioners, community psychiatric nurses and relatives of clients were less common but much more numerous than those from other sources such as district nurses and voluntary organisations.

Most services to the elderly with dementia were offered in a hospital inpatient setting in acute geriatric (21%), geriatric rehabilitation (20%) and continuing care departments (20%). Psychogeriatric locations accounted for 17% of cases. Outpatient services were provided in day hospitals (29%), by domiciliary visits (20%) and in private and local authority homes (43%). This is perhaps an indication of the need for services to extend into the community. Districts which can only offer an 'on-request' service are probably not providing for the elderly in the residential care setting.

Therapists contributing to the RCSLT survey were asked whether elderly clients with dementia were routinely reassessed: 48% of therapists answered positively and 52% negatively. Where clients were routinely reassessed this was mostly within a four- to six-month time period. This raises questions regarding the provision of ongoing services and monitoring of clients with what is essentially a progressive neurological disorder.

In terms of the management of elderly clients with dementia, approximately 60% of those with mild impairments were offered some form of management, reducing to 10% for those with severe impairment. Individual face-to-face treatment accounted for only 25% of clinician–patient contact time with many clinicians specifically commenting on the need to work directly on neurological symptoms, e.g. dysarthria and dysphagia in multi-infarct dementia. Group therapy, counselling and advice and education of carers and other professionals accounted for the majority of therapy time. Only a small number of therapists had a research commitment and most were self-initiated projects without outside funding. Therapists expressed a need for continued training in this field, with requests being made for information on differential diagnosis, assessment and management of dementia and research updates.

The RCSLT position paper on the elderly with dementia (1993) concludes that EMI services are not seen as a priority by most districts, yet where specialist provision is available, the service is well utilised, and the therapists highly motivated, professionally satisfied and well respected. The position paper therefore reflects the wide implementation gap between perceived need and service provision. The paper concludes that:

> ...the aim for service development must be comprehensive rather than frag-
> mented and that services must be planned and developed in response to
> clearly identified needs of the elderly mentally infirm and their carers (p. 11).

Guidelines for good practice

The aims and principles for service delivery are set out in *Communicating Quality* (Royal College of Speech and Language Therapists, 1991). These are:

1. to provide assessment and intervention for clients presenting with dementia. The service will consider their communicative need and evaluate the quality of their functional communication abilities;

2. to deliver services with and through significant others within the
    client's environment;
3. to offer advice and support to carers/relatives/significant others in the
    client's environment;
4. to work within a multidisciplinary framework – sharing goals of inter-
    vention and where appropriate preparing joint goals with other
    professional/carers;
5. to enable carers and other professionals to have a clear understand-
    ing of the communication strengths and needs of each client and
    provide the opportunity for carer/professional to develop the appro-
    priate skills in facilitating the client's communication.

The current emphasis by government in the UK on services for the
elderly being transferred from institution to community settings has
presented a need to reconsider speech and language therapy service
provision for the elderly. What has not been provided is a framework for
restructuring the service away from being hospital-based towards
community care, particularly to reach those elderly who are in residential care. Whether or not this will lead to an improvement of the provision of services for people with dementia remains to be seen. (The
management issues that need to be considered when developing
services for people with dementia are discussed in Chapter 4, and working in the community is discussed in Chapter 8.)

As recently as 1989 Griffiths and Baldwin described the value of
including speech and language therapy in the multidisciplinary team for
old-age psychiatry. This illustrates how new the discipline is as a recognised specialism. The account of a service given earlier in this chapter
also illustrates this. Griffiths and Baldwin (1989) outlined the speech
and language therapist's role as contributing to:

*   assessment;
*   advice on management;
*   research;
*   teaching.

The importance of open referral was also emphasised. This is important as many elderly people with dementia or related illnesses may not
be seen by psychogeriatricians and so the routes to speech and
language therapy referral may be variable. Baseby (1989) discussed
the role of the speech and language therapist in the care of the elderly
with mental illness. She emphasised the importance of speech and
language therapy to the diagnostic process where knowledge of the
effects of dementia on communication can be important in differential
diagnosis. Baseby outlined the speech and language therapist's role
as:

- continuous assessment;
- direct speech therapy;
- group work;
- counselling;
- advice;
- referral to other agencies;
- education;
- environmental considerations ;
- research.

The role of the speech and language therapist in research in old-age psychiatry is now receiving greater attention. Stevens (1994) outlined the contribution of speech and language therapists to memory clinics where language assessment has a vital role to play in the differential diagnosis of different forms of dementia, depression and the effects of normal ageing. The speech and language therapist's work has a dual role of clinical service and research from which other speech and language therapists can benefit. A study by Tanner and Daniels (1990) also provides an example of the interrelation between clinical service and research. They examined the communication strategies of carers of people with dementia. As a result of their research, they were able to run workshops to help carers become more aware of communication skills.

The benefits of respite care for people with dementia and their carers are widely recognised (Griffith, 1993; Homer and Gilleard, 1994). As respite care becomes more available, speech and language therapy will need to develop a more flexible role in providing appropriate continuing care to people with dementia and their carers which can cross boundaries of 'home', 'community' and 'hospital' provision.

Bebbington (1991) reported that speech and language therapists who worked with the elderly for more than 50% of their time were significantly more likely to have a positive attitude towards the elderly. This suggests that there are advantages to developing specialist services for the elderly and supports the need for newly qualified therapists to have the opportunity to work with the elderly in order to develop more favourable attitudes.

The role of the speech and language therapist in the management of feeding problems in clients with dementia is also under discussion (Kaatzke, 1992). The reliance upon 'high-tech' approaches such as video-fluoroscopy needs to be carefully considered given the reduced access of elderly clients in the community to such procedures and the ethical problems of attempting to utilise such procedures in people who may be confused or agitated. The term dysphagia has become almost synonymous with problems of swallowing itself. However, it is important to consider eating problems more widely in relation to people with dementia. Problems may be associated with factors such as ill-fitting or missing dentures, difficulty in getting food to the mouth, dry mouth as a side-effect of drugs or difficulties in concentrating on eating (Musson et al., 1990). Similarly the social and communicative importance of mealtimes is an important factor to consider in both home and residential care settings.

Educating other staff

Education of other staff is also an important role for speech and language therapists. This may extend to:

- other members of the multidisciplinary care team;
- carers;
- staff in the residential sector;
- referring agents such as GPs and health visitors.

The role of the speech and language therapist will, it is hoped, continue to develop as services become more developed generally for people with dementia. For example, community homes with respite, long-term care and volunteer schemes are reported as having indirect benefits on the levels of communication acheived by clients (*Community Care*, 1994). Similarly it is now recognised that mental stimulation can actually improve the level of mental functioning in people with dementia (Koh et al., 1994). This may mean that activities such as conversation groups, previously dismissed as palliative, may be worthy of properly constructed research to measure outcomes and establish the value of different forms of speech and language therapy intervention in different groups of elderly people with pyschiatric illness.

The measurement of therapy outcomes for elderly people with dementia is now considered important in order to estimate service needs and to assess whether resources have been fairly distributed. Leibovici, Curtis and Ritchie (1995) describe a simple method of quantifying levels of disability to provide indicators of service needs for dependent elderly people. The Confinement and Disability Index uses the interaction between ability to perform everyday tasks such as shopping and reading, levels of social support and living conditions to classify elderly populations into four dependency groups. If such scales or similar ones became recognised then they could be applied to assessing whether needs are being met by the services provided. Similarly, methods of evaluating outcome measures of community-based services are being developed. Ramsay, Winget and Higginson (1995) examined 81 potential outcome scales. They concluded that none of these was entirely satisfactory for assessing outcomes in community-based services for people with dementia, although some positive indications for further research were identified. (Audit of speech and language therapy services for clients with dementia is discussed in Chapter 12.)

The value of speech and language therapy to clients with dementia has been described in the literature. An extensive survey by Bourgeois (1991) of communication treatment for adults with dementia concluded that the literature reviewed supported the potential for positive outcomes from communication treatment in elderly individuals with diffuse degenerative diseases. Therapy was seen as being primarily important in maintaining function and reducing symptoms. Bourgeois suggests that speech and language therapists need to develop rigorous, maximally effective and comprehensive treatment packages. An important point made by Bourgeois was that speech and language therapy literature contained very few references to treatment for clients with dementia. Most references were to articles discussing diagnosis, whereas articles on treatments that effected change in communication were found in psychology, social work, nursing and gerontology journals. Perhaps this reflects the point raised by the RCSLT position paper that services for clients with dementia may not viewed as a priority area? Speech and language therapists appear to be reluctant to report on their work, perhaps reflecting a lack of confidence in their value or the difficulty of publishing work to which traditionally accepted methodologies are not applicable.

There remains an enormous need for speech and language therapists to report their work with clients who have dementia and other psychiatric disorders associated with ageing, and for qualitative as well as quantitative measures to be considered as acceptable methods of measuring communicative gain both within the profession and by other professionals.

Chapter 8:
Working in the Community – Care and Legislation

DEIRDRE RAINBOW, CHARLOTTE PAINTER
AND KAREN BRYAN

Introduction

A model of speech and language therapy service delivery to elderly clients in the residential sector is presented here. The speech and language therapists have reorganised their time and resources to provide a more effective service, with each stage of the reorganisation being carefully evaluated. Purchasers of speech and language therapy are increasingly seeking evidence that services are effective and therefore offer value for money. Some client groups easily lend themselves to such analysis. This is more difficult, however, with the chronically impaired, older population in long-stay settings, such as hospitals or nursing homes, where the majority of residents experience a communication disorder. The new delivery of service to the elderly clients presented here addresses the management of complex, long-term communication and swallowing impairments within existing resources.

Background

In 1991, an increase in staffing was secured to provide a service to two long-stay units within Islington Health Authority, each establishment receiving one day per week. Unit A is a small hospital specialising in the care of highly dependent frail older people with a range of medical problems. Unit B is a group of residential and nursing homes providing care of a similar level to unit A. Both units were previously covered by the domiciliary speech and language therapy service.

During the initial 18 months, a speech and language therapist worked in each unit one day per week. She was responsible for:

1. Initial screening of all residents to construct a profile of the type and severity of communication problems within each unit. Problems

identified included: dementia, dysphasia, dysarthria, confusion, hearing loss, cognitive impairments and psychiatric disturbance. In addition, the majority of residents experienced a degree of sensory loss, e.g. poor hearing, visual problems, absent/ill-fitting dentures.

This information indicated that patient care should develop in two directions. These were:

(a) a more detailed assessment of those clients with specific communication and/or swallowing problems and provision of individual management programmes for care staff to carry out. These ranged from written recommendations to aid communication skills, to the introduction of remediation programmes for dysphagic client;
(b) a weekly communication group aiming to support and train unit staff gradually to assume responsibility for these sessions;
2. assessment of the communication and swallowing skills of all new residents admitted to the wards and homes.
3. the introduction of a staff education programme. The management in unit A requested open sessions for staff, whilst the input to unit B, coordinated by their training officer, took the form of workshops focusing on specific communication impairments;
4. becoming involved in quality initiatives, such as care planning meetings, when invited by the unit management.

Critical evaluation of the service

The service was regularly reviewed throughout the first 18 months, culminating in a major evaluation in February 1993, which revealed the following:

Individual therapy

Direct individual work using intact skills as the foundation for therapy appeared to have benefited the specific clients involved, particularly the dysphagic caseload. The more recent introduction of speech and language therapy programmes and checklists proved popular with nursing staff, and steady carryover of the recommendations given was noted. A possible reason for this may be that swallowing is a more concrete area for nursing staff to understand and something which they readily recognise as part of their duty of care to residents. Additionally, progress in swallowing skills, as opposed to specific areas of communication, is more evident to both residents and their carers. This approach, however, targeted only a small number of residents in each establishment.

Groupwork

Fawcus (1983), in discussing the merits of communication groups, reported that they provide one of the most effective antidotes to the serious social dilemma facing the elderly. A number of other authors, most notably Barnett-Douglass (1986), Bryan and Drew (1987), Gravell (1988) and Jordan et al. (1993), suggest that groups provide an effective method of targeting large numbers of residents, particularly those presenting with multiple communication problems. The screening conducted in units A and B confirmed the high incidence of both specific and multiple communication problems, for which group work appeared to offer an effective treatment. Assessment of the impact of this approach with our clients, however, did not replicate the positive results of the studies listed above. The functional and specific communication skills of those residents participating showed little response to group treatment. The groups were therefore discontinued.

One factor in the limited success of the groups may be related to their frequency. The groups were run on a weekly basis over six weeks. Perhaps the outcome would have been different if they were run more frequently over a longer period. Many residents were not appropriate for group therapy, for example, those with behaviour problems or a significant hearing loss. From the remaining residents (with disparate communication problems) it was difficult to create a cohesive group. This is likely to have been a significant factor in the limited effect of the groups.

Care staff, although initially expressing an interest in attending the groups, did so sporadically and in decreasing numbers. Other aspects of patient care took precedence, particularly when staffing levels were low. Our expectation that carers might be able to assume responsibility for the groups was not realised. Finally, identifying suitable accommodation and portering arrangements presented continual difficulties.

Staff training

The success of individualised programmes carried out by staff may have been, in part, attributable to their role in carer education. A programme of staff training was implemented aiming to give staff basic information about specific speech and language problems, and strategies to deal with the difficulties they may encounter with communicatively impaired residents, as well as detailing the benefits of reminiscence and stimulation approaches. In providing carers with a larger knowledge base we may be facilitating closer examination of individual residents' needs, or, as Jackson (1990) proposes, staff may identify their training needs in relation to their immediate problems with patients, rather than in respect of communication disabilities as a whole.

Staff in unit B who attended formal teaching tutorials gave largely positive feedback about the content of such sessions, frequently requesting further opportunities to discuss their particular residents in detail. Some sessions were, however, poorly attended, whilst open sessions in unit A failed to attract any participants. We were aware that even when training is available and staff are interested, covering for others' absence from the ward is problematic. It is also possible that not all staff want training.

We concluded that our input was most effective in two areas, namely:

(i) staff training sessions;
(ii) programmes for individual residents.

This directed us to the need for an alternative model of speech and language therapy provision for older people living in these residential homes which would:

(a) influence the care of all residents whatever their communication or swallowing disorder;
(b) be tailored to the needs of each individual unit and its residents;
(c) permit all interested carers to attend regular training sessions. Jackson (1990) argues that 'on the job' training is essential, ensuring that it is integrated into everyday nursing duties, because Stockwell (1972) found that nurses felt simply talking was not nursing.

A modified model of service delivery

The model detailed below has evolved from delivery of this approach to each of the wards in unit A, and two homes in unit B. On each occasion the approach was modified in the light of feedback from both the therapist and home/ward staff. It is anticipated that we will continue to develop the model.

Aims

Although the fundamental aims of the new model are largely unchanged from the previous approach, it is considered important to restate them within the context of our new ideas. They are:

1. to provide a high-quality, cost-effective service to all clients and carers in units A and B;
2. to provide staff education which will equip carers with a basic working knowledge of communication and/or swallowing difficulties;
3. to promote communication and swallowing issues as a higher priority to staff;
4. to facilitate staff's identification of factors which may help, or pose a

barrier to, effective communication and safe, enjoyable eating and drinking, paying particular attention to the environment and opportunities;

5. to support staff in their attempts to improve residents' environment and opportunities

Structure

The most significant difference between the original model of speech and language therapy service delivery and the revised approach relates to the frequency of the therapist's visits. Intensive blocks, of up to four weeks, are offered rather than a single day per unit per week. The total number of speech and language therapy days (45 allowing for annual leave and bank holidays) remains unchanged. Each unit is offered two to three intensive blocks per year, aiming to cover the three wards in unit A, and the three principal homes in unit B. In unit A, as the wards are on the same site, it has proved beneficial to combine the input to more than one ward which is also more cost-effective in terms of the speech and language therapist's time.

Ward/home-specific input

It is considered fundamental to the project that the speech and language therapist spends time building up a picture of the specific needs of the ward/home concerned. This is achieved by:

- assessing carers' knowledge (see evaluation);
- learning about the daily routine of the home;
- understanding the practical difficulties faced by its staff with regard to residents' swallowing and communication difficulties.

From this analysis, training sessions are devised to target the key issues for that home/ward. The training sessions are heavily supported by videos of the home, staff and residents, which illustrate both positive and negative aspects of daily interaction.

Videos of a familiar environment and people have proved much more successful than using footage of standard examples of specific communication disorders or staged interactions.

Video consent forms have been devised for each home/ward and no resident is involved without his or her consent or that of next of kin (or advocate where there is no relative). Staff are understandably often reluctant to be videoed, therefore, prior to filming, the therapist visits the unit to explain the rationale for using video, and to answer any questions. We have found that careful preparation is essential.

Training sessions

Small-group training sessions are provided each afternoon. In order to minimise the problem of staff absence from the wards, the workshops are timetabled for times when two shifts overlap. In restricting the duration to 15–20 minutes, it is possible to provide two 'tutorials' each afternoon to further increase the opportunity for attendance. As outlined above, the content is specifically designed to address the needs of that home/ward and its residents, employing video footage and practical exercises to reinforce key points.

The speech and language therapist stresses to the staff that she is available as a facilitator, rather than aiming to tell them how to run their home/ward.

Topics covered

A core of training topics has developed:

- the communication environment;
- communication skills;
- communicative opportunity;
- stimulation;
- choice;
- communication difficulties in older people – theory and strategies to help;
- hearing aids.

The detection and management of swallowing disorders also feature in the course. Wherever possible, communication is highlighted in these sessions, for example during 'experiential feeding' where staff feed each other.

Teaching methods employed

Video footage is an essential element of the training because it serves to illustrate aspects of the home/ward, and the behaviour of residents and staff which may help or hinder communication. Initially videos were shot for the majority of training sessions but more variety has now been introduced so that videos are used in a maximum of half the sessions. The video clips last up to one minute. Some examples of their use are detailed below:

(a) Tanner et al. (1990) suggested the benefits of using observational checklists and tape recordings to work on interaction between clients and carers, hence in the session on 'The Communication

Environment' staff are asked to watch a video of their ward/home and, on a sheet provided, list positive and negative points relating to the environment. The group then collates their observations, concluding the session with a summary of areas they would like to change.

(b)'Choice' commences with the therapist handing out drinks to staff – some are offered no choice; others have apparent, but not real choice (e.g. 'orange?'); and the rest receive a true choice of drinks. The group establish the different level of choices and then comment on a video of choices given to their residents.

All sessions involve a practical, participative exercise. The session on hearing aids provides carers with an opportunity to experience what it is like to wear a hearing aid. Low-tech amplification devices, such as hearing wands, are also available to try out. At the conclusion of some sessions, staff are given exercises to take away and trial on a resident. For example, the 'Choice' session also includes a questionnaire which can then be placed in residents' care plans.

A training pack is provided for each home/ward at the end of the course which includes:

1. a summary of each session, noting in particular the action points identified by staff;
2. supplementary handouts, such as those detailing the communication difficulties encountered by a dysphasic or demented resident;
3. a copy of the training video.

To acknowledge the value we attach to training, and the importance of staff contributions to the sessions, each participant is given a certificate detailing the sessions he or she has attended.

Individual residents

Assessment and provision of individual programmes for new residents, those whose management requires updating, or those presenting with a deterioration in their communication or swallowing abilities are the therapist's principal duty each morning. A small minority of residents may be seen for intensive speech and language therapy. The speech and language therapist is also available each lunchtime to assess and advise on swallowing difficulties and this provides an excellent opportunity to model communication strategies. Communication and/or swallowing advice sheet(s) are provided for insertion into each resident's nursing care plan.

Individual sessions continue to be offered for patients who require assessment/management between intensive blocks. This is particularly important in the case of extra-contractual referrals, i.e. a contract made between the service provider (speech and language therapy) and the organisation holding a budget for that client's care (usually the health authority in which the client is or was resident, or a fundholding GP), and also for dysphagic patients. The training sessions have, however, equipped care staff with more skills to carry out programmes with clients, hence the therapist's role has become more one of monitoring than being a provider of treatment.

Carryover of the training topics

In being available all day over a number of weeks, the speech and language therapist can facilitate 'on-the-spot' problem solving with staff, particularly around the issues of opportunity to communicate and the impact of the residential environment. As she spends an intensive block of time on the ward, carers appear to relate to her more as a member of the team than as the visiting 'specialist'. The speech and language therapist also reports that she feels more of a team member, even when returning to the unit some months after the intensive block.

Evaluation

The effect of speech and language therapy intervention for individual clients continues to be measured utilising standardised assessment batteries and the service's outcome measures (in the development and pilot phase at present).

Any evaluation of the training sessions has to be easy to administer, in a form which can be translated into meaningful information for management and purchasers alike. Questionnaires appear to fulfil these requirements. Two questionnaires (see Appendix 5) are currently in use. Of the whole service, it is this area which has undergone the most significant modification during the past 15 months.

Quantitative measurement

True/false questions were utilised to measure staff's knowledge about specific topics, such as the normal communication process, hearing aids and clinical signs of dysphagia. This questionnaire was administered prior to the training and, in combination with the observations of the needs of that individual home/ward, the results are used to plan the training package. Pre- and post-training results can be compared to evaluate any change in the staff's knowledge.

Qualitative measurement

A second questionnaire was developed for the home/ward managers to gain more qualitative information about the training. This includes suggestions from the managers regarding modifications to the speech and language therapy service. This questionnaire is relatively new, and it is anticipated that it will evolve in the future.

Additionally the speech and language therapist notes any changes which have taken place in the unit as a direct consequence of her training sessions. Examples have included the removal of soft toys and excessive furniture from a day room in order to arrange seating for residents in such a way as to increase communicative opportunity. In another unit, alternatives to the constant use of the television were debated at length.

Variations of the model

This model of delivering speech and language therapy to continuing care units should not be seen as fixed. It is essential that the model is flexible to the changing demands of the NHS and it is the responsibility of speech and language therapists constantly to question the effectiveness of the approach and modify accordingly. Two variations which have been used recently are described below:

Altering the configuration of the training weeks

To meet the needs of unit B it was agreed to incorporate a break into the intensive blocks. Thus a two-week break followed the initial videoing and training sessions. The speech and language therapist involved also endorsed this approach, reporting that the break enabled her to return refreshed for the final two weeks, and avoided isolation from her clinical base and colleagues.

Student placements

Recently, we agreed to take two final-year students who undertook the patient assessment and care plan writing. The students and the speech and language therapist were able to complete the 'individual resident' aspect of the service within four consecutive days, as opposed to the normal 15 sessions (7 half-days). The speech and language therapist then attended the home in the afternoons, only to run the training sessions and facilitate carryover of key points. The advantages were that:

(a) the students were provided with a placement which gave them significant experience in assessment of this client group and writing care plans;

(b) a more cost-effective service is provided whilst retaining a high standard of care;

(c) the speech and language therapist avoided isolation from her clinical base;

(d) it provided additional student placements.

We will be exploring the value of this approach further in the future.

Benefits of this approach for speech and language therapy staff

The model of speech and language therapy described in this paper aims principally to improve the service to clients and their carers, but must also serve the needs of therapists themselves.

Older clients in residential settings experience a range of chronic disabilities which are generally slow to respond to conventional speech and language therapy. Even those approaches designed specifically for the institutionalised client (group work, staff training sessions etc.) proved unviable in units A and B. Speech and language therapy staff working in these units are generally newly qualified, with limited experience in dealing with such a complex client group and, when intervention fails, they may quickly become demoralised.

By clearly defining the role of the speech and language therapist, setting out not only the aims but also the method of service delivery, recruitment and retention of staff working in residential settings may improve.

Further support for the speech and language therapist's role can be found in the professional guidelines of the Royal College of Speech and Language Therapists (1991), which are briefly:

• ensuring that the communication/swallowing needs of clients are fully considered within their day-to-day management;
• guiding carers on how to maximise interaction with clients during everyday activities;
• providing strategies to aid communication/swallowing;
• gaining commitment of home staff;
• staff training;
• health promotion.

The post responsible for providing this service is split between unit A, unit B and a unit providing rehabilitation for older patients. Within the original approach, therefore, the speech and language therapist practised at a different site for the first three days of each week. She was unable to implement any intensive therapy regimes with clients or follow projects through.

The new approach minimises the piecemeal nature of the job, whilst maintaining the variety which the member of staff reports she enjoys. Whilst involved in the long-stay project she can focus on it fully, and between these periods she is able to consolidate her skills in working in elderly rehabilitation.

Devising and implementing this approach left the rehabilitation wards significantly understaffed for two-fifths of the year, instigating an evaluation of the responsibilities of all the speech and language therapists in the team. As a result, a number of posts have become less fragmented as staff assume new responsibilities, providing an opportunity to develop new skills.

The main thrust of the project is staff training, equipping them with strategies to deal more effectively with their particular residents. For the speech and language therapist too, the course is educative. Foundation skills introduced during training in effective explaining and lecturing can be expanded. Specific instruction regarding the use of video equipment and editing techniques ensure high-quality audio-visual materials for each workshop, and furnish the speech and language therapy team with a new expertise.

Benefits for care/nursing staff

The profile of training is increasing within the health service as managers recognise the importance of a skilled workforce. Our workshops are a locally agreed arrangement, but staff may choose to use them towards gaining formal qualifications. For example, care staff are being encouraged to participate in work-based National Vocational Qualifications (NVQs), which take previous experience and training into account. Trained nurses are now expected to maintain a personal log of courses attended.

In future it may be appropriate to hold discussions with the education and training establishments, particularly the School of Nursing and our Trust's training and development department, to agree the status of our workshops within specific ENB (English Nursing Board) and NVQ courses.

One home in unit B is currently working towards attaining British Standard 5750 which, if they are successful, will demonstrate the high standard of its nursing care. The speech and language therapist felt that staff found two areas of the training particularly difficult, namely problem solving and their power, especially among the unqualified staff, to implement the improvements to the environment which they had identified in the sessions. The home manager plans to address these two areas as part of the work towards BS5750, and reported the value of this feedback to the speech and language therapy service manager.

Management issues

Any manager working within today's health service must recognise the importance of purchasers – health authorities and fundholding GPs. London health authorities are subject to weighted capitation, annually reducing their budgets in line with government policy to allocate resources on the basis of population. In consequence, purchasers are forced to prioritise the services they can afford. Treatments which are proven value for money will be the only ones to survive. It is therefore incumbent upon service managers to evaluate continually the health care they provide.

The approach outlined in this project, in:

(i)   clearly defining its aims and method;

(ii) building in a means of evaluating its effectiveness; and

(iii) providing a service which addresses the needs of greater numbers of residents within existing resources, should prove attractive to purchasers. It illustrates the speech and language therapy department's commitment to improving services for the benefit of the clients (here residents and staff) within financial constraints.

In future, purchasers may dictate our style of therapy. For example, it is speculated that speech and language therapists may be directed to offer only assessment and advice, rather than ongoing treatment. Our approach builds this into the care of patients, such that they are reassessed during each intensive block and management guidelines for carers updated. Many purchasers inform trusts of the number of client contacts they expect them to make each month. Planned, intensive periods of input to long-stay units assist the prediction of patient numbers. The approach detailed in this chapter describes a specific package of care to elderly people living in continuing care settings, with built-in outcome measures. Speech and language therapy delivered in this way may be attractive to purchasers.

The general framework of the method may be applicable to the work of other professions allied to medicine, for example physiotherapists. We were approached by the psychologist working in unit A a week prior to commencing our input, who was interested in joining forces on the project. Preparations were too far advanced to include her at that stage, but in future it may be more effective to involve a number of disciplines in the training process.

Summary and conclusions

This chapter outlines how a speech and language therapy service to older people in long-stay units was reviewed and revised. The new approach offers a cost-effective but more efficient service, which ensures equality of service for all residents.

We have shown that by training nurses and care staff to detect and manage communication and swallowing problems, the traditional role of the speech and language therapist working with older people can be radically altered.

By empowering the people in daily contact with the residents to deal with the difficulties arising from communication/swallowing disorders, more effective use of limited resources is made. This applies not only to speech and language therapy services, but also to the frequently over-stretched resources in continuing care.

This new method of service delivery is flexible, and will continue to develop in response to feedback from therapists, managers and care staff.

Whilst the future of the NHS remains uncertain, we hope that this method of service delivery will prove viable and long-lasting.

Discussion of service provision in the community

As early as the 1960s there was concern about the increasing reliance upon residential care for elderly people and the resultant draining of resources from domiciliary care (Ministry of Health, 1963). However, until the mid-1980s the dominant paradigm of welfare for the elderly was a continuum of care, where increasing difficulty was served by a progression from domiciliary to residential to geriatric nursing care. This continuum reflected a progression from social to medical provision.

Subsequently community care is seen as a reflection of the right of elderly people to live as independently as possible in familiar surroundings. The Department of Health (1989a) defines community care as:

> providing the right level of intervention and support to enable people to achieve maximum independence and control over their own lives. For this aim to become a reality, the development of a wide range of services provided in a variety of settings is essential. These services form part of a spectrum of care, ranging from domiciliary support provided to people in their own homes, strengthened by the availability of respite care and day care for those with more intensive care needs, through sheltered housing, group homes and hostels where increasing levels of care are available, to residential care and long-stay hospital care for those for whom other forms of care are no longer enough. (p. 9)

As such, there is almost universal acclaim for the concept of community care but other factors, such as the need to cope with ever rising numbers of elderly people within the population and the need to curb government spending on health and social service, have led to much suspicion about the fate of provision for the elderly.

Community care began with moves to close institutions and to move residents back into the community, particularly in the mental health and adult learning disability fields. There was also growing concern about the rising numbers of elderly people when there were moves to reduce

the number of NHS long-stay beds and to close or privatise local authority residential homes. Changes to the supplementary benefit regulations
made it possible for low-income residents of private and voluntary
sector homes to claim their fees from the social security system without
assessment of the need for this care. These two factors encouraged a
significant increase in the private residential and nursing care sectors.
The number of places rose from 46 900 in 1982 to 161 200 in 1991
(Laing and Buisson, 1992), with the vast majority of these places being
for the elderly. This produced a concomitant rise in spending on private
institutional care from £10 million in 1979 to £1872 million in 1991, at a
time when the government wished to prioritise the development of
domiciliary services.

The Griffiths report in 1986 was the outcome of a review of the ways
in which public funds were used to support community care. Griffiths
suggested the following proposals relevant to community care for the
elderly:

- a minister of community care should be appointed to guide the
  development of services;
- social services departments should take the lead role for identification of need, creation of packages of care, coordination of a mixed
  economy system of services responsive to local needs and the regula-
  tion of private and voluntary sector residential and nursing homes;
- health authorities would continue to be responsible for medically
  required community health services and to be involved in both the
  assessment of need and the delivery of packages of care;
- GPs would be responsible for informing social services departments
  about non-health care needs;
- residential and nursing home residents would receive financial
  support only after assessments of both care needs and financial
  means managed through social services departments;
- in the future individuals should be encouraged to meet the cost of
  their own elderly care needs.

The Griffiths report was not without its critics although it was generally
well received, particularly from a social services perspective (Means and
Smith, 1994). The main recommendations from Griffiths (with some
notable exceptions) were contained in the White Paper *Caring for
People: Community Care in the Next Decade and Beyond* (Department
of Health, 1990), implemented on 1 April 1991. The government's
proposals list six key objectives for service delivery:

- *to promote the development of domiciliary, day and respite services
  to enable people to live in their own homes wherever feasible and
  sensible.* Existing funding structures have worked against the devel-

opment of such services. In future, the government will encourage the targeting of home-based services on those people whose need for them is greatest;

- *to ensure that service providers make practical support for carers a high priority*. Assessment of care needs should always take account of the needs of caring family, friends and neighbours;
- *to make a proper assessment of need and good case management the cornerstone of high-quality care*. Packages of care should be designed in line with individual needs and preferences;
- *to promote the development of a flourishing independent sector alongside good quality public services*. The government has endorsed Sir Roy Griffiths's recommendation that social services authorities should be 'enabling' agencies. It is to be their responsibility to make maximum possible use of private and voluntary providers, and so increase the available range of options and widen consumer choice;
- *to clarify the responsibilities of agencies and so make it easier to hold them to account for their performance*. The government recognises that the present confusion has contributed to poor overall performance;
- *to secure better value for taxpayers' money by introducing a new funding structure for social care*. The government's aim is that social security provisions should not, as they do now, provide any incentive in favour of residential and nursing home care.

Social services departments were confirmed as having the following key responsibilities:

- carrying out an appropriate assessment of an individual's need for social care (including residential and nursing home care), in collaboration with medical, nursing and other caring agencies, before deciding what services should be provided;
- designing packages of services tailored to meet the assessed needs of individuals and their carers. The appointment of a case manager may facilitate this;
- securing the delivery of services, not simply by acting as direct providers, but by developing their purchasing and contracting role to become 'enabling authorities';
- establishing procedures for receiving comments and complaints from service users;
- monitoring the quality and cost-effectiveness of services, with medical and nursing advice as appropriate;
- establishing arrangements for assessing the client's ability to contribute to the full economic cost to the local authority of residential services.

The role of health authorities included the following new responsibilities:

- *Assessment*: Health authorities will be expected to make the necessary contribution to these procedures by ensuring that health experts such as clinicians, community nurses and therapists are made available to take part in assessment.
- *Collaboration with local authorities*: Effective joint working and planning will continue to be essential.
- *Production of community care plans*: Health authorities will be expected to prepare plans setting out their community care policies and the provision they intend to make for community services and community care.

The NHS and Community Care Act was passed in 1990 but the timetable for implementation was delayed until April 1992 for community care plans to become a statutory requirement and until April 1993 for the transfer of funds for residential care from the Department of Social Security to local authority social services departments. This allowed extra time for planning of services for what is now acknowledged to be an enormous restructuring of health and social service provision for the elderly. Many health authorities or parts of health authorities have now become health care trusts. Trusts are expected to fulfil the same responsibilities but the resulting increase in the number of providers has contributed to the growing diversity of services. The main tenet of the new funding regime is the concept of care management.

Care management

The Department of Health policy guidance (1990) stated that a care management system should cover three distinct processes:

- assessment of the user's circumstances in the round, including any support required by carers;
- design of a care package in agreement with users, carers and relevant agencies, to meet the identified needs within the care resources available, including help from willing and able carers. Any preferred solutions which prove unavailable either because of resource constraints or because the services have not been developed will be fed back into the planning process;
- implementation and monitoring of the agreed package, review of the outcomes for users and carers, and any necessary revision of service provision

The concept of care management comes from the USA and should provide a system to guide people through the multiplicity of social services and health care agencies and to act as an advocate between the client, service providers and more informal carers such as family and local support groups. Early studies were positive. For example Challis et al. (1987) described the Gateshead project where frail elderly people were able to benefit from well-planned and coordinated community care under a care manager who has budgetary control. Outcomes were measured in terms of social/emotional needs such as morale and going out/social visits, and care needs such as need for personal care and need for help in daily household care. The outcome for the elderly people was as beneficial as that of entering residential care and was greater than that achieved through provision of domiciliary care without the care manager's coordination. Some 31% of the clients were said to be moderately or severely confused at the start of the study, but there was no separate assessment of the value of the care for this group. Other studies have excluded clients with dementia so that the applicability to this client group is unclear.

Means and Smith (1994) discuss how far social services departments have reached in implementing this system. They state that further work is needed to:

- stimulate a mixed economy of care with many more innovations in service provision in state, voluntary and private sectors;
- organise purchaser and provider arrangements within social services;
- develop assessments which are needs driven and acceptable to a wide range of agencies;
- prioritise services in line with resources;
- allow a wide range of staff within and outside social services to become care managers.

Progress in community care

The framework for community care for the elderly as defined by government papers is only partially implemented. This is not surprising in view of the Audit Commission's (1992) statement that: '...a process of change has been set in motion which will turn organisations upside-down' (p. 19). Hardy (1992) studied 24 authorities and concluded that the slow development of alternative suppliers of care services was due to a number of factors including:

- paucity of alternative suppliers in domiciliary and day care – the unwillingness of some potential alternative suppliers to alter their roles;
- many alternative suppliers are underdeveloped in terms of management capacity;
- the increasing paucity of volunteers.

In 1992 the British Medical Association published a report on priorities for community care, and the following concerns were raised in relation to the elderly:

- numbers of elderly people are rising;
- delays in the implementation of legislation have done nothing to slow the increasing use of nursing and residential homes, especially for the over-75s;
- pressure is being put upon doctors and upon elderly patients to move such patients into residential and nursing care in an attempt to curb hospital bed blocking;
- many health authorities are transferring the entire responsibility for continuing care of elderly people to the private sector, where access to the entire range of rehabilitation services available in NHS long-stay provision is rarely available;
- gaps are occurring in the provision of services for elderly severely mentally infirm patients, many of whom are settled in nursing homes without psychiatric assessment;
- there is a lack of coordination of services for the elderly on a local level.

The British Medical Association then made a series of recommendations for the implementation of community care as envisaged by the 'Caring for People' policy.

Despite the general consensus that community-based services are preferable, the effects on care for the frail elderly are causing concern. Implementation has not been completed in some areas and 'research continues to demonstrate the lack of coordination and liason in day to day practice, with resulting service duplication and overlap' (Henwood, 1992, p. 27).

Access to services has remained controlled by professionals and contracted-out services often merely replace previously in-house services so that choice of services has not become a reality for many elderly clients, and social services departments have found it difficult to change from being 'providers' to 'enablers' (Wistow et al., 1992). Collaboration between agencies and the professionals who provide care has not always been established (Hudson, 1987; Dalley, 1991). There has also been an enormous diversity in the response of local authorities to the community care legislation (Osborne and Rees, 1992) so that it is difficult to generalise about levels of service and exact forms of provision for the elderly.

A further factor limiting the effective implementation of community care has been the growing tension between consumer demands and financial restrictions (Hudson, 1990) and disputes about boundaries of responsibility between health and social care provision (Henwood, 1992a). Questions about the equity of provision in community care also arise. These concern different client groups, income groups, generations and localities (Challis and Henwood, 1994).

In response to concerns such as these, innovative projects have been set up which provide ideal models of care. An example is a project in Darlington involving care managers located in a geriatric multidisciplinary team to provide an alternative to long-stay hospital care. The care managers were employed by social services and had devolved budgets (Challis et al., 1991a). Elderly clients could be referred by any member of the multidisciplinary team. They would then be screened by the care manager as suitable for the project in terms of carer participation, suitable housing, etc. Full assessment would then take place involving medical and paramedical input and a home visit. The care manager would then produce a care plan and manage both the discharge and subsequent monitoring within the multidisciplinary team. The care manager was also responsible for deploying the home care assistants who were recruited for the project. The home care assistants were given training including SLT input and were expected to act as assistants to professional where appropriate.

The project provides a model for care management which brings together the two key agencies of health and social services and is based within a multidisciplinary team. The cost and effectiveness of this care was evaluated in detail (Challis et al., 1991b). The evaluation showed that frail elderly people receiving community-based care had a higher quality of life with no evidence of greater stress upon their carers. The cost of the service was cheaper overall than long-stay provision and costs appeared to remain relatively stable over time.

However, the majority of social services departments have not developed such models and are not likely to do so in the immediate future (Henwood, 1992b). A further point made by the authors in relation to the elderly with dementia is that the service model was most effective in managing the problems of uncomplicated physical frailty, but would have greater difficulty in coping with more complicated clients where problems of mental disorder and family stress are more prominent. This suggests that such schemes need to be evaluated in relation to elderly people who present with dementia and/or other physical and social problems. This is particularly important as the number of very old people is expected to rise, resulting in a greater number of elderly people with complex problems, such as dementia (Evans et al., 1989), for which care provision will need to cater.

A survey of all elderly residents in the London Borough of Waltham Forest examined the prevalence of dementia, depression and physical disability in the elderly population in residential homes, long-stay NHS wards, private and voluntary homes, sheltered housing or those in receipt of augmented domiciliary services (Harrison, Savla and Kafetz, 1990). The survey showed that almost all the people with dementia were in residential care, with the bulk of this being health service or local authority provision. This study casts doubt on the appropriacy of community care for elderly people with dementia particularly when the dementia reaches the moderate and severe stages. Speech and language therapy services for clients with dementia might then remain primarily hospital based, as they are now, with expansion into the residential sector where necessary. If it becomes evident that clients with dementia are cared for primarily in the early stages of the disease process at home, then speech and language therapy input into community care via carer support might be expected to be an important service development.

Another innovation described is that of NHS nursing homes. A study by Donaldson and Bond (1991) showed that high-quality nursing care with a full range of multidisciplinary input could be provided at a cost which is no greater than for hospital care. The NHS nursing homes were found to be more costly than private sector equivalents but were found to cater for a less able group of people. It is important that such provision does include a full range of rehabilitation services, but this does not always appear to be the case.

An interesting study by the DOMINO group for domiciliary rehabilitation in Nottingham looked at rehabilitation after stroke (Gladman, Whynes and Lincoln, 1994). However, the majority of patients were referred from departments of health care for the elderly. The results showed that use of day hospitals for frail elderly patients led to better outcomes including lower rates of entry into institutional care. Increased age, living alone, more severe strokes and cognitive impairment were risk factors that might indicate benefit from day hospital attendance. This study supports the notion that outcomes as well as costs need to be evaluated (Fletcher, Dickinson and Philp, 1992). Initial higher spending to increase the level of support for elderly people might also be necessary in order to prevent later high costs of institutional care.

There has, however, been concern over the reduction in available day-care provision for the elderly (Rickford, 1993) and there are suggestions that decreased hospital contact may be associated with problems such as abuse of elderly people (Marchant, 1993; McCreadie and Tinker, 1993) and disruption to care due to financial factors such as closure of a residential home (Hallewell, Morris and Jolley, 1994).

For speech and language therapists the changes in service provision that are emerging suggest that there will be a greater range of working practices for speech and language therapists who work with the elderly. Some evidence of this is provided by the services described in this chapter and in Chapters 4, 5 and 7. In the future, this may involve greater opportunities to work in domiciliary and community-based settings and involvement in care management schemes within either a health or social services setting depending upon local arrangements. Little evidence of changes in speech and language therapists' working arrangements has yet emerged in the published literature. The need for professionals to take their expertise into the community and the ways in which this might be accomplished are being discussed by a number of professional groups. For example, Greveson (1994) outlines the scope for the development of the geriatrician's role in the community. This might include:

- greater availability of domiciliary visiting for frail patients;
- consultant clinics in primary care settings such as GPs' surgeries;
- more flexible arrangements for the assessment and follow up of patients in residential or nursing homes (see also MacPherson, Donald and Ludbrook, 1992);
- clinical services to social services particularly for assessment but also for advice on patient management;
- participation in 'hospital-at-home' schemes;
- a contribution to service planning for the elderly in both health and social services sectors;
- participation in training and education in residential, voluntary sector and carer group areas as well as traditional areas such as student training.

Most of the above would be relevant to any professional working with the elderly including speech and language therapists. As most SLTs working with the elderly with dementia have been based in hospital departments, the same type of changes in working practice might be expected to occur. (The speech and language therapist's work in day hospitals is described in Chapter 5.) The other area relevant to community care where there is already input from speech and language therapists is the residential care sector. At least 50% of residents present with communication problems, a large proportion of these being associated with dementia (Brodie, 1986; Bryan and Drew, 1989).

Bryan and Drew (1987) described a programme of intervention in local authority residential homes which involved a rolling programme of staff training and experimental group work to encourage communication in two homes. An example of the type of input needed is provided in a handbook for care assistants working with the elderly mentally infirm (Bryan and Maxim, 1991). Lester (1994) describes a project which was jointly funded by health and social services to evaluate the role of the speech and language therapist in residential homes. Action for Dysphasic Adults is currently producing a training pack for care homes which aims to educate care workers on how to encourage communication and how to cope with a range of communication disabilities including dementia (ADA, 1995).

Research into communication within residential environments is also yielding interesting information which can be directly applied to clinical practice. Kaakinen (1995) found that the nursing home environment appeared to foster negative communication and that residents had their own motivations for talking or not talking. Additional factors that play a role are staff attitudes, architectural barriers, family expectations and resident frailty. Kaakinen then described six major strategies for assisting elderly residents in sustaining conversations in the nursing home:

- reminiscing;
- matching talkers with talkers (and including residents with communication disabilities in such initiatives);
- providing more resident-to-resident communication opportunities;
- altering inhibitory rules, e.g. allowing discussion of death and allowing residents who cannot sleep to socialise at night;
- establishing 'mentoring' schemes;
- altering the physical environment.

Orange et al. (1995) described the application of a communication enhancement model to encourage and develop communication between care staff and elderly residents with Alzheimer's disease.

Shadden (1995) described the application of discourse analyses and discourse-based interventions to focus communication intervention and to measure outcomes effectively within a residential setting. (Outcome measurements and service audit are discussed further in Chapters 3 and 11.)

This chapter has outlined a model of speech and language therapy input to residential care which provides an example of how a high-quality, cost-effective service to all clients and carers in two different residential settings can be provided by defining the therapist's role and by managing therapy time in order to allow the therapist to become an active member of the care staff team.

Chapter 9:
Language, Cognition and Communication Assessment of Older People with Psychiatric Disorders

LINDA ARMSTRONG

Introduction

This chapter describes current issues for speech and language therapy assessment of the communication ability of the elderly person with psychiatric disorder. Heritage and Farrow (1994), who visited centres of excellence in the care of this group of people, consider that assessment provides a 'significant role for all the therapists as part of their contribution to the overall care and management of clients' (p.15). The purposes of speech and language therapy assessment will be described before possible processes and procedures are discussed and evaluated. Several contrasting direct and indirect methods will then be described.

Purposes of assessment

Why should the speech and language therapist be involved in the assessment of an elderly mentally infirm person? According to Gilleard, Boyd and Watt (1982), symptoms related to communication problems in EMI people contributed significantly to indices of dependency, demand and disturbance. These indices represent groupings of problems, e.g. 'dependency' subsumes problems of dressing, feeding, communication, washing, being not safe outside or left alone. They discuss the outcome of a carer questionnaire (including problem checklists) in which almost half of the carers reported difficulties with communication. In this sample, inability to hold a sensible conversation ranked fourth among the 25 problems. Continual questioning was also reported by 36% of respondents, a symptom commonly reported in people with dementia. Similarly, in Rabins, Mace and Lucas (1982), half of the families of people with some variety of dementia identified communication difficulties as a problem to them. More recently, the communication problems associated with mental illness in the elderly population have received some attention in the literature (see Chapter 3 for a review). Whilst carers identify the communication difficulties of their EMI relative among the constellation of their problems, speech and language therapists now have relevant knowledge and experience of working with this elderly client group to bring to assessment.

The process of assessment is, in fact, integral and central to all aspects of the therapeutic role. Bayles and Kaszniak (1987) describe four responsibilities for the speech and language therapist in the management of a person with dementia:

- diagnosis;
- monitoring;
- therapy;
- counselling

These responsibilities can be extended to other forms of psychiatric disorder and all require assessment for their successful implementation.

The primary purpose of assessment, as with all client groups, must be the description of a person's communication needs, strengths and weaknesses, and that person's ability to repair language and to use alternative strategies when communication via spoken language fails. This description will aid diagnosis (and differential diagnosis) and should help to answer the following questions:

- Is the person's communication normal for chronological age?
- If not, is the problem mild, moderate or severe?
- Does the difficulty seem very specific, e.g. limited to one modality or to one process?
- Is communication the only problem or the primary problem?
- Is communication with carers easy, difficult or impossible?
- Is the communication disorder caused by a psychiatric disorder or by a specific neurological condition?

Once a diagnosis of communication difficulty has been made, a choice of action(s) will be based on the assessment, on factors which relate to the person's medical diagnosis and other relevant factors. The therapist may decide that no intervention is indicated, but that the communication status of the EMI person will be monitored over time for change. This monitoring procedure will, by its nature, require that the initial method of assessment is repeated.

Should the therapist, on the other hand, decide that a period of therapy may be beneficial, the programme will be based on initial assessment results, as for any client group. Either communicative strengths or weaknesses illuminated through testing may form the focus of direct intervention. If an indirect approach to communication difficulties is more appropriate, then counselling and/or advice to the elderly mentally ill person and/or carers will be based on the initial assessment. Methods of alleviating word-finding difficulties, for example, could be discussed with home carers.

Another crucial aspect of communication assessment for this client group is as a contribution to multidisciplinary evaluation of all aspects of the EMI person's behaviour. Overall assessment here is seen as the precursor to care planning and long-term management decision-making. Assessment has to be a coordinated exercise. All parties involved should be included in pre-planning. Good planning will ensure that the most efficient approach to a comprehensive overview of the individual being assessed will be achieved. *Communicating Quality* (Royal College of Speech and Language Therapists, 1991) is a set of professional standards for the speech and language therapy profession. It advocates this principle of joint assessment and liaison with other members of the multidisciplinary team when working with elderly people. Assessment (with a written report of findings) may sometimes be the only direct contact between the speech and language therapist and the client although he/she may be involved also in management planning.

Other members of the care team (who assess mobility, cognitive function, mood and personality) may find that the communication assessment helps them in their administration and subsequent interpretation of assessment results. For example, the inability to understand long and complex instructions may be at least a partial explanation for non-compliance in the test procedures of other professionals.

Focus of assessment

For pragmatic reasons, speech and language therapy assessment is likely to focus on functional communication, i.e. on how the EMI person communicates in everyday situations. The first reason is a paucity of specific knowledge of how communication is affected in this client group. Few detailed descriptions exist of the effects on the structure or function of communication associated with mental illnesses in elderly people (Bayles and Kaszniak, 1987; Maxim and Bryan, 1994). Because of the lack of such literature, Griffiths (1991) suggests that the primary aim of assessment will be a 'detailed description of communicative behaviour'.

Second, broad-based methods of assessing functional communication can be easily borrowed from other communication-impaired client groups and applied to the EMI person.

Third, face-to-face formal assessment may not be possible (for reasons which are discussed in the next section). The therapist may therefore assess functional communication through the carer(s) or through observation, both techniques used routinely with other client groups.

Fourth, this approach offers a very appropriate method of assessing communication needs.

The challenge of formal assessment

Ideally speech and language therapists want to achieve formal assessment with elderly mentally ill clients, but this is not an easy or straightforward aim. Ripich (1991) describes the assessment of symptomatology in the dementia syndromes as a 'complex challenge'. Such a summary is equally true for the wider range of mental illnesses found in elderly people. The two main problems for successful and informative assessment of communication are the EMI person's two essential characteristics: advanced chronology and medical diagnosis!

Issues for communication assessment which are associated with normal ageing processes are discussed in Gravell (1990), Armstrong (1993a) and Maxim and Bryan (1994). These include sensory changes, lack of normative data and the effect of drugs on normal performance. Individual differences in this age-group should also be taken into account: scores in the pathological range may reflect typical performance for some normal elderly people (Walker, 1982; Armstrong and Greig, 1992). Lack of normative data may lead to the over-diagnosis of communication pathologies in a group of people whose 'normal' performance is not well documented. The specific effects of mental illness in elderly people (such as short-term memory loss, poor concentration and disorientation), added to the problems associated with normal ageing, have profound significance for testing.

Speech and language therapists have to be very conscious of the need to take account of the effects of normal ageing and of psychiatric disorder in their assessment. Modifications to test materials and test administration may be necessary, but these modifications will depend on the needs of the individual client. Possible modifications include:

- increased time allowed to reduce anxiety, to gain and maintain rapport;
- test administration over several short sessions;
- repeated explanation of the purpose and need for the assessment;
- allowance for longer processing time and response time;
- repetition of test instructions and stimuli;
- enlargement of picture and word test items.

The testing environment also requires careful consideration. A more valid and useful assessment is likely to be achieved when the client feels relaxed and comfortable. If possible the therapist should try to assess the client in familiar surroundings (e.g. at home) rather than in a new and unfamiliar place (e.g. the clinic office).

Formal assessments currently available are The Arizona Battery for Communication Disorders of Dementia (ABCD) (Bayles and Tomoeda, 1993) and the Functional Linguistic Communication Inventory (FLCI) (Bayles and Tomoeda, 1994). The ABCD was developed specifically to 'identify and quantify the linguistic communication deficits' associated with Alzheimer's Disease. It combines language and memory tests and consists of four screening measures and 14 subtests. The latter include:

- reading words and sentences;
- picture naming;
- describing an object;
- defining words;
- repeating anomalous sentences;
- answering yes–no comparative questions;
- following commands;
- mental status;
- retelling a story (immediate and delayed);
- recalling and recognising words;
- copying;
- drawing.

The battery is lengthy to administer, uses American vocabulary and examines structural rather than functional aspects of language. The scoring profile provides quantitative but not qualitative analysis and the battery contains little on writing ability. British norms and modifications to vocabulary, instructions and some picture stimuli are available. UK subjects score very similarily to the US standardisation sample (Armstrong et al., in press). Whilst some of the UK subjects commented on the cultural bias of some of the test stimuli, these did not produce notable effects on test performance and so alterations to test materials are not required for the test to be used with validity in the UK.

However, the very low mean scores of the moderate Alzheimer's disease subjects used in the UK validation study suggest that this test is too difficult for the type of dementia patient usually referred for speech and language assessment in the UK.

The FLCI aims to quantify the functional linguistic communication skills of individuals with moderate or severe dementia: The FLCI has ten parts and considers:

- greeting and naming;
- question answering;
- writing;

- sign comprehension, e.g. toilet, entry/exit and object-to-picture matching;
- word reading and comprehension;
- ability to reminisce;
- following commands, i.e. one and two part;
- pantomime;
- gesture;
- conversation.

Nine stimuli are repeated throughout the tasks, e.g. testees are asked to name, write down and understand the written form of the same words. People who are able to perform on ABCD will produce near ceiling scores on the FLCI. The authors suggest that test results on FCLI can be used to determine functional communication abilities, to decide about patient management and to plan functional maintenance programmes. They can also be used to predict 'communicative functions that will be vulnerable as the disease progresses' and as a basis for counselling professional and personal caregivers.

Assessment validity

There are many potential pitfalls in the use of formal assessment with the elderly mentally ill person. The first concerns validity, i.e. does the assessment measure what it purports to measure? Factors which are said to influence validity include:

- unclear instructions;
- inappropriate difficulty levels;
- poorly constructed or inappropriate test items;
- too few items;
- improper order of items (Hatch and Farhady, 1982).

Only two formal assessment batteries for one section of this client group exist (as described in the preceding section). The speech and language therapist may therefore need to use assessments which have been designed for other client groups such as functional communication profiles designed for aphasic clients. However, we must seriously question the validity of the use of assessments designed for and standardised on other ages and client groups. Non-standard test administration, such as: enlarging stimuli to compensate for visual difficulties; repeating instructions for clients with hearing difficulties; not recording response times when tests require this, invalidate standardised results but these modifications may be necessary if the speech and language therapist is to extract useful information from the assessment.

Assessment reliability

The second potential problem concerns reliability. The known daily variation in the abilities of, for example, the depressed elderly person or the elderly person with dementia will have implications for the administration of a formal assessment which cannot be completed at one sitting. This variation will also have implications for the building (and rebuilding) of rapport, the test–retest situation and for inter-tester reliability, should the person be tested by another therapist for purposes of monitoring or review. Whilst test length is an important variable in reliability (Hatch and Farhady, 1982), Sullivan (1991) asks how often formal assessments are administered in full to elderly clients.

Assessment practicality

Allied to validity and reliability, practicality must be considered in the assessment of the elderly mentally ill person. Most published test batteries which aim to assess speech and language in adults are long and examine structural aspects of language such as the ability to generate a grammatically correct sentence rather than language content or language use.

Ability and motivation to comply with the testing procedure is required for results to be valid and for them to provide meaningful information to the therapist. Because of confusion, poor attention and other factors resulting from psychiatric disorder in elderly people, compliance may be difficult, if not impossible to achieve. Another practical issue relates to resources: is there a therapist available at the optimum time of day for the person who is to be tested? This optimum time will be influenced by medication and aspects as mundane as travel arrangements should the client attend a day care facility. Finally, test outcomes can be influenced by the therapist's knowledge of the assessment procedure, of normal effects of ageing on communication and of the effects of mental illness on communication in older age as well as his or her level of familiarity with the client group.

In summary, at present none of the formal assessment batteries available to the speech and language therapist is adequate for use with this client group. Formal assessment therefore may not be the method of first choice for speech and language therapy assessment of the elderly person with mental illness. With increased knowledge and experience within the profession, this situation may change to some extent in the future. The profession's position paper on *Speech and Language Therapy and the Elderly with Dementia* (RCSLT, 1993) suggests that, in the absence of 'a conceptually strong, and clinically useful evaluation', research should 'continue to emphasise refining descriptive and/or differential diagnostic evaluations' (p.7). This suggestion applies equally to the wider client group of elderly people with mental illness.

However, the difficulties for testing which are associated with the effects of normal ageing and of mental illness will remain. What, then, should be the form of speech, language and communication assessment offered to the elderly mentally ill person?

Form of assessment

Communicating Quality (RCSLT, 1991) offers advice on procedures for the assessment of communication in elderly people and people with dementia. The battery of possible assessment types includes:

- observation;
- discussion with significant others;
- screening;
- informal assessment;
- formal assessment.

Broader aspects which should be considered are motivation for communication, insight and communicative environment.

RCSLT's advice can be broadened to the present client group. The first part of the assessment will be case-history taking. At this early stage, the therapist will be interested in gathering information about the client's medical/psychiatric history, including: diagnosis; client knowledge of diagnosis; most recent medical assessment; drug regime; current assessment by other members of the multidisciplinary team, as well as personally gathering information specifically about communication.

It may be possible for the speech and language therapist to acquire accurate information from the person who has been referred for assessment. However, often therapists will have to rely on carers for biographical information and for information which relates to the nature of the communication problems and the effect they are having on everyday life.

Bayles and Kaszniak (1987) propose a set of criteria as characteristics for a good test of communication in dementia:

- it assesses the integrity of the contents and processes of semantic memory;
- it analyses communication beyond the sentence level;
- ecologically valid test paradigms are adopted;
- it tests communication processes that are non-automatic;
- generative and creative communication abilities should be assessed.

Heritage and Farrow (1994) describe the forms of assessment which are currently used in the field. These comprise selected sections or subtests of formal assessments normally used with people who have language deficits following neurological damage, e.g. The Boston Diagnostic Aphasia Examination (Goodglass and Kaplan, 1983), Test for Reception of Grammar (Bishop, 1983) and Psycholinguistic Assessments of Language Processing in Aphasia (Kay, Lesser and Coltheart, 1992), observational checklists and carer questionnaires. They note that responses (especially the types of errors made) were more informative than the actual test scores.

Ideally, then, the assessment of the elderly mentally ill person will take place over a period of time, so that rapport can be built up with the person who has been referred for assessment and with his or her carers. A multi-contact assessment also ensures that a comprehensive view can be established. The speech and language therapist will not carry out the assessment in the isolation of the clinic office, but will view the elderly mentally ill person's communication in its normal context. Similarly, the assessment should involve others, so that a clear and reliable picture can be built up of how the person communicates in everyday settings.

The form of assessment, whether it is direct or indirect, which is selected for a particular client will depend on the individual person and his or her circumstances. The use of formal assessments may be problematic, as discussed earlier. At present, it is possible that therapists will use indirect assessment as their primary method of choice. However, both observations made by the speech and language therapist and carer responses from checklists and questionnaires are subjective. Therapists can observe:

- level of motivation to communicate;
- attention and concentration;
- social uses of language;
- possible sensory impairments;
- degree of appropriateness of content of spoken language;
- form of spoken language (Seaman, 1990).

The structuring of questions can help to organise carers' observations but can also distort possible responses.

Finally in considering the form of assessment, the reality of the clinical context cannot be ignored. It is likely that the speech and language therapist will see elderly clients with psychiatric disorder among a more general caseload (RCSLT, 1993). Assessment of this client group will therefore be influenced by:

- the limited availability of therapist time;
- the availability of tests and other resources;
- the therapist's knowledge and interest;
- the availability of more specialised colleagues from whom to receive help and support.

At present, an eclectic approach to assessment of communication in elderly mentally infirm people is indicated. The speech and language therapist is likely to use a combination of different forms of assessment (including observation, formal and informal assessment, checklists and carer questionnaires) to provide an adequate view of an individual's communicative abilities, disabilities and needs. Seaman (1990) considers that 'for most clinical purposes, a combination of observational techniques and informal language assessments is both appropriate and adequate' (p.8). The following sections review some methods of assessment which have been reported in the literature. They consider formal assessment leading to differential diagnosis, direct and indirect methods of describing communication abilities.

Differential diagnostic assessment

The speech and language therapist, when working with elderly people who may have mental illness, is faced with several possible questions of differential diagnosis. Correct diagnosis is essential for appropriate medical, paramedical and social management. Although there are limits on the formal assessments available, speech and language therapists now have adequate information and a range of clinical resources available to play a meaningful role in this early part of the therapeutic process.

Differentiating normal ageing from dementia

The differentiation of normal ageing from mild forms of dementia (especially Alzheimer's disease) is particularly difficult. Bayles and her colleagues have been especially interested in this problem for some years (Bayles and Boone, 1982; Bayles et al., 1989). Bayles et al. (1989) employed an earlier form of The Arizona Battery for Communication Disorders of Dementia (Bayles and Tomoeda, 1993) to successfully distinguish normal elderly subjects from people with mild Alzheimer's disease on all 14 of their measures. The tests whose scores best discriminated between the groups were (in order):

- delayed story recall;
- mental status task;
- pantomime expression;
- Peabody Picture Vocabulary Test (Dunn, 1959).

When asked to retell a short story after a delay of 60–75 minutes, the subjects with mild Alzheimer's disease scored a mean of less than 1, from a possible total of 25, compared with the normal elderly group's score of 18.9.

Many studies have employed picture naming as a central task in attempts to distinguish normal elderly people from those with mild dementia. A very early paper (Barker and Lawson, 1968) showed that people with dementia took significantly longer to name pictures than normal subjects, especially for low-frequency words. Word fluency (naming words within a category) is sensitive to early dementia (Hart, Smith and Swash 1988; Bandera et al., 1991) as is spelling (Rapcsak et al., 1989).

Stevens et al. (1992) report the discriminative effectiveness of several tests of language which were employed as part of a battery of assessments in their memory clinic. They found word fluency, using the category of animals, was not helpful in their differential diagnosis. In that study overall, the Boston Naming Test (Kaplan, Goodglass and Weintraub, 1983) proved more discriminative at detecting cognitive deterioration than either the 'Mini-mental status examination' (Folstein, Folstein and McHugh, 1975) or word fluency (including production of words beginning with the letter 's').

In the 'Set test' (Isaacs and Akhtar, 1972; Isaacs and Kennie, 1973), participants are asked to name ten colours, animals, fruits and towns. The authors claim that this is a useful test in discriminating normal ageing from dementia that is easy to administer. However, in Armstrong's (1993b) pilot study three of the nine subjects with dementia produced scores which exceeded the suggested cut-off score of 25 (out of a possible score of 40).

Armstrong (1993b) concludes that on tests of picture naming, reading aloud and writing single items to dictation, subjects with probable Alzheimer's disease produced an error profile which greatly resembled in quality that of the normal elderly control subjects. However, on tests which require no access to word meaning (reading aloud and repetition) these groups did not produce significantly different scores. As in Bayles et al. (1989) very poor scores on delayed story recall characterised the subjects with dementia as did lack of success in recognising from a list words that they had just read aloud. On this basis, in order to identify early dementia, clinicians should employ tests which require active lexical search (e.g. picture naming and word fluency), rather than those which have little cognitive effort (e.g. word repetition and reading aloud) as well as tests of verbal memory (e.g. delayed story recall and verbal recognition memory).

Differentiating aphasia from dementia

Another question of differential diagnosis which is of clinical interest to the speech and language therapist is that of distinguishing fluent aphasia from the language of early Alzheimer's disease. These two disorders can mimic each other in severity of breakdown when tested using published formal assessments for aphasia.

Direct comparisons are difficult because the literature reveals that group studies aimed at distinguishing these two patient groups have used different materials (new tests, aphasia test(s) and a modified aphasia test) and different sets of subject groups (Alzheimer's disease and other unidentified types of dementia, aphasia of various types, right-hemisphere brain-damaged adults and normal controls of varying ages, community or institution-based). Bayles and Kaszniak (1987) report several such studies. Others include Thompson (1983); Murray et al. (1984); Bayles et al. (1989); Fromm and Holland (1989); Horner et al. (1992); and Stevens (1992).

Reviewing group studies

The most original of the test batteries in these studies was also the shortest (Stevens, 1992). Whilst test brevity is an attractive characteristic in a test for use with elderly mentally infirm people, some very brief tests (Kendrick, Gibson and Moyes, 1979; Weeks, 1988) have been criticised on the grounds that little information can be gained in five to ten minutes. Long tests often require assessment to be completed over several sessions, a procedure which has inherent problems in terms of likely performance variability, as noted earlier. Whilst very long tests or a combination of tests can provide a large amount of information, a balance is required so that sufficient and correct information is gathered. In the set of studies reviewed here, length of test was not always associated with accuracy of discrimination.

It has already been argued that tests designed to assess aphasia are not appropriate as assessments of other communication disorders. Stevens (1992) presented a battery specifically designed for differential diagnosis, whilst Thompson (1983) and Bayles et al. (1989) used batteries designed to assess communication function in dementia. Other studies have employed aphasia batteries.

Stevens (1992) used small groups of nine elderly subjects with Alzheimer's disease and eight moderately dysphasic elderly subjects. The dysphasic subjects were linguistically selected via their scores on responsive and confrontation naming sections of the Boston Diagnostic Aphasia Examination (Goodglass and Kaplan, 1983). A mix of community- based and institutionalised people were tested. All but one of the subjects were correctly classified by Stevens' subjective graded scoring system using full test and retest scores, in which dysphasic-type errors were rated positively (e.g. literal paraphasia scored +7) and Alzheimer's disease-type errors negatively (e.g. visual misperceptions scored -4). All subjects, however, produced both dysphasic-type and Alzheimer's-type errors: some 18.2% of errors were not produced by the expected group. Two tests (description of a drawn action and verbal description of object use) were found by regression analysis to be discriminative. Of particular note is that her battery does not include any test of episodic memory, which is known to distinguish the groups. One difficulty with the results is that they appear to be based on groups with different degrees of communication impairment. Another problem is the absence of a normal elderly base-line group.

Bayles et al. (1989) used large groups of healthy elderly, mild and moderate Alzheimer's disease, non-fluent and fluent aphasic subjects (130 subjects in total). Of particular interest here was the finding that three tests proved effective in distinguishing normal elderly, fluent aphasic, mild and moderate Alzheimer's disease subjects by their mean scores:

- story-retelling (immediate and delayed);
- delayed verbal recognition memory;
- sentence disambiguation.

Several more of the test performances showed significant differences between fluent aphasic and mild Alzheimer's disease groups:

- delayed spatial recognition memory;
- mental status;
- pantomime expression;
- drawing.

However, discriminant function analyses were not undertaken to classify aphasic and dementia subjects as some of the aphasic subjects did not complete all the tasks.

Thompson's (1983) battery consisted of 31 subtests. Performances distinguished among different groups of psychiatric and neurological patients on the basis of test scores. Error analyses were not extensively used. Data presented were cross-sectional and longitudinal in nature, with emphasis on younger subjects with dementia. This long and unpublished battery was 86.7% accurate in classifying subjects with aphasia and dementia.

Horner et al. (1992) attempted to differentiate subjects with Alzheimer's disease, left hemisphere and right hemisphere stroke and neurologically normal adults using the Western Aphasia Battery (WAB) (Kertesz, 1982). Discriminant analysis produced correct classification for 29 of 40 (72.5%) subjects, including 19 of the 30 patient-group subjects (63%). Of the groups, Alzheimer's disease subjects were the second least well classified. Not surprisingly, all Alzheimer's disease subjects demonstrated 'anomic aphasia' using WAB's taxonomy. These results were slightly better than those achieved in an earlier study (Horner, 1985), but still one-third of the patients were misclassified.

Fromm and Holland (1989) gave the Communicative Abilities in Daily

Living (CADL) (Holland, 1980) to groups of normal elderly, mild and moderate Alzheimer's disease, depressed and Wernicke's aphasic subjects. Although moderate Alzheimer's disease and Wernicke's subjects were not distinguished by mean score, error types showed group differences. The dementia subjects' responses were irrelevant, vague or incomplete, whereas the aphasic subjects produced perseverations, paraphasic substitutions, jargon and had auditory comprehension problems. This study serves to show that group differences can be masked when test scores alone are considered and elucidated when error distributions are observed.

Murray et al. (1984) used a combination of scores on a formal and functional test to successfully classify their dementia and aphasia subjects, by means of discriminant function analysis. They employed the CADL and The Porch Index of Communicative Ability (PICA) (Porch, 1971). The dementia subjects had multi-infarct senile dementia and were mainly resident in nursing homes. Type or severity of aphasia are not documented as selection criteria. PICA results showed superiority of score by the dementia group, whilst the aphasic group performed significantly better on CADL. This finding was said to reflect a basic difference between the groups, i.e. people with aphasia communicate better than they speak, whereas people with dementia speak better than they communicate. Additionally, it was reported that the dementia group had difficulty with the simulated nature of CADL which is designed to assess communication using role-play situations.

One of Armstrong's (1993b) main aims was to develop a clinically useful screening test battery which would distinguish fluent aphasia from the language associated with probable Alzheimer's disease (and both from the language of normal ageing) using measures of language expression and verbal memory. Tests were drawn from single-word processing tasks and modified versions of the three tests (delayed story retelling, delayed verbal recognition memory, and sentence disambiguation) which discriminated between the three groups in Bayles et al. (1989). Methodology, especially selection criteria, was explicitly developed from the literature reviewed here.

A pilot study provided useful indication of the discriminating power of 12 language and memory tests and resulted in the reduction of the battery to the following set:

- *Mini-Mental Status Examination (MMSE)* (Folstein et al., 1975): orientation, language, registration/recall and attention/calculation. Scores out of 30. A score of less than 20 indicates pathological performance.
- *Picture Naming*: 50 black-and-white line drawings are presented to be named to confrontation. Semantic and phonemic cues are provided as in the administration of The Boston Naming Test (Kaplan

et al., 1983). Testing is discontinued after five successive failures to name, even after the provision of cues.

- *Reading Aloud*: 30 words and five non-word letter strings are presented individually to be read aloud.
- *Verbal Recognition Memory*: subjects are presented with a list of 20 words and asked to indicate which ones they have just read. The list contains five real word targets, each with semantic, phonetic and unrelated distractors.
- *Writing Single Items*: 12 words and three non-word letter strings are dictated individually, stimuli given alone and (for the real words) in context.
- *Delayed Story Recall*: subjects are asked to recall a story heard after the picture naming test and before the reading aloud test.

The battery was given to 25 normal elderly people and groups of 20 people with anomic aphasia or probable early Alzheimer's disease. A subset of the subjects were given the battery twice in order to examine longitudinal patterns. A discriminant function analysis which used a synthesis of test scores and error behaviour best distinguished the aphasic and dementia groups.

No significant relationship was found between the distributions of error types produced by the patient groups although they shared mainly the same types of errors. The distinction was very clear in terms of the numbers of phonemic paraphasic errors and neologisms produced where only aphasic subjects produced such sound errors. Although phonemic errors are said to occur in Alzheimer's disease (Bayles and Kaszniak, 1987), these only become apparent later in the disease process, when the present differential diagnostic question would not be raised (i.e. when more general behaviour differences would easily distinguish the groups). A positive error type discriminator for the dementia group was at the picture-recognition stage of picture naming. Dementia subjects did not recognise the stimulus and made errors of visual perception significantly more often than anomic subjects (but in the same proportion as the normal group).

Similar patterns of error behaviour were found on reading aloud. More than half of the errors made by the anomic group were phonological or suprasegmental compared with less than 10% for the dementia group. So for the anomic group, retrieval of the phonological form was difficult: although the target was correctly identified and its name recognisable, it was distorted, e.g. stress placed on the first syllable of 'cigar' rather than on the second. For the anomic group, there was no corresponding increase in the number of error types as the number of reading errors increased. On the other hand, for the dementia group, there was a significant relationship demonstrated so that the dementia subject who made more errors tended also to produce more error types.

The dementia subjects consistently showed that their difficulty with the reading aloud task lay in reading aloud non-word letter strings (novel stimuli). On writing single items to dictation, the largest discrepancy in frequency of error types made by the patient groups lay in the 'no response' category. The anomic subjects were aware of their spelling problems and tended to be unwilling to attempt to spell words which they recognised as very difficult. The dementia group rarely displayed this behaviour.

Error analysis was also illuminating for the verbal recognition memory test, in which subjects are asked to select from a list of words those which they recognise as stimuli in the immediately preceding reading aloud test. Overall the dementia subjects selected most distractors, i.e. they showed most evidence of inaccurate recall of words just read. Some reported that they selected randomly among the words to carry out the task as requested as they could not remember any of the words they had just read. Others simply admitted they could not remember any of the previous stimuli. The remainder appeared to attempt the task and selected both correct and incorrect words.

Apart from general behaviour, the choice of distractor reponses also provides insightful information. Dementia subjects consistently selected more phonetic and unrelated distractors and fewer semantic distractors than the anomic group, i.e. a more even distribution of distractor types. This more random selection, along with their mean score and range on this test, are indicative of the known short-term memory deficit associated with Alzheimer's disease. The anomic group generally demonstrated more intact verbal recognition memory, through the selection primarily of semantic distractors, which indicates degraded representations of target responses.

Performance on some of the sections of MMSE (Folstein et al., 1975) distinguished the groups. The anomic subjects scored significantly better on orientation and registration/recall than did the dementia subjects (Armstrong, 1994).

Other aspects of performance, such as cueing responsiveness in picture naming, word type and stimulus length effects and error consistency added to the strength of the group distinctions.

The dementia subjects benefited equally from semantic and phonemic cues, whereas anomic subjects benefited more from phonemic cues. The anomic response patterns suggest that people with anomic aphasia recognise the pictures and access the required semantic information. Their poor success rate following semantic cue, together with accompanying behaviour (e.g. 'yes, I know that'), can be taken to indicate that the recognition function of the cue was complete. Their difficulty lies in accessing the word form itself. The equal success of the two cueing strategies for the dementia group indicates a more general inefficiency:

sometimes the problem lies in identifying the particular picture and sometimes in finding its name.

Reaction to different word types in the reading aloud test also distinguished the patient groups. Words such as 'cigar', which does not rhyme with any other word, proved most difficult for the anomic group to read aloud. The dementia group did not show this pattern. Anomic subjects' errors were on low-frequency rather than high-frequency words.

Length of words influenced anomic group performance on all three single word processing tasks but not at all for the dementia group. This disparity can be explained by the dementia group's intactness of phonological processing.

On all three tests, the anomic group showed some error consistency over time on longer, and therefore more difficult, stimuli. On the other hand, the dementia group produced very low degrees of error consistency similar to the normal group.

In summary, the main areas of difference between anomic aphasia and the language associated with early Alzheimer's disease lay in:

- distribution of error types;
- cueing responsiveness;
- awareness of difficulty;
- sensitivity to word length;
- sensitivity to word type.

The most successful discriminant analysis (which produced 100% correct classification) included both test scores and error data. Thus, together the two types of data proved more discriminating than one alone (although separately both types yielded very accurate classifications).

Armstrong (1993b) therefore showed that this battery of tests can provide an objective differential diagnosis, but so far it has only been used with people whose medical diagnosis is certain. Field trials are now in progress to ensure that it can successfully diagnose people who are referred to the speech and language therapist for differential diagnosis. The battery, although a formal assessment, was developed specifically for this one purpose. Normal elderly people are able to achieve almost ceiling scores thereby ensuring that error responses can be more certainly assigned to pathology. Following differential diagnosis, further assessment is necessary so that the communication difficulties can be more fully explored and described in an appropriate manner for therapy planning.

Differentiating depression and dementia

A third differential diagnostic set of questions concerns depression and dementia. Several writers have shown that it is possible to distinguish these groups using measures of language. Weeks's (1988) Anomalous Sentences Repetition Test (ASRT), for example, was designed to diagnose dementia or depression in people over 55 years. Its stimuli consist of six test sentences, all of which are morphologically intact but semantically abnormal with the final two also being syntactically abnormal. There are four parallel forms of the test (to allow for repeated testing), which is able to be used by a wide range of professionals. The author suggests that a concurrent mental status assessment (such as a depression scale) should be used with the test. The standardisation and validation data are impressive and demonstrate the test's possible use with a range of patient groups. On this test, people with dementia will have difficulty, whilst those with depression will not.

Fromm and Holland (1989) found that although their depressed subjects' functional communication was not normal for their age, it was superior to that of their subjects with mild Alzheimer's disease. Qualitatively, the depressed subjects produced incomplete utterances, whilst the dementia subjects' style was more irrelevant, vague and rambling. Maxim (1991) assessed and compared the performance of groups of normal elderly people and elderly people with mild dementia, depression or fluent aphasia on a picture description task. Several useful differentiating features were found among measures of the well-formedness of language produced, production errors and language-monitoring abilities. The aphasic subjects produced more sentences than the subjects with dementia and made more repairs. The dementia subjects abandoned more utterances than the depressed subjects and were the only group to make value judgements. They also produced more linguistic errors than did the depressed group. The depressed subjects were not distinguished from the normal subjects on any measure. Similarily, in Stevens et al. (1992), depressed patients showed little evidence of language deficits on the naming tests used.

Describing communication abilities

Complementary to formal procedures such as the ABCD and FLCI, Ripich (1991) suggests that a complete description of communication impairments in Alzheimer's disease requires assessment of 'a range of pragmatic and discourse features' as well as of linguistic aspects (phonology, syntax and semantics). She describes the Discourse Abilities Profile (DAP) (Terrell and Ripich, 1989) as a quick method of structuring observations of 'naturally occurring interactions' between patients and clinicians or carers. Three types of discourse are considered:

* narrative (e.g. relating a past event);
* procedural (e.g. describing a simple task);
* spontaneous conversation initiated by the tester.

The fourth part of the profile rates coherence, paralinguistic and non-linguistic behaviour (such as use of intonation and eye contact) as observed in all three discourse situations. Scoring is based on rating for presence/absence of certain features in the three discourse types and for the quality of the behaviours described in the fourth section. Whilst this method can be used solely to describe discourse abilities in an elderly person with mental illness, Ripich (1991) also compares results gained on DAP by normal elderly people and people with Alzheimer's disease. This method of assessment is much less confrontational than traditional formal assessments. In fact it could be used as an indirect method where the clinician observes communication with a carer without intervening. Discourse analysis, as a method of assessment, is still relatively new in speech and language therapy, but presents a useful way of examining communication skills, especially in people who are unable to comply with test situations.

Indirect assessment

Indirect assessment through interaction profiles, communication check-list and carer questionnaires can be used as a basis for planning remedi-ation. Whilst direct therapy may not be indicated for many elderly people who have communication difficulties as a result of mental illness, the speech and language therapist has a useful role in advising carers on how to maximise and maintain communication in face-to-face conversa-tion and, more generally, on how to make the most of the communica-tive environment. The Revised Edinburgh Functional Communication Profile (Wirz et al., 1990) was designed specifically for elderly communi-cation-impaired people for whom formal assessment was not appropri-ate and therefore is ideally suited for the purpose of profiling functional communication in elderly people with mental illness.

Carer questionnaires

Many therapists will already have their own personally constructed or adapted carer questionnaire for use with other client groups. The Communication Assessment Profile for Adults with a Mental Handicap (CASP) (van der Gaag, 1988), for example, has three parts, one of which is a carer questionnaire. This questionnaire has been designed for a different client group, and would require modification for use with any other. Essentially, these questionnaires should vary according to the problems known to occur with different communication pathologies and to the age of the client group.

Alongside the project mentioned above which collected British data for the ABCD (Armstrong et al., in press), a comparison between test result and carer perception of the communication problems was attempted (Armstrong and Borthwick, submitted). Some examples (from one subject) of answers received from a home carer and from day care staff which did and did not relate to test results are provided in Figure 9.1. These preliminary data show that test result and carer perception do not always equate and that the ABCD is not designed to elicit important communicative behaviours, such as repetitive questioning.

Powell, Hale and Bayer (1995) used a carer questionnaire to investigate the prevalence of 32 communication symptoms as perceived by

Subject	Test and score	Carer perception
ER	Reading comprehension single words 8/8 sentences 0/7	Local paper 'delivered – whether it is read, we doubt it. No magazines, books etc'. (home carer)
		'Does read newspaper in the day hospital.' (day care staff)
	Following commands 7/9 (failed three-part commands)	'She understands but is incapable of retaining given answer.' (home carer)
		ER 'does have have difficulty in understanding some information and does look vague on occasion.' (day care staff)
	N/A	'repeats question...she latches on to conversational questions and keeps repeating them.' (home carer)
		'tends to...confabulation and is repetitive.' (day care staff)

Figure 9.1: Comparison between test results and carer perception

carers of elderly dementia patients and healthy elderly subjects. Areas which most clearly distinguished the groups were:

- asking the same question a number of times;
- difficulty following conversation in a group;
- trouble keeping a conversation going;
- struggling to think of the names of people and places.

They did not, however, attempt to measure whether these perceptions were accurate.

Both types of information are considered important. They are complementary and together they provide a more rounded view of the communication skills and abilities of individual clients. Assessment by a speech and language therapist may be more objective than carers' perceptions. However, carer knowledge is based on possibly many years of communicative experience with a person, whilst professional assessment is based on theoretical and clinical knowledge of a client group and interaction with an individual for a relatively short time.

Interaction profiling

Tanner and Daniels (1990) used an observational checklist to assess whether carers were using specific strategies for communication, whether these were effective and which were counter-productive. They visited eight carers and their relatives with dementia to build up a picture of the carers' communication with their relative. Both verbal and non-verbal behaviours were observed (e.g. redundancy and forced alternatives; touching and gesture) and the communicative function of the particular behaviour was noted (e.g. getting attention, responding). Their results showed that carers were often using effective strategies, but not always intentionally. Therefore a programme of early education was indicated to 'increase their awareness of how they themselves communicate generally, and thence to monitor how they communicate with their relative'.

Communicative environment

Communicative environment is a term made popular by Lubinski (e.g. Lubinski, 1981, 1991; Lubinski, Morrison and Rigrodsky, 1981). Armstrong and Woodgates (in press) developed a measure of social communicative environment and applied it to the comparison of two day care facilities for people with psychogeriatric problems. The methodology was based on Adelson et al. (1982) with an emphasis specifically on interactional behaviours. A checklist method of data collection was employed (see Figure 9.2) to collect and organise sampled observations of conversations occurring throughout the day. The categories of interest included the communicative partners, whether the conversation occurred spontaneously or as a result of a planned activity, conversational topic, how long the interaction lasted and, by subtraction, periods of silence.

The results demonstrated the relationship between:

- time of day and the amount of conversation occurring;
- patterns of communicative partners (staff–staff, patient–staff, staff–patient and patient–patient);
- the range of topics discussed and the extent to which conversations were spontaneous or designed (e.g. by quizzes).

More qualitative observations were also made, based on Gravell's (1988) list of opportunities and barriers to communication, which itself is based on Lubinski (1981). Clear quantitative differences were apparent between the two settings. In one location most conversation occurred early in the day and in the other at lunchtime. In one location most of the interaction occurred between staff and clients whereas in the other most interaction was between staff. Periods of silence also distinguished the settings (41.25% compared with 8.2% of total time observed). Health-related issues (health, smoking and death) were discussed more often in one setting whereas there was more conversation about individuals' interests and past lives in the other. Furthermore, analysis of individual environments highlighted areas of good practice (e.g. use of themed-activities) and areas of concern (e.g. amount of silence).

Whilst this method of observational assessment is perhaps lengthy, it can provide very useful information both for groups of EMI people and for the individual, where observation would focus on one person rather than be sampled for a group as in the study described. It could be used in institutional as well as home settings and would form a sound basis for staff training. Monitoring assessment of communicative environment could then be implemented through the repeated use of the checklist.

Summary

Speech and language therapy assessment of elderly people with mental illness is as yet an imprecise procedure. The profession is still learning about the associated communication impairments and developing methods of assessment, which either directly or indirectly examine aspects of language in this new client group. The future holds promise as more

TIME	COMMUNICATION PARTNERS (Patients/staff/visitors)	SPONTANEOUS/ PLANNED ACTIVITY	TOPIC OF CONVERSATION	LENGTH OF INTERACTION	SILENT PERIODS

Figure 9.2. Checklist of verbal interactional behaviours.

clinicians become interested and more posts are funded in this ever-increasing area of the communicatively impaired population and as more work is completed in the development of conceptually strong tests and a range of other less traditional methods of assessment.

Chapter 10:
Multi-Infarct Dementia –
A Special Case for
Treatment?

KATE SWINBURN AND JANE MAXIM

Introduction

Why is multi-infarct dementia, a special case? Because it is not necessarily progressive, there may be improvement of function during the course of the disease, certain forms of multi-infarct dementia may respond to medical intervention and, as will be described in this chapter, specific language impairment may respond to remediation.

Multi-infarct dementia (MID), sometimes called vascular dementia, is caused by multiple small infarcts which leave lacunae (small holes) in the white matter of the brain and the brain stem in about 70% of cases, and is often associated with hypertension. The infarcts are largely from the heart and atheromatous plaques in blood vessels outside the cerebrovascular system. There may also be larger cortical infarcts in about 20% of cases and a mixture of cortical and subcortical lesions in the remaining 30% (see Brun, 1994 for a review of pathological findings). As with Alzheimer's disease, there is considerable debate as to whether the variation in symptoms and disease progression in MID represents heterogeneity within a single disorder or a number of separate syndromes.

A major issue for health-care professionals is the differential diagnosis of vascular dementia from multiple strokes which is not necessarily easy at a clinical level. Where the medical diagnosis is made on clinical features alone and without neuro-imaging information, misdiagnosis can occur. Where a major aspect of the presenting clinical features is aphasia, tests of cognitive function which are verbally mediated will show deficits which do not reflect cognitive damage but are due to specific language impairment.

The first part of this chapter describes an intervention programme for a man with a diagnosis of multi-infarct dementia who showed both cognitive and linguistic deficits but nevertheless responded to treatment of his language deficits only. In the second part of the chapter, the heterogeneity of clinical features and specific clinical syndromes within the vascular dementias are described. Recent research, for example, has begun to divide the vascular dementias into those with cortical versus subcortical features. Careful search through the literature shows a paucity of clinical descriptions, both for groups and single case studies of the speech, language, communication and cognitive ability in multi-infarct dementia. There is a methodological difficulty because the pathology of the disorders or group of disorders which cause this dementia produces more variation in symptomatology than, for example, Alzheimer's disease.

Making irrelevance relevant: treating a client with multi-infarct dementia

This therapy study is of a client (KM) who had a fluent aphasia with evidence of associated cognitive deficits. He had been described by a number of therapists and doctors as having multi-infarct dementia.

KM was treated using two different therapy regimes: the first was semantically based whilst the second focused on increasing the relevance of his verbal output. It is the latter stage of 'relevance therapy' which will be the focus of this study and which, it is hoped, will convincingly demonstrate the efficacy of treatment with a client who has multi-infarct dementia and whose output was poorly controlled and fluent. There will also be consideration of how to analyse discourse from picture description in a quick and repeatable way.

KM was 77-years-old at the beginning of treatment, married with no children. He had previously been a foreign exchange bank manager in the City in London. He enjoyed gardening, reading the *Daily Telegraph* and travelling within Britain. He sustained two strokes within a three-month period. CT scanning revealed a left thalamic infarct and multiple small cortical lesions.

Language presentation

Detailed cognitive neuropsychological testing was carried out which showed that KM presented with an atypical fluent dysphasia. Table 10.1 shows KM's performance on various tests based on a cognitive neuropsychology framework. He had preserved auditory and visual analysis: lexical decision tests were 90% or above in both modalities. His semantic system was impaired: auditory modality single-picture recognition Biber 'is it a...?' was at 78%, auditory modality Pyramids and Palm Trees (Howard and Patterson, 1992) at 57%, low imageability synonym judgement 'do safety and security mean the same?' at 68%.

There was evidence that access to the output lexicons may have been impaired. On a syllable judgement task, when the therapist said the word, KM was near perfect, showing that he understood the task.

However, when making a judgement on the number of syllables for himself from a picture, his performance reduced to 28% correct, suggesting he was not able to access the output phonology unaided. Repetition was preserved at non-word, word and sentence level (95% for words and non-words, 103/107 for short phrases). It should be noted that his written route in all areas was superior to his auditory route.

He therefore had an atypical fluent aphasia in that repetition was preserved and his acoustic analysis was intact. On a more functional level, however, his output was typically fluent. There was a press of speech, he made many literal and verbal paraphasias, there would be frequent pauses, reiterations and backtracking as he spoke. The cognitive neuropsychological tests give a feel for KM's linguistic deficit. However, to exemplify the treatment effects, reference will be made to more general linguistic parameters such as confrontation naming, relevance of verbal output and summed scores from the Boston Diagnostic Aphasia Examination (BDAE).

In addition to his linguistic deficits, the following cognitive and perceptual difficulties were present:

- right homonymous upper quadrant hemianopia;
- visual inattention to the right;
- short-term memory problems;
- constructional and visuo-spatial difficulties;
- personality changes.

KM had short-term (working) memory problems. He forgot events and people. He was unable to remember what had happened that day and he mistook staff for family friends and relations. He had constructional and visuo-spatial problems, getting lost repeatedly on the ward. He had difficulty dressing and made many visual misperceptions on object and picture comprehension. He also demonstrated personality changes. His wife reported he was uncharacteristically lethargic, unmotivated and short-tempered.

Table 10.1: Cognitive neuropsychological assessment

Lexical decision	Spoken	19/20	(95%)
	Written	18/20	(90%)
Biber (Is it a...?)	Spoken	25/32	(78%)
Pyramids and Palm Trees	Spoken	30/52	(52%)
Synonym Judgement (low imageability)	Spoken	26/38	(68%)
Syllable Judgement	Therapist spoken	37/40	(93%)
	Pictures	6/20	(28%)
Word/Non-word Repetition		76/80	(95%)
Phrase Repetition		103/105	(98%)

Despite his cognitive and linguistic problems, it was felt that KM might benefit from therapy. As a preliminary test of learning ability, KM was given information about the therapist's family and friends and tested each week on his recall of this information. He was able to recall a significant amount of this information, up to 85% from week to week. Therefore, though he had demonstrable memory problems, he was registering and storing information at some level and 'learning' could therefore be demonstrated. His linguistic deficit was the deficit that he, his wife and the therapist all identified as being the most intrusive feature of his communication problem, rather than the extra-linguistic cognitive features. He was therefore taken on for therapy on a very strict test–treat–retest basis.

Stage 1 treatment – semantic therapy

Treatment started with work on single-word semantics. The test results suggested that reduced semantic specification via the auditory route was leading to poor auditory comprehension and a concomitant anomia. The hypothesis for treatment was that enriching the specificity of the semantic knowledge that KM had available to him via the auditory route would lead to improved auditory comprehension at the single-word level and possible corresponding improvement in his spoken naming.

Therapy was very structured and repetitive, using black-and-white line drawings taken from Snodgrass and Vanderwart (1980). KM was asked 'do you recognise the pictures?' He made visual perceptual errors and this initial part of the activity was an attempt to reduce the influence of these misperceptions in therapy. If his response indicated failure to recognise the picture or an error of recognition, KM was corrected. KM was then asked a series of yes/no questions of increasing semantic specificity. For example, if the target word was 'penguin' the questions might be:

- Is it a piece of furniture?
- Is it an insect?
- Does it live in cold countries?
- Can it fly?
- Is it a pelican?
- Is it a duck?
- Is it a penguin?

KM was only required to answer yes or no and was not asked to name the picture. Any words that he did not understand in this task were written down. Information gained so far was reiterated, so for the penguin example a reiteration might be 'It's a bird that lives in cold countries that can't fly.' This phase of therapy lasted seven months, with treatment taking place once or twice a week.

Following treatment all the semantic indicators had improved:

- Biber 'Is it a...?' increased from 78% to 90%.
- Synonym judgement increased from 71% to 85% .
- Functional comprehension was now excellent.

When examining more generalised language indices, the results can be seen in Figure 10.1. The scores obtained from the BDAE subtests have been summed to give comprehension and expression quotients. A non-standardised confrontation naming test (black-and-white line drawings taken from the remainder of the Snodgrass and Vanderwart collection) and the Boston Naming Test were also used. This graph shows an improvement in comprehension was followed by an improvement in naming.

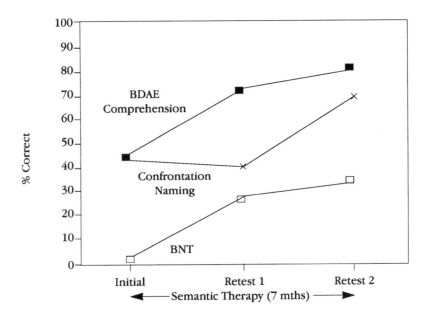

Figure 10.1 General linguistic change: summed % of BDAE and confrontation naming

Figure 10.2 shows an analysis of the relevance of the verbal output from picture description. KM was now able to access more words (total words increasing from 144 to 215) and the relevance of these words was increasing (relevant words increasing from 15% to 26% to 45%).

KM now had excellent functional comprehension and his access to semantics was good enough for him to name 75% of a selection of noun pictures on confrontation, although there was still an anomia as shown by the results of the Boston Naming Test. He was saying more

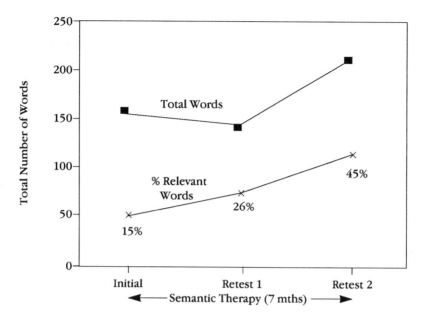

Figure 10.2 Change in verbal output: Relevance analysis of BCT picture

and relevance had improved, but he was still only 45% relevant in his picture description (see Figure 10.2). Observation of his spontaneous conversation confirmed that it was the fluency and irrelevance of his output that was the most intrusive feature of his communication, and not his anomia. The focus of therapy therefore changed for the next stage.

Stage 2 treatment – monitoring therapy

When speaking in phrases or sentences, KM had difficulty distinguishing between the relevance or irrelevance of his own verbal output and in editing out irrelevant speech. The hypothesis for treatment was that by improving his self-monitoring and editing skills, we could facilitate increased relevance of his output and reduce the total amount of verbal output at a sentence/functional level. Black-and-white LDA and Winslow Press photo cards were used. Therapy was less structured than in the previous stage and was an eclectic mix of techniques, all of them designed to encourage monitoring and editing of his own verbal output.

KM was requested to gesture from a single action picture. This task had two functions:

- It showed whether he had understood the picture as he frequently had difficulty with interpretation of action pictures if the action was inferred, e.g. clapping
- It also focused his attention on the main action within the photograph.

He was then required to say the verb. After a few weeks, therapy moved on to allowing a full sentence description but again restricting the output to a description of the most salient feature. After this, a three-picture sequence was used, with KM describing each individual action picture first and then summing up the whole activity in one sentence.

If the task was difficult, a number of strategies were used to help:

- As well as KM using gestures as a cueing mechanism, he was given a gesture to act as a prompt.
- A delay was imposed before KM could speak.
- During the pause he was instructed to think of the main action before saying anything.
- His output was audio-taped and played back to him for him to make judgements on and to correct if necessary.
- His verbal output was transcribed and KM then corrected it in terms of what was of direct relevance to the picture and what could have been omitted

This period of therapy lasted for four months and the results, shown in Figures 10.3 and 10.4 and in the Cookie Theft picture descriptions, demonstrate that treatment was successful. The percentage of relevant words had continued to improve from 45% to 84%. More significantly in terms of efficacy of therapy, there had been a reversal of the previous trend and the total number of words had reduced dramatically as predicted by the hypothesis. On a chi-squared test, there was a highly significant difference in relevance pre- and post-relevance therapy ($p = 0.001$). As can be seen in Figure 10.3, other indicators (the comprehension and anomia indices) all stayed static over this period where spoken output showed increasing relevance.

Pre-therapy Boston Cookie Theft Picture Description

This little girl is having some pupils ... trained to he ... she has just ... mm ... oh dear ... she has been ... rewinding ... sh–sh–sh oh damn I can't get the idea she's rewinding ... there's one here is talking to somebody on the pl–pl–platforms ... she's just talked to somebody ... rewound ... rewound ... the um talk to ... talked ... I can't quite see ... on the ... I don't know what the mistake is ... on the ... um ... it seems as though she's dropped something ... she might have had that in the ... night ... well ... be ... she might have had that in the ... night ... well ... be ... that thing

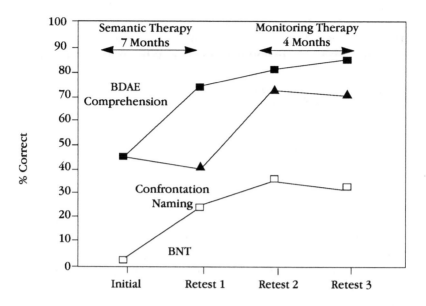

Figure 10.3 General linguistic change: Summed % of BDAE and confrontation naming

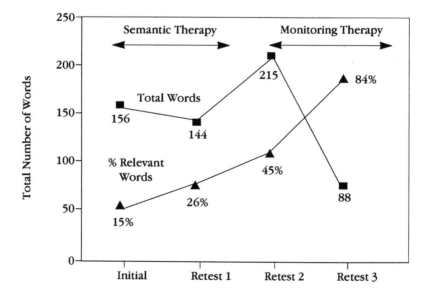

Figure 10.4 Change in verbal output: Relevance analysis of BCT picture

should have come for and there ... instead of that it didn't I think this wasn't very interested in the piece that was coming ... oh gosh this of course that'll be a picture and it's gone wrong (points to cookie jar) because the ... yes ... here you have the ... that has gone wrong first of all (points to stool) that this has been looking at the bibe well bidlpeds whatever they are (pointing from boy to girl) and she has been correctly assume them to be these things there.

Post-semantic therapy Boston Cookie Theft Picture Description

Well first of all the boy is going through the cookie jar and he's taking out a cookie because it has or has not get ... anything to identify it ... from what he's got any rate ... the man is standing on a slippery ... /s/... chair and er there is no ... nothing on the chair to stop him slipping down if he wants to ... yes ... he will fall backwards by the way the chair will go down backwards and he because he's on the chair and back is facing the way it's going he will go down backwards as well ... the girl is attracting the boy for some reason she's got she's asking I think for one of the cookies ... she's taking them out of the tin um the mother has er taken the ... iron pot ... from the ... somewhere ... washed it and is just drying it up again ... prior to putting it back clean and dry ... meanwhile the ... cold water tap has been kept going in to the ... sink ... the ca ... cold water is going from the ... ca ... canister over the top of the ... something what it is I don't know and its going down a hole in the floor ... in front of the baths .. a hole that is going down in front of the ... yes ... I know it sounds daft but it's true.

Post-monitoring therapy Cookie Theft Picture Description

A boy and girl are looking at a pound cookie jar ... the boy has taken out one cookie and is proffering to the girl who is not taking it because ... no forget because because out ... the girl has obviously asked for a cookie ... she has not been given one ... the boy's stool is slippery ... the girl ... well ... no ... no... I'm afraid now the woman is doing nothing but a bit of washing-up which she isn't doing very cleverly because the sink ... ugh ...the sink is draining to the floor below.

The therapy process: conclusion and comment

The first stage of therapy (semantic therapy) improved auditory comprehension and then word finding. The second stage (monitoring therapy) enabled KM to monitor what he said more effectively and become less verbose. He was better able to get his message across by using fewer, more relevant words. This last stage produced the dramatic crossover between relevance and number of words whilst other indicators remained stable.

Level of analysis

Detailed cognitive neuropsychological assessment was used to produce a hypothesis about the focus of linguistic breakdown at the single-word level. This was crucial to suggest appropriate intervention for the first stage of treatment which was semantic therapy. However, this form of single-word, detailed linguistic assessment was of little use in the treatment planning or analysis of the second stage of treatment, that of monitoring therapy at the sentence level.

The method of analysis used for this stage was devised by the first author and is quick and easy to administer, reasonably accurate and repeatable so that it can be used for standard clinic practice. It is not intended to be a measure of functional communication, and at present has only been used on picture description and not in other types of discourse. It involves transcribing the sample, counting all the word units and then discarding any irrelevant words or information (precise details of adminstration are available from the first author). A total word count and a relevance percentage are then obtained. This level and method of analysis quantified what was demonstrated by the language samples and KM's spontaneous speech.

Treatment of multi-infarct dementia

It is often suggested that those who have dementia should be assessed only and then they or their carers offered support and advice. It is rarely suggested that they should receive direct therapeutic intervention as the memory deficits associated with dementia are thought to negate the benefits of therapy. KM had been diagnosed as having multi-infarct dementia. On the Stevens screening test (1992), which makes a differential diagnosis between dysphasia and dementia, he was classified as having dementia. All doctors who had assessed him after his second admission had diagnosed him as such. He did have short-term memory problems, made visual misperceptions frequently, was disorientated in time and place and had poor visuo-spatial skills. However, his language difficulty was the deficit that he, his wife and the first author identified as being his main disability. As previously discussed, learning ability could be demonstrated.

Figure 10.5 shows data from Ravens Coloured Progressive Matrices (Ravens CPM) which is a non-verbal reasoning/IQ test and the Rivermead Behavioral Memory test (Rivermead BMT) which tests functional performance memory. Figure 10.6 shows the language indicators previously described: the summed Boston Diagnostic Aphasia Examination scores (BDAE), the response naming and the relevant word count. As can be seen in Figure 10.6, his language improved whilst cognitive measures remained static or deteriorated.

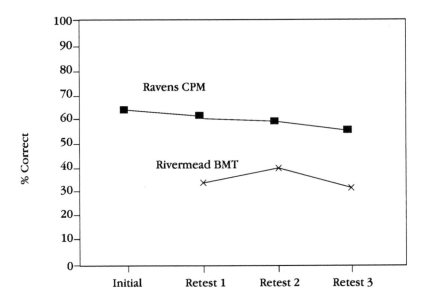

Figure 10.5 Cognitive change

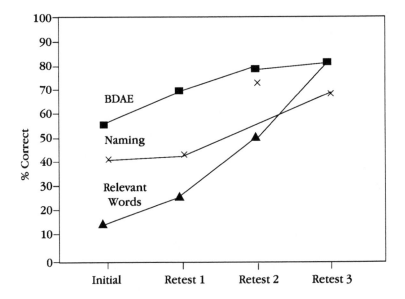

Figure 10.6 Language change

Thus if the client has awareness of his or her linguistic deficit, feels handicapped by it and learning ability can be demonstrated, then a structured test–treatment–retest regime could be tried where the linguistic involvement is the major disability within the disorder of multi-infarct dementia.

Differentiating multi-infarct dementias from Alzheimer's disease

MID is the second most common cause of dementia after Alzheimer's disease in North America, Europe and Australia but is the most common cause in Japan and China (Bannister, 1992). Prevalence estimates vary considerably between 9% and 46% in European and North American surveys, the highest estimate being from an area in the USA with a large black population (Folstein et al., 1985). Results from the Rotterdam study (Ott et al., 1995), a large population-based cross-sectional study, suggest that MID accounts for 16% of the dementia cases. Unlike Alzheimer's disease where the increased incidence with age is well documented, the Rotterdam study found only a small increase in MID with age.

Hachinski et al.'s (1975) 13-point ischaemia scale helps to differentiate vascular dementias from primary degenerative dementia and is now widely accepted as a useful tool in the diagnosis of MID. High scores suggest MID whilst lower scores suggest Alzheimer's and other non-ischaemic dementias. Features which score most points and therefore make a diagnosis of MID more likely are:

- abrupt onset;
- fluctuating course;
- history of strokes;
- focal neurological symptoms and signs.

The fluctuating course of MID may include at least some recovery after an episode and MID is considered to be amenable to a range of treatments (Roth, 1981). A complication of medical diagnosis in MID is the high incidence of both MID and Alzheimer's disease in the same people. Tatemichi (1990) suggests that a dementia can result from cerebrovascular disease because the location of cerebral injury is in a region which can affect many cognitive functions such as the association areas of the posterior cerebrum. The volume of the cerebral injury may reach a point where compensation is no longer possible because the number of injuries have an additive or multiplicative effect. There may be an interaction of Alzheimer's disease and stroke where stroke adds to the effects of early Alzheimer's.

Loring et al (1986) concluded that neuropsychological testing alone could not reliably distinguish between MID and Alzheimer's patients but there is some evidence that more specific language testing may be able to do so (Kontiola et al., 1990; Sasanuma, Sakuma and Kitano, 1990). Sasanuma et al. (1990) carried out a longitudinal study of MID and Alzheimer patients and found that those with MID had preserved recent memory, more diverse language profiles and less decline in their scores over time than the Alzheimer patients.

In MID, there is simplification of structural aspects of sentence production with retained sentence content and empty words are used less frequently than by Alzheimer's patients (Hier et al., 1985; Mendez and Ashla-Mendez, 1991). With increasing severity of MID, sentence length and syntactic complexity are further reduced and sentence fragments become more common. Powell et al. (1988) compared the language and speech characteristics of a group of MID subjects with those of an age- and severity-matched group of Alzheimer subjects. They conclude that MID is associated with a clinically distinguishable pattern of speech and language disturbances. Motor-speech disturbance was present in nearly all of the MID subjects but few of the Alzheimer subjects so that a diagnosis of Alzheimer's disease should be questioned in a patient with melodic or articulatory disturbance. Language abnormalities were not as evident in MID subjects who had fewer characteristics of fluent aphasia. Instead, the MID subjects produced fewer, shorter, less syntactically complex utterances than Alzheimer patients.

Patterns of impairment in the multi-infarct dementias

The patterns of language, cognitive deficits and behaviourial changes are determined by the specific arteries affected and the location and extent of infarcted tissue (Mahler and Cummings, 1991). Because of the variability in motor speech, language and swallowing deficits, careful assessment of MID patients is necessary.

MID patients with lacunae infarcts who show cognitive deficits may also have decreased spontaneity and initiative, response inhibition and mental set shifting deficits (Ishii, Hishahara and Imamura, 1986) whilst another MID group with presumed stroke-related white matter degeneration are more likely to exhibit decreased spontaneity, decreased speed of information processing and elaboration (Gupta et al., 1988; Junque et al., 1990). Control of hypertension may stop deterioration in some patients and there may even be limited improvement in cognitive function. In hypertensive subjects, cognitive function can improve with controlled hypertension whilst in normotensive patients, performance can be improved by daily aspirin and giving up smoking (Meyer et al., 1986, 1989).

Cortical and subcortical forms of MID have been described, having different pathologies and symptomatologies. Subcortical MID, as might be expected, is likely to be associated with a dysarthria, emotional lability, gait disturbance, bradykinesia and depression whereas the cortical form is more likely to produce an aphasia, apraxia or agnosia and other focal cortical signs. Depression is often a specific complicating feature in MID and may not be amenable to medication (Kramer and Reifler, 1992).

Binswanger's disease, for example, is a subcortical form of MID, caused by multiple infarcts of the white matter of the cerebral cortex with lacunar infarcts in the subcortical areas of the basal ganglia and the thalamus but sparing of the cortex and subcortical arcuate fibres (Bennett et al., 1990). More than 80% of the patients are over 60 years of age, with men and women equally affected. Clinical features of the disease are a history of hypertension, vascular disease and possibly acute strokes. Neurological symptoms are:

- a prominent motor disturbance and associated gait disorder;
- pseudobulbar palsy with associated dysarthria;
- history of incontinence;
- behavioural and mood changes including agitation, depression, irritability and euphoria.

There is also a memory disorder which is difficult to assess due to inattention (Caplan and Schoene 1978). Parkinsonism is a common finding (Kotsoris et al., 1987). Renewed interest in the disease is evident because the white matter infarcts can be clearly seen by MRI scanning. Binswanger's disease is essentially progressive but, if high blood pressure is controlled, patients can have periods of relative stability and may be able to benefit from treatment for speech and language deficits (Cummings and Benson, 1992).

Despite the high incidence of MID, there are very few studies of language impairment, perhaps due to the problem of reporting fluctuations in performance which may include partial recovery of function. Language impairment may be similar to specific aphasia syndromes (Benson, 1979) but there may be a co-occurring dysarthria. Lesser (1989) described a patient with MID whose language profile was similar to that seen in transcortical sensory aphasia. This man had preserved oral spelling and repetition but severe anomia and poor semantic comprehension. His spelling suggested a dissociation between his semantic system and his store of written word forms (graphemic output lexicon).

Hachinski et al. (1974) say that early features of MID are a dysarthria and dysphagia with associated weakness, slowing, a small-stepped gait and emotional lability. Pseudo-bulbar dysarthria is the most common form of speech disturbance. Because of the focal nature of the damage, there is no characteristic pattern of behaviourial deficits in the earlier stages of the disease but language deficits may be present if there is specific left hemisphere damage and dysprosody has been reported where there is right hemisphere damage (Ross, 1981).

Conclusion

Language function has not been studied adequately in MID, perhaps because it can be described as a researcher's nightmare. The MID population is more variable than that in Alzheimer's disease. When a multi-infarct dementia begins and multiple CVAs stop is not an easy clinical decision. The disease progression and disease pathology are diverse. Studies which contrast MID with other dementias often have poorly controlled and diagnosed MID groups. Yet this group of patients can benefit from both medical intervention which can improve cognition and, as the single case study of KM in this chapter shows, from specific intervention which can improve language.

Chapter 11:
Management Approaches Involving Carers

NIKI MUIR

Introduction

Speech and language therapists have an undeniably vital role to play in care of the elderly with mental health problems (Griffiths and Baldwin, 1989; Heritage and Farrow, 1994). Access to speech and language therapy services is increasing for this client group (RCSLT, 1990), but as people are living longer, the problems are outstripping the provision and we need to adopt different models of service delivery to meet need (Seaman, 1990). Such a change in practice for this care group is likely to take the form of working with the carers and thereby making the best and most widespread use of our skills by adopting a more 'consultative' role. Rather than trying to spread the service even more thinly and maintain the traditional models of delivery, speech and language therapists will now be looking to the wider issues of how to assure efficacy and to audit quality outcomes in this area of work.

Because in this field we are not in the business of being able to measure outcomes by 'cure' and complete discharge is unlikely, we must address ourselves to the task of how best to maintain the skills of our clients and continually adapt to changes and deteriorations brought about by the illness process. Caring for an elderly person with a mental health problem is a 24-hour task and therefore the input needs to be tailored towards strategies which will enable a greater range and depth of coping. Once-weekly therapy or even periods of intensive work will be unlikely to have the same generalising effects as giving carers the tools which will equip them to manage a little better in what is likely to be a long-term, distressing and challenging battle against the frustrations of the disease process and the alienation and loss brought about by the resultant degradation of communication in all its many forms.

Even as speech and language therapists with all our acquired knowledge and insights, we are likely to be continually amazed by the complexity of the linguistic process and the range and depth of communicative interaction. We are therefore unlikely to take these abilities for granted. For many people there is an assumption that communication is a natural gift and this can lead to an under-rating and undervaluation of the ablility – until something goes wrong. Communication changes can be the first sign that all is not well (Gravell and France, 1991). Losses in communication can lead to a range of psychological, psychosocial and relationship problems because it is so central to what and above all who we are. Communication is a skill and an activity which thrives on feedback and if that is lost it can begin to atrophy. Studies by Greene et al. (1982), Rabins, Mace and Lucas (1982) and Gilleard (1984) amongst many others show that loss of meaningful interactive and conversational skills are more distressing to carers than the developing of behaviours upon which many professionals focus their attention, e.g. 'aggression', wandering and incontinence. These findings are constantly being supported by first-hand reporting from carers themselves. They talk to us of the 'multiple bereavements' of skill loss and most of these are related to communication or to personality change expressed through communicative change. Bowlby (1981) talked of bereavement in terms of four distinct phases, these are seen to be alternate numbness and intense distress, yearning and searching, disorganisation and despair and finally a measure of reorganisation. The speech and language therapist wants to be able to contribute to the final reorganisation process for the client and carer but must pay heed to the other phases of the process via effective management.

The elderly with mental health problems can and do enjoy communicating at whatever level is available to them and relatives and other carers need to achieve whatever levels of reciprocal communication are possible in order to continue to interact meaningfully (Tanner and Daniels, 1990). We cannot underestimate the sadness and loss experienced by carers. Mulhall (1988) refers to the words of a wife on the occasion when her 69-year-old husband with dementia was admitted to hospital for respite care for the first time. There was relief coupled with a sense of failure and a sorrowful recognition that this was 'probably the end of the most important chapter in their mutual lives'. Speech and language therapists working as part of a team of health care professionals with the elderly need to acknowledge the guilt, the sadness, the frustration, the confusion, the loss and the anger likely to be experienced by relatives. In a study by Malone, Ptacek and Malone (1970), which related to the attitudes of the spouses of those with dysphasia following CVA, there was 100% reporting of having experienced guilt, unrealistic attitudes, rejection, overprotectiveness and withdrawal. It therefore follows that relatives of those with the mental health problems of ageing, particularly dementia, are likely to mirror those experiences. Indeed the feelings could take on a greater intensity owing to the misplaced stigma of mental health disorder and to the deteriorating nature of the illness, as well as the many other so-called 'normal' changes of ageing which may have gone before. These are most certainly retirement, possible losses of status, income, family, mobility and feelings of self-worth.

It is important not to place demands on carers which they are unable to carry out. Should we do this we run the risk of increasing guilt and feelings of helplessness. It is equally important not to place the carer in a role which demands unsustainable or potentially harmful changes in their relationship. He or she is already facing a great many of these. Imagine, for example, the wife who for 50 years has never had to manage any of the financial aspects of the marriage and the home, being placed in the situation, through the onset of her husband's dementing illness, of having to take on this aspect of their lives. Added to this and to the many other enforced role changes of their previously close partnership, she is also being asked to become her husband's therapist and carry out tasks and 'homework'. By asking the wife to become teacher and to attempt to complete exercises linked to some form of cognitive neuropsychological programme of language intervention, or to a facilitation programme for dysarthria, the therapist could be prompting quite a significant role change. Looked at in terms of a transactional analysis model (Berne, 1966, discussed further in the counselling section of this chapter) the interplay between the two would be less on an adult-to-adult level and more on an adult-to-child level. Limits should perhaps be set on these exchanges unless the wife can be made aware of the dangers and can manage the interactions and the boundaries well. She should be encouraged by the therapist not to impose a regimen which constantly appears to demand a 'performance', and should be helped to satisfactorily address the feelings both she and her husband may experience should he fail in tasks.

Quite apart from the alteration of her perception of herself in relation to him is the risk of intensifying his painful insight and confusion. There is the risk of increasing anger and further endangering relationships. Overemphasis on linguistic retraining when working with elderly clients with degenerative mental health problems can be fraught with dangers, not least those of raising unrealistic hopes of improvement and change. Working through carers needs to be delicately balanced, realistic and personalised, taking into account pre-morbid factors as well as likely prognosis. Strengths need to be built on and managing the needs of the carers as a priority, rather than adding in any way to their burdens, can be central to maximising quality of life for the client.

The aim of this chapter is to look at ways of providing the 24-hour packages of flexible and appropriate management of communication which will enable relatives to cope with greater insight into both the person that they care for and their own feelings. It also looks at using improved communication strategies as a way of maximising the care offered by other professionals, whose service delivery to this client group is going to be more intensive and ongoing than that of the speech and language therapist.

Information

As previously stated, communication changes can indicate that all is not well. Carers are not aware of what underlies these changes and will often show their bafflement in statements such as 'he(she) can do it if he(she) tries' or 'he(she) is only doing it to annoy'. When clients manifest both behavioural and personality changes as they are most likely to in dementia of the Alzheimer's type, subcortical dementia and depressive illness, the carer can see a 'changed person'. The person with dementia may behave in a way that is totally out of character and may be withdrawn, disinhibited or swinging between both these mental states. They may use abusive language where this was never previously the case. All the familiar frames of reference for that person may change. As it is human nature to personalise things, the carer may only be able to think of these changes in terms of 'being awkward', 'being hurtful' or 'being attention seeking'.

It is a vital role for the speech and language therapist to ensure that carers are given clear information as to the process of communication, highlighting the reasons for possible inconsistency and loss of conversational skills, attentional deficits, comprehension and memory impairment or changes in personality and behaviour (Powell, Hale and Bayer, 1995). Quality information in appropriate format, e.g. leaflets, packs and talks, can begin to raise the carers' awareness of the complex communication process. They can begin to see how language and communication is on many different levels and can perhaps begin to make distinctions between the functions, i.e. hearing/vision versus perceptual loss or receptive language versus expressive language. Information should provide genuine insight so that the carers can begin to unravel some of the complexities and inconsistencies. Grasping some of the theory and being able to process it on their own terms can help carers to be a little more objective and positive. This goes a long way to relieve frustration and to begin to allow for more realistic expectations. Information is often, for all of us, the initiation of change and the 'fitting of the key to the lock'.

Looking more closely at the kind of information that is to be given to carers, the starting point is often with some basic neurology of speech and language. A simple diagram of the brain supported by a clear and easily understood text or talk is often very effective in drawing attention to the complexity of the communicative process, as is a good representation of a 'speech chain' or simple cognitive neuropsychology model. These should show the stages of function required for communication to be intact. For example:

- hearing;
- perception;
- understanding;
- processing;
- storing;
- retrieving;
- organising;
- motor programming;
- production;
- functional ability.

This will need to be accompanied by written and/or verbal explanation in a clear form as to what types of communication breakdown occur at each level, how the processes can be identified and how they are linked.

Once a knowledge base is provided and there is an awareness of why and how communication breaks down, the role of the speech and language therapist is to provide information and demonstration on the skills which the client retains rather than on those which are 'lost'. There are many valuable leaflets available from associations such as the Alzheimer's Disease Society, the Stroke Association and Action for Dysphasic Adults, which provide essential 'rule-of-thumb' guidelines. If these are supported by personalised information packs as to exact stimulation and cueing techniques which have proven value for that individual client, then the relative can feel more in control. Many speech and language therapy services for the elderly with mental health problems devise their own pamphlets and handouts which can be constantly revised as the 'state of the art' changes or as individual needs dictate.

The speech and language therapist will also need to have access to the full range of information about local services. It is hoped that this will be something that each team has readily available and constantly updated but, as the communication specialist, it behoves the speech and language therapist to be fully conversant with information relating to local and national societies, support groups, respite facilities, specialist advisers, social services and even benefits. It may be simply for purposes of repetition to the carer or it may be that the team or the carer has identified the speech and language therapist as the most appropriate key worker. For whatever reason, having relevant information of all types to hand is good and truly holistic clinical practice.

Advice

In mental health care of the elderly, the role of team members as 'consultants and advisers' is paramount. This can demand significant changes for the individual therapist with regard to his or her role. It may demand a shifting of perception of self as therapist and a restating of what, in this context, therapy means. Major areas for the speech and language therapist to take on an advisory role are those of the communicative environment and of sensory needs, thus working with and through the carers in order to promote a higher level of preserved communication. We have to look at where the client has to communicate, what militates against it being of maximal quality and how it is undertaken by the carers.

Advice to all carers, whether relatives or other professionals, needs to be sensitively handled. Lubinski, Morrison and Ridgrodsky (1981) talk of the 'communication impaired environment in institutions'. Griffiths (1991) states: 'the Speech and Language Therapist can influence the level and quality of interaction by helping to clarify the role of care staff with regard to communication.' Working in an advisory capacity means walking the tightrope between constructive and negative criticism. It means taking time to build rapport and trust with carers and it means identifying practicable areas for change and working within constraints.

There are likely to be inevitable frustrations in this alternative model of care but it represents an enormously worthwhile challenge for our skills. The speech and language therapist will have to be creative with locations and look to adapt and to maximise them, given that these are the environments in which the client and the carers are having to cope on a daily basis. The following list represents some of the major areas for adaptation of the communicative environment on which the speech and language therapist may advise:

- seating;
- noise levels;
- proximity;
- stimulation – over/under;
- use of written/pictorial labelling;
- memory aids;
- verbal and non-verbal cueing strategies.

Advice both written and verbal may be needed on identifying and/or management of visual, attentional, hearing or perceptual difficulties. The carer will need to be advised on how to make appropriate changes in the home and other environments in order to foster greater communicative ease, make the best use of residual abilities and maximise strengths, for example picture boards, notebooks, colour coding or simplified labelling to act as a memory aid or to enable the elderly person to make a choice.

A further area in which advice may be required is in the assessment for and choice of a system of augmentative or alternative communication. This might be the choice and use of a communication aid or the selection of an appropriate system of signing, should either of these be indicated. Carers often find it difficult to accept a different communication modality and will be naturally hopeful of a return of verbal functioning, so clear advice may be needed to circumvent any resistance. The specific advice needed may be on the value of alternative manual systems, as for example Makaton (Walker, 1979) or perhaps Amer-Ind (Skelly, 1979), which is an iconic and easily decoded system of signing for those with reduced vocabulary and confusional states. Advice may also be given on computerised systems as an adjunct to the spoken word, for example a Lightwriter or a Canon communicator. Both of these are basic keyboard designs but do not have more sophisticated functions. Also, practical help such as accompanying the carer and client on visits to the recognised communication aids centres and outlets, reinforcing the information and advice they are given there and helping to decipher instruction manuals can be of support as they develop confidence and come to terms with the required adaptations and training necessary to understand and retain the basics of a well-used and ideographic system of signing or to grasp the intricacies of a 'machine'. It should be borne in mind that the latter may prove a particular difficulty if the carer is of a generation who have a degree of technophobia.

Another major advisory area will be that of feeding and swallowing. As with alternative communication and hearing requirements, it is likely that the speech and language therapist will offer advice but also access the advice of other professionals. Correct diet, posture and facilitation techniques will need to be arrived at in consultation with dieticians, occupational therapists and physiotherapists and all advisory leaflets will need to reflect this liaison as well as reflecting current dysphagia management guidelines from the professional bodies. Table 11.1 is an example of the sort of reminders that carers may need in written form.

In all instances where an advisory role is undertaken there should be an aim to be both prophylactic as well as reactive, and it will of necessity be ongoing.

Table 11.1: Guidelines for carers in managing feeding and swallowing

---

1. Ensure the person is sitting upright, with head symmetrical, chin slightly down to chest
2. Ensure the person is fully awake and concentrating
3. Take into account the tastes/likes/dislikes of the person
4. Do not forget the importance of colour and texture
5. Consider temperature, quantity, flavour, smell and presentation of food
6. Avoid mixed textures, floppy textures, acidic foods, food items with husks/skins
7. Offer drinks before and after, NOT during a meal
8. Use all methods of communication to explain to the person being fed
9. Feed from the front
10. Give small spoonfuls

Education

One of the greatest ways to educate could be said to be by demonstration. Being prepared to put one's own skills on the line is often a good way of stating one's role in the team and of gaining the trust of carers and therefore their greater acceptance of the advisory role discussed here. The speech and language therapist needs to be a role model for carers on how to manage communication impairment. This may mean having to work in less than ideal situations so that staff carers as well as relatives can observe both directly and indirectly. Several major areas of educative practice and need will be discussed below:

Audio- and video-taping: clients, environments and specific interactions on audio and/or video recorders and use of a two-way mirror are ideal means of offering opportunities for training via observation. They can offer a degree of self-monitoring or self-evaluation to the client or the carer. If used judiciously they can provide much needed insight into behaviours and allow for problem solving and change of both communicative and environmental features. However, they are seldom widely available except in the most modern, proactive and well-funded units and departments.

Mainstream speech and language therapy techniques: Specific education on the use of recognised therapeutic approaches and techniques will often be required, giving carers accessible information and training on the use of more mainstream speech and language therapy techniques for maximising attention and in using cuing strategies such as associative cues, forced alternatives, run-ins and phonemic cues to promote improved comprehension and elicit both verbal and non-verbal expressive output. Alongside this may be the need for training in management strategies for facilitation techniques as well as for feeding and swallowing. The Winslow Press *Working With* series (Fawcus et al., 1986; Stokes and Goudie, 1990) are of great practical value. The speech and language therapist can educate carers on how much to enrich the linguistic environment, for example by building structured communication and memory tasks into everyday activities such as meals, baths etc.

Reality orientation: The strategies of reality orientation (RO), as set out by Holden and Woods (1988), are not the sterile, prescriptive interventions that many have taken them to be. Day and date boards are only a part of this technique, whereby the carer can be encouraged to use time, place and person reminders and cues in order to bring structure to the daily lives of the confused elderly.

Reminiscence therapy: It has been suggested that for many elderly people reminiscence therapy (Norris, 1986) is a very positive experience. Hughston and Merriam (1982) indicate that it can improve cognitive function for some time. It is certainly the experience of the writer that it reduces depression and promotes improved communicative attentiveness and output. The carer will learn to use shared or cued memories of the past to form the basis for topics and interaction. Even if not in the here and now there is still great value in the fact that this technique can enable meaningful or more meaningful communication. Carers should, however, be alerted to the fact that not all people, elderly or otherwise, will wish to reminisce. For some it may be too painful, touching on unresolved life events or conflicts. For others there may be no wish or need to go back.

Validation therapy: Feil (1982) introduced this technique which encourages acceptance by the carer of their relative or client's 'fantasy world' and use of what is being said, as well as the behaviours produced, to form communicative links and bonds. She suggests that the cognitive impairments of the confused elderly person often allow them to function only from the deep subconscious and that here the functioning may be intact. Whatever opinion one might hold on this theory, it is undeniably true that to 'go where the client is' and try to establish an interaction in response to their communicative statements and behaviours, rather than to set one's own agenda for what is normal and acceptable, is a valuable and often remarkable therapeutic tool. For carers, knowledge of the prompts and responses offered by the validation can provide structure and help them to act on the moment rather than see each seemingly aberrant behaviour as a cause of further regret for skills lost.

Resolution therapy: Knowledge of and training in this technique are likely to foster in the carers a greater understanding of the feelings and cognitive processes which may be underlying and triggering the seemingly anomolous or even meaningless output (Goudie and Stokes, 1989). Whilst it may be embarrassing if an elderly person is asking for his or her mother all the time, a recognition of the fact that this sentiment may be coming from anxiety can help give meaning to the behaviour and offer possible options for managing it in a sensitive and appropriate way. As speech and language therapists we may be aware that a paraphasic error results in a plea for mother rather than daughter or wife, but the underlying anxiety, fear and confusion are going to be the same and should not be devalued or avoided.

Hearing impairment: An understanding of hearing mechanisms and the resulting impairments can help the carer to maximise residual hearing by use of improved communication. The carer will need to learn which is the better ear and how to position him- or herself correctly as well as how to make the best use of light, natural acoustics, voice and non-verbal skills. The carers will also need to be taught to manage the hearing aids or any speech amplifier that is being used as an alternative, e.g. Sarabec, Telemik, etc. There could be the assumption that wearing the aid or using the amplifier all the time will provide an answer to much of the confusion and it is important to teach that such aids are not a universal panacea and may in fact add to the confusion if used where there is too much noise. It will also be important to help the carer to recognise the difference between hearing loss and auditory perceptual deficit.

Sensory stimulation: This is a form of intervention whereby the carer can offer therapeutic input which will help to maintain the various sensory pathways. Along with true Sensory Integration Therapy (Ayres, 1972), which will extend this in a controlled way and to a neurological model to activate brain mechanisms and promote adaptive responses, stimulation can allow for genuine elements of structured interaction. Learning how to use these techniques may alter carers' perception of themselves and of the often frustrating routine tasks, rendering them less of a duty and responsibility and more of a fostering of a measure of independence; for example, a carer could be taught to use a sponge along the muscle lines to stimulate facial musculature during routine face-washing.

General educative tips: One must exercise some discretion in teaching carers to promote and maintain greater levels of independence in their relatives or patients. A study by Goodlove, Richard and Rodwell (1982) gives credence to the belief that carers, particularly staff, prefer to look after dependent clients as their needs are more predictable and frames of reference for the carer therefore more stable.

Snowden, Griffiths and Neary (1994) offer evidence in their study of 'semantic dementia' of the importance of the client's own experiences and own things as facilitators of recall and naming. It will be of great benefit to carers to learn of the contribution of autobiographical and personal relevance to the preservation of meaning, because they are going to be ideally placed to furnish the necessary linguistic adaptations and cueing materials. The importance of educating carers in strategies to gain and maximise attention and how to develop good listening skills when interacting with the relative or patient cannot be stressed too highly – as too must be the value of scaling down output, keeping it in the 'here and now' and making it non-ambiguous and interest related, with appropriate use of visual aids, genuinely supportive gestural cues and use of the written word.

Formal training

Sessions may be undertaken for small groups of staff or relatives in all the key areas mentioned above. The range, type and level of this training should be dictated as much by the needs and availability of the carer as by the need of the client as perceived by the therapist. The speech and language therapist working in mental health care of the elderly needs to be prepared to offer and undertake a great deal of formal training. This may be to pre- and post-registration nursing and other students, to care staff in nursing and residential homes, to colleagues within the team, to volunteers and to staff from care agencies and societies as well as to relatives' groups. A varied level of handouts to support these training sessions is essential and research suggests that role play is a particularly effective formal training tool (Koury and Lubinski, 1991).

Also important is ongoing training and constant updating for the speech and language therapist personally. This can be achieved through allowing time for reading, gaining membership of special interest groups and, when possible, attending some of the increasing number of relevant courses being offered in this field.

The task of educating carers serves to stress the vastness of linguistic and communicative function. It is a task which can overwhelm the speech and language therapist by its immensity, so it can certainly be imagined how overwhelming it could prove for the carers themselves. Sessions may need to be 'little and often'. The carers may need to identify their own priorities for training, perhaps by the use of questionnaires offering a choice of topics with some short explanation of content. In some rare cases, no amount of education is going to succeed in equipping individuals to manage change and adapt to new techniques. In these cases the speech and language therapist should acknowledge the impossibility and, if viable, seek alternative approaches which will be less stressful to all concerned. These alternatives may involve focusing on another key carer or looking to implement the major changes in the environment rather than in people. They may involve facilitating social and respite opportunities rather than active, assertive interventions, or the client may require referral on to other services.

Assessment via carers

Assessment of the elderly with mental health problems can be quite problematic. Whilst batteries, or at least subtests, of standardised aphasia tests such as the Aphasia Screening Test (Whurr, 1974), the Boston Diagnostic Aphasia Examination (Goodglass and Kaplan, 1983) or the Western Aphasia Battery (Kertesz, 1982) have value and assessments offering a degree of differential diagnostic information as, for example, the Middlesex Elderly Assessment of Mental State (Golding 1989), the Clifton Assessment Procedure for the Elderly (Pattie and Gilleard, 1979) the Severe Impairment Battery (Saxton et al., 1993), have an even more significant worth, they are scarcely fully representitive. Carers may become anxious or confused by standard scores and think only in terms of pass or fail criteria. They are more likely to respond to measurements of what they may consider real-life behaviours. Carers can provide wide-ranging information on behaviour and performance across many situations and areas of linguistic and communicative function which a 'one off' test would neglect. Communicative and behavioural rating scales and questionnaires can be adapted or devised for the carer to complete thus giving a more broadly based picture – even allowing for inevitable subjectivity and inaccuracies. This approach can allow the carers a measure of objectivity in judging the performance of the person in their care and can help them to realise strengths and preserved skills as well as weaknesses and needs. It can therefore be a learning experience. A very basic measure appears in Table 11.2.

Personal preference checklists can be of great value in devising client-centred therapy programmes and it will be to the carer that we turn in gaining this information on family, hobbies, pets, places of relevance, life events, likes and dislikes, etc. These areas of personal information can form the basis of language intervention programmes and also be used for reality orientation approaches and reminiscence sessions. Personal information and preferences can also be cued in group situations as, for example, social skills groups (Trower, Bryant and Argyle, 1978), which can have a value in mental health care of the elderly, or in interpersonal skills groups (Burnard, 1990). An example of a personal preference and information sheet appears in Table 11.3.

Assessment via carers will also likely lead to timely re-evaluation of needs, in that the carer may be able to indicate changes in behaviours which may lead the speech and language therapist to wish to reassess on a more formal basis and perhaps to adjust or redirect all or some elements of the therapy and management. As on many occasions the management approach is directly through the carer, another area for assessment is that of the individual carer's own attitudes, feelings and behaviours in interaction with their relative.

Mulhall (1977) devised a Personal Relations Index which will yield a unique profile of a relationship between a person with aphasia and his or her spouse. Data can be abstracted from an interview situation in which one spouse describes his or her own feelings as well as how he or she sees their partner's behaviours. A questionnaire can be prepared from the information that has been gained. A representational 'graph' can then be prepared which can almost paint a picture of the interrelated feelings and behaviours and can highlight 'vicious circles' and areas of stalemate. In this way it may become apparent that a wife sees herself as being very loving but sees her husband's response to this, since his illness, as irritability, which in turn she is construing as being a rejection. Looking to assess the carer's behaviours and needs can form the base-line for accurate support and counselling interventions as

Table 11.2: Social and communicative behaviours

Column A	A applies	Between A and B	B applies	Column B
1. Tries to avoid conversation				Happy to engage in conversation
2. Very short answers to questions				Gives full answers to questions
3. Very slow to respond				No delay in response
4. Seldom initiates conversation				Regularly initiates conversation
5. Speech very hesitant				Speech flows well
6. Avoids eye contact/eye contact innapropriate				Eye contact appropriate
7. Limited (or inapropriate) facial expression/gesture				Appropriate facial expression/gesture
8. Highly distractable, poor attention skills				Good attention skills
9. Poor conversational content, e.g. frequent topic changing, recurrent themes, words used inconsistent with topic				Good conversational content
10. Articulation of speech unclear/slurred				Articulation clear

Source: NJM (1993).

Table 11.3: Communication information form

Present/recent interests and activities
Present social links/friendships
Place of birth
Place(s) with strong associations (e.g. holiday venues)
Family information (parents, siblings, husband/wife, children, grandchildren, other relations, particular friends)
Any pets (past/present)
Previous jobs
Wartime experience
Hobbies and interests
Food and drink likes/dislikes
Reading likes/dislikes
Television likes/dislikes
Other topics of relevance
Any topics to be avoided because of painful association

discussed later in this chapter. Allowing carers to gain insight and to evaluate their own behaviours from a more objective viewpoint can help them make the necessary changes and adaptations in a self-directed way, rather than expecting the greatest change in the person they care for and having to confront the issues over time.

Management via staff carers

Working with other staff within the multidisciplinary team is likely to involve much of the information and advice giving previously discussed, as well as the elements of education. There is much evidence in the literature that the attitudes and behaviour of staff often change when they are involved in specific therapy programmes and interventions (Powell-Procter and Millar 1982). An understanding of the aetiology and management of speech, language and communication difficulties and an involvement in their remediation, or at least their maintainance, can lead to better focus and greater satisfaction for staff.

Many qualified mental health professionals have little or no training in neurology and therefore may be unaware of the many discrete disorders which can result from a dementia or other disease process. A knowledge of the presence of an agnosia or a dyspraxia, for example, will be of value to them and will serve to highlight the need for individualised management and the necessity for continual differential diagnosis. If this insight is provided by the speech and language therapist it may help prevent staff consigning all behaviours to the categories 'confusion' or dementia and thus feeling that these behaviours are irremediable.

In order for the speech and language therapist to adopt a management approach involving staff carers, the multidisciplinary team needs to be sound and needs to be constantly nurtured. There must be flexibility and a recognition of constraints, with only realistic demands being made. To some extent it could be said that the speech and language therapist will be adopting the same 'clinical' approach to assessing the team, its needs and its 'care plan' as will be used with the client. Rather in the same way that untangling the component parts of an elderly client's difficulties is like the speech and language therapist as detective, so is the overview that needs to be taken of the team. Who are the members as individuals? What are the dynamics of the group? What are the constraints? What are the service issues?

Good communication is as essential for a good multidisciplinary team as it is for work with the clients and their relatives and perhaps in this the speech and language therapist can also be a role model. There are many barriers to effective team work (Pollock, 1986) and these could significantly affect the readiness of staff carers to become involved in management of the direct communication needs of clients. Some major barriers could be those of organisational factors and/or role conflicts. There may be intra-professional differences or philosophical differences, e.g. cure versus care or the medical model versus a more consensus model of approach. The elderly with mental health problems are likely to be multi-handicapped and therefore they require multiprofessional input. However, this in itself can lead to many 'grey areas' where ownership of certain perceived roles becomes less clear and a great many core skills can be said to be within the remit of the whole team rather than the specialist function of one professional group.

Core skills need to be identified and agreed upon and the specific areas of specialist skills need to be made clear as part of a formal or informal team-building exercise in order to have trust and mutual respect within the multidisciplinary team. When this is present there can be role sharing and a blurring of boundaries without too much threat and territorialism. This can lead to a true skill mix whereby management is enhanced and there is reinforcement of the expertise and efforts of each team member.

Improving communication in a general sense is a core aim for all team members and the speech and language therapist is likely to have very specific skills and techniques to impart to other staff in order to make their interaction with the client more effective and therefore, by definition, offering the staff member greater satisfaction from the encounter. These skills are going to be mainly the subjective communicative acts of active listening and the use of repair strategies (Erber, 1994). It is not a question of getting another member of the team to do one's work, but a recognition of their central and more 24-hour role and a suggestion that this may be improved for themselves and their clients by taking on board elements of a communication programme and an improved communicative environment and approach.

Support and counselling

Many speech and language therapists may feel anxious about working in this more psychotherapeutic way and may feel that their skills are not adequately developed. However, undergraduate training is likely to have included many elements of counselling, and postgraduate skills courses are much more widely available. It is the opinion of the writer that speech and language therapists, by virtue of their trained listening skills and their unique combination of knowledge in the areas of psychology, neurology and linguistics, are ideally placed to broaden their skills and offer valuable therapeutic input by adopting a support and counselling role in working with the carers of the elderly experiencing the many communication deficits that can be resultant from mental health problems. Carers can often be unable to cope with their confusion and grief at the onset of cognitive and communicative changes. This may actually be compounded by the amount of detail they are often asked to take on at the time of diagnosis and leave them feeling helpless.

Mental health professionals are now much more aware of the rights of relatives and most are very prepared to offer information and advice. However, it may be that the relative needs time to adjust to being given a diagnosis and, on occasions, an ensuing poor prognosis. They may be unable to listen with full attention, feel bombarded with information or be unable to process and problem-solve the full implications. A relative may 'over-react' owing to extreme distress, or conversely 'under-react' owing to blunting of their feelings. The opportunity for relatives to express and share their feelings in a supportive milieu offers reassurance and a sense of being able to share responsibility (Kearns, 1986). It can also lead to them being able to come to a sad realisation at their own pace and, having reached a measure of acceptance, being more receptive to information and advice from the professionals (Parkes, 1975).

Support groups

Support as a means of service delivery via carers will be built in to intervention with the client on an individual basis to address the feelings and concerns already referred to, but the speech and language therapist may choose to run support groups. Within the safe setting of a support group, relatives and other carers can express their negative feelings, emotions and frustrations in a setting where acceptance is guaranteed. This therefore avoids the worst of the 'bottling' which can increase frustration and stress and may lead to explosive anger which can then take one round the vicious circle of guilt again.

Support groups need to meet *many* times to be effective (Whitehead, 1992) and to be of the highest quality (Gilhooly, 1984) but are strongly favoured in all the literature because they give the carer an opportunity to communicate fully, when in those areas of their lives involving their relative, that facility is becoming limited. The emotional responses, anxiety and preoccupation of the carer are likely to further diminish communication with the sufferer, unless they are addressed. Regular support groups can, to some extent, break that particular vicious circle. It should be remembered at all times, however, that many relatives are not of the generation where feelings are overtly recognised, let alone voiced to 'strangers'. Care is therefore needed in allowing a support group to go at its own pace and dictate its own agenda without undue leading from the speech and language therapist as facilitator.

Support groups have marked psychotherapeutic effects in that they result in the carer feeling less alone both in practical and social ways, as well as in the wider and more far-reaching emotional sense. They offer contact with others, a focus and structure to an often rather anarchic weekly programme and the opportunity for self-help as well as for helping others.

If the speech and language therapist is going to run a support group for carers then as much care and attention to detail should be given as for any other direct therapy group. The venue should be carefully selected so that it can foster the chances provided to relax and socialise in a cheerful and not too clinical environment. The layout of the room should be considered for maximum comfort and minimal threat. Coffee and tea are a must! The time of day should be considered and carers given a chance to choose what is most convenient for them in the light of arrangements for care of their relative during that period. Not all have ongoing or easily implemented day-care arrangements. This may be because they are feeling they should 'go it alone', or they may wish to maintain their independence for as long as possible. Provision which is acceptable to the individual carer and to the client needs to be made to enable attendance. This may take the form of finding someone to remain in the home, or offering an alternative client group in another room, or short-term day care for the duration of the session. Transport is another item which the speech and language therapist may need to arrange, so it can be seen that the therapist will need to have access to a range of resources before being able to set up a support group.

The speech and language therapist should have the aims and objectives of the group clearly defined in his or her mind before the group commences, but allow the participants to refine those aims and objectives and the routes by which they are achieved. Group dynamics should always be considered and there may need to be a 'selection' process based on an understanding of an individual carer's likely needs and the therapist's own interaction skills. This is not to say that anyone should be excluded, but that attempts to achieve a harmonious balance should be made and likely problem areas within the dynamics of the group anticipated.

Carers who are more reticent or new to the role may need smaller groups. For some, the speech and language therapist may need to effect an introduction to only one other carer, who is prepared to visit and support in the home, before any other form of support can be introduced. This can often be done through the local Alzheimer's group or through Age Concern, or even by a carer currently known to the service who would be prepared to act as a befriender. Effecting these contacts again suggests the need for a database or information pack of a variety of resources and possible models of supportive intervention.

Support groups can often avert the need for more direct psychotherapeutic interventions (Gordon, 1976). They do this by providing a format which allows carers to discuss specific issues arising within their daily lives as well as the wider and more psychological issues. The speech and language therapist may have a format for the group which continues session by session, i.e. social 'warm-up'–topic activity–social 'wind down'. Or they may elect to have a goal of gradually escalating the level of disclosure session by session. Whatever format is selected, it is suggested that it may be helpful to give a little written feedback, which can keep the supportive elements going until the next session, by providing the repetition which is so necessary to carers. It should also be recognised that there may be a need to increase the attendance at groups or to offer one-to-one sessions at times of crisis, i.e. readmission to hospital, further marked deterioration, other loss, etc.

Individual counselling

If relatives and carers cannot come to terms at all with their mixed emotions and feelings of negativity then direct and individual counselling may be needed. There could be fear, emotional disturbance or denial and this will need sensitive management. The speech and language therapist may refer the carer on to an experienced counsellor or to another therapist with fuller counselling training. Alternatively if the rapport is good and there is an adequate measure of process supervision available for the speech and language therapist, then the relative may receive direct therapy via a counselling approach and the client be seen elsewhere.

Speech and language therapists are often made anxious by the thought of taking the step towards a more psychotherapeutic approach and yet communication is of itself 'psychotherapeutic'. Parker (1983) makes it clear that speech and language therapists' ability to listen and to talk is as much part of their skill as is the more widely perceived ability to increase intelligibility. Therefore speech and language therapists are ideally placed to gain the relevant experience and to take on the formal training needed for counselling and use it to maximum effect, offering the carer the opportunity to speak to a receptive and professionally trained listener.

It is important to avoid a conflict of interests between the client and the carer (Brumfitt, 1986) and to be clear what relates to interpersonal and personal difficulties acquired since the illness and what reflects a depth of unresolved previous problems in the relationship. Therapeutic boundaries and clear goals will be needed, so that initially management can be set in the 'here and now' of communication breakdown and needs. If it becomes apparent as sessions progress that the carer has a previously unresolved experience which is causing their present reaction to be intensified, then some work in this area will be necessary if the therapist has the expertise and feels comfortable. Relevant past experiences could be death of a parent, fear of hospitals, other punitive or 'trapping' situations, etc.

Counselling will be aimed at helping the carer clarify and find solutions to this very significant life event and the approach used may be of several types, either alone or in justifiable combination. It may be psychoanalytical – after Freud or Jung – which would look to make the unconscious thoughts, motivations and drives conscious. It may be underpinned by the 'unconditional positive regard' and the techniques of reflecting back of a Rogerian psychotherapeutic approach (Rogers, 1951). It may be along the lines of Personal Construct Psychotherapy (Kelly, 1955; Button, 1986) in which the therapist suspends his or her own rationale in order to establish how the other person is construing the world and then encourages him or her in identification and experimentation with alternatives.

Transactional analysis (Berne, 1966) can also be of immeasurable benefit, as touched on earlier in the chapter. It offers a theory of social interaction that allows for a systematic analysis of interpersonal communications (transactions) of all types. The premise put forward is that all transactions come from and are responded to from one of three ego states: adult, child or parent. A mismatch of the ego state can be the root cause of all interpersonal breakdown. This theory explains why, for example, we are all from time-to-time children with our parents and consequently unable to confront, respond and change on an adult-to-adult level within this particular relationship. Indeed some of us may still become a bit 'whiny' with our mothers! For many carers, having a relative with deteriorating abilities who has to all intents and purposes changed and is perceived as being very needful of care and protection will foster the parent/child role, which can be unhealthy for both parties.

In their book on transactional analysis counselling, Lapworth, Sills and Fish (1993) discuss and develop the approaches whereby difficulties can be identified and changes made. Transactional analysis is also helpful in allowing the therapist to be aware of the ego state from which his or her interactions come. This allows for change and a measure of safeguard so that interactions do not become derailed but remain centred and healthy.

The theories and practices of Neuro Linguistics Programming (NLP) (Dilts et al., 1980; Bandler and Grinder, 1982) may be of great value in counselling because this approach is both behavioural and psychodynamic and is concerned with identifying both conscious and unconscious patterns of communication and behaviour and looking at how they interact in the process of change. It is an understanding of the unique and systematic way each individual structures sensory experience and deals with the information. Recognising and 'matching' language systems through the principles of NLP can increase rapport between the therapist and the client and can be taught to some carers as a way of enhancing communication with their relative and thus being less 'at odds'.

It may be important to change the carer's model of the world in terms of his or her communicative expectations, and many of the experiential exercises of NLP can be of great value in helping him or her achieve a measure of insight into the other person's perspective. It may also help in allowing the carer to achieve a measure of specificity when stating his or her problems, and with this comes an element of control and a chance for change.

A Gestalt approach, as discussed first by Perls (1972), may also be used. In this there can be an expression of feelings in safety without undue comment or facilitation, thus avoiding the building of an overly needy and needful relationship with the therapist or group. It can be a catalyst or a key to unlock the feelings and provide catharsis particularly for those individuals who are over-intellectualising their difficulties. Current thinking advocates blurring of boundaries between theories in order to offer an eclectic approach to therapy by integrating what is best from a variety of approaches (Harrington, 1988).

The real value of any of the recognised counselling approaches is that they increase self-awareness and foster a greater understanding of how the self and other key people in the situation function and interrelate. Above all, counselling is exploratory and provides opportunities to rethink and re-evaluate in a way that can be immensely revealing and rewarding to the carer. In an attempt to give a definition of counselling it could be said that it aims to give the client an opportunity to explore, discover and clarify ways of living more resourcefully and work toward greater well-being in terms of self, others and life events.

There are three stages to counselling: exploring, understanding and action. By exploring we can reach a measure of understanding and this understanding will enable the making of a plan for action and thus re-invest us with a degree of control. Within the exploring phase of counselling the therapist needs to paraphrase, reflect meanings and feelings, be empathic and use techniques such as open-ended probes, pinpointing, summarising and silence. In the phase that will lead to understanding for the client, the therapist will need to empower the client to self-disclose, to express what is only implied, to recognise patterns and themes, to confront discrepancies and to interpret. In the final action phase of the counselling process the therapist will be supporting the client by putting him or her in touch with strengths and in goal setting, programme choice and evaluation.

When embarking on counselling the therapist should be prepared for both anger and elements of resistance which will need skilled and flexible management. Non-directive approaches are often most beneficial, with emphasis on active listening, the appropriate use of interjection, reflecting responses and questioning in order to offer focus and promote exploration. Counselling is a re-educative therapy (Wolberg, 1977) because it is client centred in cognitive, behavioural and transactional contexts. The aim of counselling for carers is to allow them to come to terms with the social and interpersonal implications of the communication breakdown. Above all the resolutions must be of their own devising.

Family therapy

The feelings and needs engendered by the onset and progression of a mental health problem are not solely confined to the elderly person's immediate carer. Although we are no longer a society where the extended family is the norm, many other family members may have concerns and wish for an involvement. Distance and separate lives may cause their own cycle of guilt and blame, and fragile relationships may founder in the face of such a major crisis.

Gravell (1988) suggests that speech and language therapists should not consider offering family therapy unless they have accredited counselling qualifications. This would certainly be the case if the family dynamics are particularly complex and the effects of any particular behaviours, disagreements or breakdowns are having far-reaching implications. However, there is much to suggest that as another type of non-directive therapy, which is also re-educative, family therapy can be a valuable and logical progression from or extension of counselling.

Many families who are carers of clients now in long-term hospital or other residential settings need to feel included in 'treatment'. They are able to provide valuable information on the client's background and role in the family and the patterns of communication which preceded the illness. Improving communication between family members can often help the main carers to come to terms with the illness and to build towards a more positive future where there is more open communication, improved relationships and greater mutual assistance and support.

Basic family therapy (Barker, 1986), along the lines of proven systems which are psychodynamic and allow for analysis of communication, can be of great benefit and can be undertaken by the experienced speech and language therapist either alone or with another mental health care professional. For family therapy, as for any other psychotherapeutic activity, adequate process supervision should be available for the therapist.

Conclusion

Management of clients by genuine involvement of their carers demands creativity and innovation. It also requires more fieldwork and research from within the profession to evaluate its worth objectively. However, subjectively and through use of informal service evaluation questionnaires the benefits of this kind of approach as a means of maintaining and supporting this client group with its multiplicity of need is proven.

Carers learn through the practical support, guidance, encouragement and empathy of contact with a speech and language therapist as well as through the direct intervention of counselling and training. What they learn is how to redefine their own means of communication so that they can adapt and interact with more flexibility and success.

In this area of work it seems mandatory that speech and language therapists should be prepared to move away from what may be considered more traditional roles and expand and extend their knowledge and skills in order to do full justice to all that is encompassed by the term communication. Professional assurance and confidence are required to fulfil the role of 'consultant'. The therapist needs the personal ability to take risks and to move into a more fully psychotherapeutic model of care.

The linguistic and communicative effects of a dementia and of the many other mental health problems of ageing are devastating to all concerned. By developing fully both personally as therapists and professionally as a specialist service and as core team members we will be able to fulfil our central role, that of playing a full part in the enhancement of quality of life – of the carer as much as the client.

Chapter 12:
Analysis of Current Service Provision and Service Audit

SANDRA WALKER

Introduction

Although in the last 20 years we have been uncomfortably aware of the increasing problems imposed by the growing numbers of people with dementia, sufferers, the issues have engendered comparatively little professional attention and minimal change in planning priorities. Neither has there been significant public or professional demand for altered policies or reallocation of limited resources. Within the profession, indeed, we have been challenged to consider whether we are 'currently trying to do too much and venturing into areas in which there is little, if any, evidence of [its] effectiveness' (Enderby and Davies, 1989, p. 328). Not surprisingly, therefore, in a survey of professionals most likely to be involved in the care of dementing people, speech and language therapists are not listed (Greene 1988). This, against the evidence that (68%) of carers report communication as impaired and three-quarters of these report it as a problem in day-to-day living (Robins, Mace and Lucas, 1982).

The dilemma is compounded for speech and language therapists who are unlikely to be included in proactive or even reactive service planning (Wade, 1992). Further, in the recent past, services for EMI patients have not been seen as a priority for most speech and language therapy managers (RCSLT, 1993).

Norman (1990) raised many questions with regard to the complex issue of sovereignty in the decision-making process for care of elderly mentally ill people. For example:

- Who assesses what the need really is? (Often it is whoever happens to receive the referral first.)
- Who decides the criteria for allocation of scarce resources?
- Who takes the final decision on the final allocation of resources in particular cases?
- Who is responsible for ensuring quality of care?
- Who decides who will be rejected as being unsuitable for care or too difficult to cope with or to manage?

These questions apply equally to the speech and language therapist: whether the concomitant communication problems for or between the client/carer will be recognised and referral to a service made; whether a service exists to meet these needs; what kind of service is offered; whether clinician and organisation standards are defined, monitored and met; and whether shared case management decision making exists.

In 1994 a Bill of Rights for patients with Alzheimer's disease and related disorders was proposed (see Table 12.1) (Troxel, 1994).

The Bill of Rights (or charter in UK terms) is not absolute. The implications for the professional to strive to adhere to it for each individual in his or her care are a challenge so that better plans of care and improved sensitivity to the individual's needs can be achieved.

Based on the Bill of Rights, the challenges for the speech and language therapist must be:

- how to provide for service access and informed diagnosis;
- what constitutes appropriate speech and language therapy care;
- what advice and training to provide for others;
- how to ensure continuing professional development in dementia for speech and language therapists.

And having met these:

- What evidence exists of a positive outcome for such investment?

This chapter considers service review and quality as the keys to ensuring growth and development of future care for this patient group and for their caregivers.

Table 12.1: Alzheimer's Disease Bill of Rights

Every person diagnosed with Alzheimer's disease or a related disorder deserves:

- to be informed of one's diagnosis
- to have appropriate, ongoing medical care
- to be productive in work and play as long as possible
- to be treated like an adult, not a child
- to have expressed feelings taken seriously
- to be free from psychotropic medications if at all possible
- to live in a safe, structured and predictable environment
- to enjoy meaningful activities to fill each day
- to be out of doors on a regular basis
- to have physical contact including hugging, caressing and hand-holding
- to be with persons who know one's life story, including cultural and religious traditions
- to be cared for by individuals well trained in dementia care

---

Source: Troxel (1994).

Dilemmas in care

Health professionals in the new NHS face many philosophical, ethical and moral dilemmas on a daily basis. Issues such as allocation and provision of care for progressive disorders versus acute care; prioritisation versus the return for society; intervention or management; efficacy and outcome are all debated.

In dementias these choices are further complicated if we encompass the World Health Organisation sequelae of disease: Impairment, Disability, Handicap and Distress (Enderby, 1992), recognising that the disabling, handicapping and distress factors may shift the focus from the sufferer to the carer.

Concept of care

Throughout history there has been a succession of specific care groups for whom provision of services has generated more moral ethical decision and latterly financial decision making than others: the learning disabled (mental handicapped) in the1950s; the elderly in the 1960s; organ donation and transplantation and IVF in the 1970s and 1980s; HIV/AIDS into the 1990s. During these decades the 'silent epidemic' of dementias was spreading until, at the point of greatest recognition in the mid-1980s, the question was raised as to whether we should (or more particularly would be able to) work with yet another group who were in all likelihood close to the end of their lives and who, though previously contributing and active members of society, were unlikely to make a further contribution. The assumption prevailed that intervention can be justified if it benefits the individual or those caring for that individual whether or not there is a return to or for society.

The therapeutic philosophy

Degenerative diseases also bring dilemmas for care professionals, especially those in the therapies, implicit in whose care aims is a positive bias towards rehabilitation, improvement, alleviation or problem resolution. Implicit also in the term *therapy* is an expectation to alleviate the linguistic and cognitive sequelae of the disease.

A major conceptual change has been to adopt the more umbrella terms of intervention or management. These might include:

- specific therapy techniques in a therapist–patient model;
- direct or indirect individual or group techniques;
- evaluation and advice;
- counselling and training of others to manage and facilitate communication.

This range of care aims is covered, for example, by the Scottish Community Core Dataset/EPPIC definitions (see Table 12.2) which include enabling; maintenance and support; palliative care, etc. (Health Services Division Scotland, 1995).

From the therapeutic viewpoint many clinicians also view quality only against measurable gains. For them there can be no such measure for progressive conditions whose outcome for the patient is inexorably negative, because predictive outcome would be based on loss or deterioration. It will be shown later that the notion of consensus change, e.g. by therapist and carer, can still be effectively addressed even in degenerative conditions (Walker, Caird and Gilhooly, 1992). In the introduction it was suggested that the speech and language therapy profession faces three major challenges. These were also well recognised by the RCSLT Working Group in Dementia (1993):

- access to service and diagnosis;
- appropriacy of speech and language therapy care;
- training and development in the speciality.

To determine whether we can fulfill the Bill of Rights and are meeting the challenges requires a framework which can also evaluate:

- quality of service/organisation;
- quality of clinical care;
- quality of the clinician.

Haffenden (1991), in his list of carer needs, also identified three major requirements: (a) a service related to the circumstances, needs and views arrived at through consultation; (b) practical help to lighten the task of caring; (c) someone to talk to about their needs.

Table 12.2: The Scottish Community Core Data Set – care aims (the extended care aims are given in Appendix 6)

The Scottish Community Core Dataset

Care aims
Assessment*
Rehabilitation
Restorative/Problem resolution
Enabling**
Supportive care**
Maintenance care**
Palliative care**

*Assessment alone. Otherwise implicit in all areas
**Likely care focus

To determine whether all of these requirements are satisfied involves evaluation of equity of access, with systematic auditing; responsiveness to the individual's needs and changes of need; empowerment, the inclusion of clients and carers in the control of the outcome process.

As will be shown later, this might essentially fulfil the democratic approach to evaluating quality in health care.

The organisation/service quality

Proving fit for purpose, i.e. capability, inextricably links the standard of the clinician, the structure of the organisation and the measure of clinical activity.

Audit can be applied to all or aspects of each of these. For example:

* by profiling the skills and expertise needed by a clinician working with a particular client group;
* by verifying the ability of the organisation to meet the needs of the communication-impaired population as a whole, or a specific care group, and against local and/or professional guidelines;
* by evaluating outcomes of clinical, patient- or carer-centred activities.

A service can offer well-organised delivery but fail to meet patient needs because of inappropriate specialist knowledge. Similarly, patient needs may not be satisfactorily met by good clinicians who lack organisational structures and processes in which to practise. Finally, activity without verification of effectiveness of outcome may be activity for its own sake only.

There is a public expectation that patients and their carers and relatives are entitled to a service in which requisite knowledge, skills and attitudes will be efficiently applied to the management of disorders of communication irrespective of aetiology (RCSLT, 1993). The most appropriate way of determining fitness of purpose is by quality assurance of audit.

Service quality

Audit has been described as the documented systematic and critical gathering of evidence about performance of day-to-day practice and comparison of this evidence with previously defined purposes and standards to establish the level of performance. Essentially it should systematically and independently examine these components, implicit in which is the ability to identify deficiencies and take remedial action.

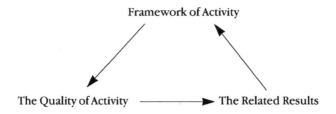

Figure 12.1: Components in clinical audit

More specifically clinical audit encompasses the activities of any health care professional with direct patient contact (see Figure 12.1). The speech and language therapy profession has embraced the basic concept of audit in clinical practice (Van der Gaag, 1993).

Audit approaches

Various approaches have been made to measure quality in health care:

1. *The traditional approach* equates quality to a superior service, with the expectation of expense, and status, but which has little relevance to welfare services.
2. *The scientific (or expert) approach* relates quality to 'fitness for purpose' according to standards set by experts. This is most commonly the choice for medical audit but it can ignore public opinion, requires significant internal policing and can lead to professional autonomy and personal preference, owing to insularity within the professional group.
3. *The managerial/excellence approach* proposes customer satisfaction as the key and involves everyone in the responsibility for (commercial) success. Its profit-driven nature and emphasis on managerial power are not suited to welfare services.
4. *The consumerist approach* empowers the consumer to have choice. However, as choice may not equal quality, and choice based only on cost may defeat quality, this leads to problems. The purchaser–provider concept of the present NHS encourages managers to make choices on behalf of patients, hence the managers become the consumers, not the patients, who then have little control.
5. A more *democratic approach* can be achieved by incorporating aspects of these previous approaches. In the health service this offers a more multifactorial approach involving the experts, managers, clinicians and patients. The purpose is not to give everyone the *same* but as *equal* chance, i.e. equity. Equity is suggested as the real test of quality for any welfare service. Thus audit, incorporating as many of these factors as possible, is proposed as the most effective method for achieving service quality.

The next section aims to consider whether a model for service can be achieved which encompasses the components shown in Figure 12.1:

- Audit of the organisation of care and its components for the EM1 client, i.e. the framework.
- Audit of the appropriacy of the therapist, in terms of personal, experiential and clinical specifications required for the job and the role *per se*.
- Audit of outcome in a progressive neuro-degenerative disease as applied to speech and language therapy/communication, i.e. evaluation of the clinical activity.

Quality of organisation

The RCSLT has provided clinical guidelines and standards for all patient groups and for clinical organisation, as well as specific recommendations for patients with dementia (RCSLT 1991, 1993). Such guidelines would support a model capable of providing open referral and access and continuing access over time. The model should address the needs of patient and caregiver on an individual basis. It should provide for appropriate assessment and management as required, and be able to demonstrate efficacy and outcome from the client, carer and service perspectives.

Enderby (1993) has outlined the organisational and clinical requirements of a 'good' service (see Table 12.3) which endorses the 'model' structure.

Specifying therapist quality

The Bill of Rights states that every person deserves 'to be cared for by individuals well trained in dementia care'. It is expected that all clinical posts carry specifications, both for the person and for the job. The working party in dementias also suggested undergraduate and postgraduate training needs as identified by therapists working with this patient group. Davies and Van der Gaag (1992) attempted to identify a consensus view on the attributes, skills and competences required by therapists working with several patient care groups including the elderly.

Their commission was to determine professional competence of speech and language therapists in terms of core knowledge base; skills and skills mix; and attitudes and attributes. Appendix 7 illustrates the distribution of agreement on knowledge base (Table 7a) the skills base (Tables 7b, 7c, 7d, 7e, 7f) and the attitudes base (Table 7g). In combination these would support a therapist profile specifying a significant breadth and depth of knowledge and experience with adults, the elderly and the elderly mentally infirm. Such a personal specification might expect the postholder to demonstrate or be working towards fulfilling a continuing professional development portfolio which might comprise the following components (see p.252):

Table 12.3: Broad care standard aim: speech and language therapy (after Enderby 1993)

Client/carers' need	Implications	Client/carers' need	Implications
To have communication problem/identified noticed.	Better awareness of speech/language difficulties in health care/medical, social services and education authority staff.	Not to be given ineffective treatment.	Treatment planning, goal setting. Standards of care. Peer review. Support of staff.
To be referred or refer self to appropriate service.	More awareness of referral procedures among staff and voluntary agencies. Improve public awareness.	Knowledge of progress.	Reassessment using objective as well as subjective methods. Good record keeping. Communication skills.
To know if one has been referred. Be sent acknowledgement of referral and appointment.	Standards should include procedure for management of clinics, prioritising of patients' communication systems and waiting list management.	To be given help with the handicapping aspects of the condition.	Counselling skills. Time for support. Involvement of carers.
Not to wait too long for appointment.	Appropriate staffing levels. Prioritisation system to identify length of waiting time.	Not to feel abandoned when treatment is completed.	Help with realistic expectations. Appropriate use of support groups and volunteers.
To see therapist in convenient location.	Comprehensive service across district and in key locations.	To be given information on alternative treatment when appropriate.	Awareness of speech therapy framework. Knowledge of own competence, and of alternative opinions.
To see therapist who has an appropriate manner.	Appropriate staff selection. Interpersonal skill training and supervision.	To have treatment carried out in organised and structured manner.	Goal setting, note keeping, professional competence.

To be assessed bearing in mind all relevant information.	Pre-registration training, continuing education and supervision.	To be assisted in a way that inspires confidence.	Adhering to standards of practice. Personal skills of therapist. Management of department.
To be referred to relevant professionals.	Familiarity with other services available.	To be discharged from treatment when appropriate.	Staffing levels, standards of care, peer review. Supervision and support.
To have information explained clearly.	Training, departmental policies, liaison with support groups, information leaflets.	To be offered appointments regularly as is appropriate but not making unnecessary unrewarding visits.	Staff levels, competence, treatment planning.
To have competent diagnosis made and explained.	Training, continuing education, communication skills.	To have treatment coordinated with others involved.	Multidisciplinary team involvement. Common skills. Management.
To understand implications of the disorder.	Training – use of other clinical experts within discipline. Development of clinical expertise. Use of support agencies. Information leaflets.	To have records kept in professional manner and confidential.	Adherence to administrative standards, office procedures, note keeping skills, secretarial support.
Realistic treatment programme with defined goals.	Knowledge of treatment, efficacy and expectations. Treatment planning, goal setting. Peer review.	To be treated in safe, appropriate surroundings, which allow for quiet and confidential facilities.	Adherence to policies on health and safety at work. Provision of appropriate facilities. General cleanliness and maintenance of facilities.

Sample: Portfolio/Package of Training

1. Open University Mental Health of the Elderly
2. RCSLT advanced course in elderly/dysphasia.

Evidence of Learning Based Activity covering:

(a) *communication in normal ageing*;
(b) considerations of *testing/managing* in the elderly: sensory/cognitive, psychological sequelae;
(c) *assessment* of communication in the dementias: aphasia model approach; global approach; situation/function; competence/performance; cognitive neuropsychology;
(d) *dementias*; dysphasias; and communication in other psychiatric disorders. To include DAT, semantic dementia, multiple systems atrophy, progressive supranuclear palsy (PSP), cortical and subcortical presentations. The relationship to genetic, chromosome and other progressive neurological conditions, i.e. Down's syndrome, Parkinson's disease;
(e) *carers*: evaluating knowledge; carers' perceptions of communication; carers' reactions of grief and loss; counselling and psychosocial support;
(f) *management and care planning*: patient and carer focus; focal neuro-concomitants, i.e. dysphagia; targeted communication tasks; group work techniques; reality orientation; reminiscence; social skills; advice and training of carers; reassessment and restructuring care plans;
(g) *service organisation and issues*: determining local needs; allocating resources; etc.

Hence this job profile expects an extensive knowledge and skills base, maturity of attitude and evidence of focused continuing professional development. In the Hay system (1994) of job evaluation in health care, these could be assessed and the specialist and specialised responsibility for such a clinical profile acknowledged. It might be surmised that the responsibility for a caseload within such a specific client group includes complex cases, multiple presentation and critical diagnosis. The likelihood of a local advisory role, with service delivery and evaluation across one's own and others' caseloads, is also likely to allocate this post to the upper clinical grade spinal points.

Quality of clinical activity

Having considered aspects of quality in the organisation and the therapist, we must address the third component: clinical audit applied to direct patient care activities. Enderby (1993) (see Table 12.3) highlights expected and acceptable clinical activities, i.e. realistic treatment programmes with defined goals. Appropriacy and quality in clinical care are considered to constitute that care which would be accepted as reasonable by a body of our peers. The Bill of Rights embraces this concept under 'To have appropriate ongoing medical care'.

Guidelines and standards of appropriacy for general clinical care are given in *Communicating Quality* (RCSLT, 1991) which is to be revised in 1996. As yet there is no prescriptive model for specificity in speech and language therapy care. Indeed the diversity and innovatory approaches described elsewhere in this book preclude such definition, except for core clinical requirements covered by organisational audit, i.e. record keeping, case recording, etc. Clinical activity also embraces (as stated earlier in the chapter) the need to demonstrate some effective outcome for the time invested in clinical activity.

Having discussed the dilemmas in the concept of care and the therapeutic philosophy in neuro-degenerative disorders, a clinical service model will be described that attempts to overcome these dilemmas, and to address and incorporate many issues of quality.

Closing the circle

The service described here was established in 1993 at the Victoria Infirmary NHS Trust in Glasgow. The service was founded on the outcome of a Scottish Home and Health Department research project grant (HSRC Grant No. K/OPR/2/2C879), which had demonstrated the potential of different intervention packages to influence caregiver well-being and perceptions (Walker, Caird and Gilhooly, 1992). The service is provided by one speech and language therapist with a recognised portfolio in adult acquired disorders with specialism in the elderly (Postgraduate degree, Dip. ACS and research).

The study referred to above provided the model for the service set out in Figure 12.2, including the assessment measures, management packages and timescale.

Additional to the care study, the service now incorporates the Scottish Community Core Dataset care aims definitions (see Table 12.2), an extended package (see Appendix 6) and a method of evaluating activity outcomes, consensus evaluation and user audit. The specific remit for the service is 'to offer those with memory problems and their professional and family carers, assessment and training in practical ways of coping with the social and verbal communication problems on an individual basis'.

The programme has three components:

Stage 1a: to assess the patient's baseline communication ability and determine his or her response to specific techniques aimed at promoting the best response and interaction;

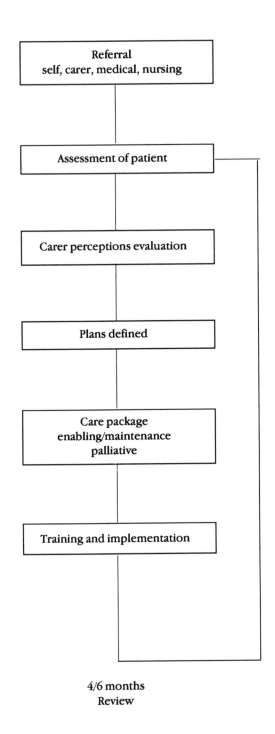

Figure 12.2: Speech and language therapy – a model for a dementia service

Stage 1b: to determine the concerns expressed by carers with regard to day-to-day communication problems;

Stage 2: to combine both 1a and 1b to form an individual management plan;

Stage 3: to advise and train carers in techniques and strategies.

Access

The service is routinely offered as part of the range of clinical speech and language therapist specialist services in a district general hospital. There is open access and open referral; however, confirmation of diagnosis and medical endorsement are sought. The service provides for both direct referral and tertiary referral from other speech and language therapists. Patients and carers are also encouraged to access the therapist on request at any time of concern or need.

Assessment and management

The patient-centred procedures are given in Appendix 8. These procedures were chosen and/or modified not only to provide baselines but also to incorporate information on potential as well as actual communication. These form the basis for goal setting (Appendix 9).

Outcome measures

An effort has been made to provide multifactorial rating of outcome for:

- level of impairment;
- level of disability;
- level of communicative burden (on carer);
- overall rating of communication (by carer);
- agreement score at each review or retest.

The outcome measure form is given in Appendix 10.

According to the care aim, i.e. maintenance or palliative, positive outcomes or expected outcomes can be arrived at from various permutations of the measures. For example: patient-centred deterioration in impairment and disability with carer-centred level of communicative burden maintained or improved would represent a positive outcome, as would maintenance of level of impairment and disability with reduced level of communicative burden.

Review, continuing care and open access

The department operates a database register which offers a system for maintaining contact with patients known to the speech and language therapy service and diagnosed as having progressive neurological disorders or other 'high-risk' aetiologies, i.e. head, neck or cranial tumours. The aim is 'to provide a structure for good practice', for these patients and for their carers.

The system provides for patients with dementia or other cognitive decline (e.g. associated with Parkinson's disease), and particularly those currently having enabling, supportive or maintenance care aims (see Appendix 7).

The register ensures that:

- the key therapist retains knowledge and maintains access to a summary record of the patient;
- therapists are provided with routine reminders of review or recall; and hence
- the prescriptive care aims are fulfilled.

User audit

A patient (or informant) questionnaire is routinely given to all patients on initial contact with the department and at the end of a period of care. This has been modified to accommodate progressive neurological case management.

By upholding and evolving the basic quality of the clinician, quality of the organisation and quality of clinical activity, we have attempted to structure a service based on the identified needs and circumstances of clients and carers. Practical management to lighten the care-giving role and a caring milieu in which to provide a forum to discuss communication and other needs is also provided. Norlin (1986) said that there are unique problems for families experiencing acquired communication deficits. He labels the phenomenon the 'metacommunication barrier'. Metacommunication is defined as communicating about communication. Families with a member whose communication is impaired are denied this opportunity. Successful coping by carers involves talking amongst family members as well as with professionals. Because of the unique nature of the communication and cognitive deficit, families are often unable to use this strategy. The inability to maintain relationships and verbally achieve problem solving locks families into a spiral of frustration and impotence. Enabling families to escape this spiral by providing opportunity and routes round the metacommunication barrier is a major goal in family intervention.

By acknowledging the contribution of the client and the carer in the process and being responsive to them and their changing needs we are working towards fulfilling fitness for purpose.

Conclusion

Norman (1990) described a 'pyramid of need' in dementia. Securing the care of the elderly mentally disordered person in the centre requires meeting the needs of everyone on all other sides. In a similar way providing a good service for any client and carer depends on addressing quality issues on each side of the same pyramid (see Figure 12.3).

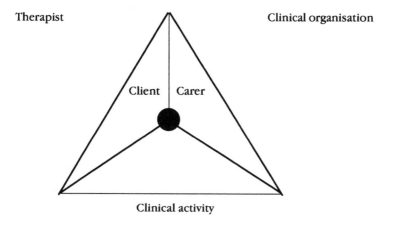

Figure 12.3: Pyramid of need in dementia.

This chapter has focused on charters, professional and clinical standards and guidelines and the experience of speech and language therapists, carers and elderly mentally ill clients. Drawing on these elements, it is possible to go some way towards meeting the challenge for better, appropriate and justifiable care for many elderly disabled people and their families.

Chapter 13:
Future Directions

KAREN BRYAN AND JANE MAXIM

Introduction

Recent changes in the NHS, particularly the move towards community care, and research advances, have produced a number of positive developments in speech and language therapy services for older people with mental health problems:

- Legislative changes have provided an opportunity for services to be reconsidered and, in some cases, restructured. Occasionally this may involve additional funding, but innovation is also evident in the flexible use of existing resources, for example, as we saw in Chapter 8.
- Clinical managers have more flexibility to consider options for the use of limited resources (although the fact that resources are limited might not be considered as positive).
- Clinical specialists in the psychiatry of old age are now recognised as necessary.
- Speech and language therapy input to the multidisciplinary team is now more evident.
- Innovations in clinical practice such as memory clinics to which people can self-refer are evident.
- Special interest groups in old-age psychiatry now exist to support clinicians and to promote research and high-quality clinical practice.
- Research interest in this area is growing, with papers on the speech and language disorders in the dementias appearing in academic journals and on conference agendas.
- The need for training initiatives for care staff in the residential and nursing care sectors is now recognised by both care staff and their managers. Speech and language therapists have the requisite skills and knowledge to carry out such training.
- Research is beginning to differentiate between different subgroups of disorders which is leading to clinically useful indicators for management, for example in multi-infarct dementia, semantic dementia and the progressive aphasias as well as in Alzheimer's disease.

- Community care has produced an increased role and an increased burden for carers. There is now government interest in and research on this burden and growing awareness of the need for carer support as a vital part of care packages.

Despite these improvements, there is no doubt that for speech and language therapy, as for other health and social services, the service to older people with psychiatric disorders is scarce, fragmented and variable owing to reliance upon local initiatives and resources.

Issues for service provision

A number of issues which have been raised and discussed elsewhere in this book are worth returning to as they are likely to be the key to improvement of services for older people with mental health problems.

Access to services

Access to rehabilitation services is not automatic for older people with mental health problems. There are a number of issues surrounding the local service:

- Is there a service to the elderly with psychiatric problems?
- Is the service restricted, i.e. assessment only?
- Is domiciliary care available?
- Are there restrictions on treatment options such as time limits or geographical constraints such as hospital-based treatment only?
- Is there efficient and effective coordination between health and social services elements of care packages?

A further issue of vital importance is whether or not there is access to services such as rehabilitation, for older people who are in residential and nursing homes. In some areas of the UK there is still no provision for older people who are in care; in other areas this is restricted to social services homes but does not extend to the private sector and in a few areas it is extended to all older people who are registered with local GPs regardless of where they live. The quality of the care offered is also variable. Given recent research findings into the dementias and the fact that treatments for dementia are likely to become available which may slow or even arrest the progression of the symptoms of dementia (Perry and Perry, 1993), the acceptability of 'assessment only' services must be questioned. Some clients with progressive disorders such as multi-infarct dementia can benefit from direct therapy (Swinburn and Maxim, Ch. 10). The continuity of care offered and the provision for training care staff, working with them for a short period of time to illustrate how to communicate effectively with a new resident and professional support for carers are all issues which need to be addressed in quality control initiatives by speech and language therapy managers.

Referral arrangements

Hall and Channing (1990) reported that many older people did not receive the help that they needed at home because they were reluctant to discuss non-specific or strictly 'non-medical' issues with GPs. Thus older people, almost invariably, consult their GPs ostensibly about some specific ailment. Their general condition may then go unregarded as doctors are often reluctant to embark on detailed questioning about functional problems in case this awakens latent fears and leads to negative thinking. Referral for services such as rehabilitation and indeed social provision such as home help and meals on wheels may then be rather arbitrary. Older people themselves may try to manage without seeking help. Studies have shown that elderly people accept a degree of impairment that they would have found unacceptable during middle age (Wells and Freer, 1988). Some older people may be well aware that they need help but may be reluctant to ask. Some doctors may not favour referral until as late a stage as possible, there may be budgetary constraints, although there is, as yet, no evidence that this restricts referral, or the doctor may just not have the necessary information to realise that extra help is needed (Hall and Channing, 1990). It may be that the present GP screening arrangements for over-75s need to be expanded or more carefully geared to allow older people to discuss their problems and worries rather than just addressing medical issues.

It may be that medical access, i.e. GP or geriatrician/psychogeriatrician referral to social services is not sufficient. At present many health care workers such as speech and language therapists would have to request referral to social services via a doctor. Although this referral might help with coordination of services, this is not always the case. Health care professionals such as speech and language therapists will often have a very clear idea of the problems that an older person has because they will have discussed daily routines, problems and priorities etc. in gaining a communicative history and in formulating an assessment of communicative needs.

Questions can be raised regarding the cost effectiveness of early referral to rehabilitation and social services. It has been shown in other areas, such as carer support, that early intervention allows the carer to cope more effectively and longer, therefore saving costs of expensive residential care (Brodaty and Peters, 1991). It may be the case that early referral to speech and language therapy for impairments such as word-finding difficulty or mild dysarthria will facilitate the preservation of independent living in older people by helping to prevent problems such as social isolation and depression. It is essential that methods of therapy audit which take account of qualitative gains, such as increase in general well-being and ability to cope with daily living, are accepted as valid indicators of therapy value.

Research involving clinical audit of services is needed in order to evaluate the most efficient and cost-effective way of ensuring adequate referral of older people to the help and support that they need.

Coordination of services

Services for the elderly mentally ill involve a range of provisions including health, social services, voluntary sector and family involvement. Problems are evident in coordinating these services (Webb, 1991) to achieve the best possible care package for the older client. An example is discharge from hospital: in a survey conducted in 1992, Neill and Williams found that one in five elderly people experienced a 'bad' discharge and that 59% were experiencing self-care difficulties. They state criteria for a good discharge which consist of:

- at least 24 hours' notice;
- an opportunity to discuss how they would manage after discharge;
- somebody with them on the journey home;
- somebody waiting for them at home;
- somebody to call and see them on the day of discharge.

Yet Jones and Lester reported in 1994 that 46% of carers could not recall discussion of the discharge taking place.

Examples of good discharge quoted above always involve visits to the home, provision of aids and adaptations prior to discharge and synchronisation of health and domiciliary provision to accomplish key tasks. This always involves expensive professional time and resources, but could allow very disabled older people to return home successfully thus avoiding expensive residential care and allowing the older person to achieve their goal of returning home. Professionals such as speech and language therapists may or may not be involved in such procedures with their clients. It may be that the role of rehabilitation professionals, such as speech and language therapists, needs to be discussed and defined, ratified by efficacy studies and then included in good practice guidelines, ensuring that high standards of service provision are generalised across the country.

Services for older people

Cassel (1994) stated that there is a need to recognise that for most elderly people the quality of life after age 75 is more important than the length of life. Therefore research and service provision need to be prioritised to address diseases that result in long-term disability such as dementia, depression, and visual and hearing disorders. Advances in preventing or delaying the onset of such disorders or in managing the resulting disabilities more effectively could greatly increase the independence and productivity of people in their older years (Cassel, 1994).

Age-based access to services is also questionable in its effectiveness at maintaining older people as independent and self-caring. In some cases, access to particular treatments might allow an elderly person to remain independent rather than needing to enter expensive residential care. Lack of rehabilitation services for the elderly mentally ill might be cited here as of particular concern. 'Ageism' is rife in the western world, and because there are increasing numbers of older people aged 85+, it is important to ensure that this increase does not lead to 'age rationing' of health resources. 'Age rationing' implies that older people are denied access to services which are of expected benefit to them; this is distinguished from cost containment where services that are not expected to be of benefit are withheld (Wicclair, 1993).

Services also need to be organised so that the elderly can benefit from them. Issues such as transport can determine whether older people can gain access to services which are provided. Speech and language therapists are starting to become involved in initiatives such as community-based services and training projects in residential homes but such initiatives need to become more widespread. The majority of specialist speech and language therapists who work with the elderly mentally ill remain hospital based, so there is a need for flexibility and outreach services to accommodate the older client and to give him or her the best possible chance of benefiting from therapy.

Perhaps therapy practices need to be evaluated in terms of their suitability for the elderly generally and for the elderly mentally ill in particular:

- Are the assessments that we use designed specifically for this client group or validated to use with this sector of the population?
- Is sufficient known about the effects of normal and pathological ageing on language and communication?
- Do we know enough about how the elderly use language and what their priorities are for functional communication?
- Do we know enough about what happens to language usage when older clients enter residential or nursing care?
- Do we have methods of therapy which have been designed for use with the elderly and/or validated with older clients?
- Do we organise speech and language therapy services for older clients to facilitate continuity of care for clients with needs which progress and result in changing needs such as entering day care and later full residential care?

The answer to most of the above is, sadly, only partially yes. But improvements are being made and increasing awareness is resulting in those issues being afforded greater prominence.

Future speech and language therapy services

We need to consider what an ideal health and social service for the older person would consist of, and then how speech and language therapy services would fit into this. An important starting point is health screening.

Under the new GP contract (Department of Health, 1989b) patients over the age of 75 were to be offered an annual assessment. It was envisaged that such screening would be carried out by practice nurses (UKCC, 1990) but there has been debate as to who should be involved (Nocon, 1992). The practice nurse would seem to be well placed to carry out the screening as he or she has the required skills (Mackereth, 1995) and the process would be time-consuming for a GP. The screening could therefore consist of a home visit by a trained practice nurse who is part of the team from the local GP's surgery. The nurse would use a structured questionnaire to interview the older clients. She or he would try to address general concerns such as housing, coping with activities of daily living, social isolation etc. as well as carrying out some basic health screening such as blood pressure and tests for diabetes. The nurse practitioner would then report to the GP and would be able to make referrals directly (in consultation with the GP) to social services, geriatrician or psychogeriatrician, physiotherapy, speech and language therapy and any other services deemed necessary. Once the referrals were implemented, reports would come back to the nurse practitioner via the GP. At this early stage, a key worker should be appointed if the elderly client has complex problems or if there is no regular carer available to check on arrangements, etc. At present, key workers for clients in the community are primarily social workers. It may be appropriate for other professionals to become involved in this role, for example a physiotherapist for someone whose primary problem is physical difficulty and a speech and language therapist if an elderly client has difficulty in communicating. The role of key workers with regard to advocacy for people who are unable to make their needs known should be clarified. Perhaps key workers need to have a client-representing role that is divorced from service provision concerns. This would then leave social workers to assume a more clearly defined care-manager role where matching needs to local service availability will be necessary.

The elderly person should then receive the required treatments following the health screening. It is essential that treatments are available in the community, perhaps being day-hospital based with outreach for elderly clients who do not need to attend hospital. Current research into drug treatments (Farlow et al., 1992) to slow down or even partially arrest the decline in dementia is promising. It would then follow that a larger number of relatively well older people will be based in the community and these people will require help and support from health care professionals for extended periods of time.

All professionals would report back to the nurse practitioner via the GP. She or he would then ensure that the elderly client has a review of their progress at a recommended time and that any treatments are followed through. Because many elderly people have multiple problems which necessitate contact with many agents, in both the professional and voluntary sectors, it may be necessary for contacts to be logged, especially where language or cognitive problems may make it difficult for the client to report on recent visits. A health log book could be used so that all contacts are recorded. The nurse practitioner would then have a way of easily checking on the client's level of support.

The nurse practitioner might review the elderly client regularly if problems are ongoing or would revert to annual review if the problems were acute and responded to remediation. This would give the system some continuity so that a nurse going back to an elderly client would notice changes in the person's circumstances, or the onset of a condition such as depression which might not be so obviously evident on an initial visit. The majority of over-75s will be essentially fit and well so that the review process will not be time-consuming. Resources can then be targeted at those who need help. A further advantage is that if an older person has had several annual reviews prior to developing problems, they will have a contact, a person that they know and who will, it is hoped, be seen as non-threatening and sympathetic. This may assist in enabling elderly people to seek the help that they need at an early stage rather than after a crisis such as hospitalisation following a fall that could have been prevented.

As the older person develops medical problems or needs more help with activities of daily living, care might be transferred primarily to either:

- medical care under a geriatrician or psychogeriatrician;
- social services care under a care manager or social worker.

In either case, for as long as the elderly person remains in the community, the nurse practitioner needs to remain involved and to monitor the situation, with the GP being alerted when problems are occurring. Perhaps the nurse practitioner should assume the key worker as 'advocate' role once care is not entirely GP based. The nurse would be in a strong position to be an 'advocate' as he or she would know the elderly person, would have detailed records on their previous care, social situation etc. and would provide the elderly person with some continuity of care. Also the key worker would be informed of changes in care such as discharge from hospital which require careful coordination. The nurse could also alert the GP to any problems that were occurring after discharge from hospital and could carry out routine monitoring for the GP. The nurse practitioner would therefore still be involved with the care of older people with multiple or complex problems, but this would be more contained so as not to duplicate efforts.

Many elderly people, even those with multiple problems and severe levels of disability, can remain in the community if sufficient help and support are locally available. Others will need to enter residential or nursing home care, the majority of which is now in the private sector. At this point the nurse practitioner would have a vital role. She or he would be able to give the residential or nursing home staff information about the elderly person and his or her care. If the home was local, the elderly person would probably remain under the GP's care, so the nurse practitioner's monitoring and key worker 'advocate' role could continue. If transfer into residential care involved a change of GP, then the nurse practitioner could refer the person to the relevant doctor's nurse practitioner, again being able to transfer information and provide some continuity of care.

Advantages to a nurse practitioner scheme are that:

- nurses are cheaper to employ than GPs and screening may not be the best use of a GP's time where there are no significant medical problems;
- if the nurses could provide a primarily home-based service, then this might be much less threatening for elderly people. There are also some indications that elderly people might be more comfortable with the idea of speaking to a nurse rather than 'wasting the doctor's time';
- regular reviews would allow older people to get to know the nurse, in the case of the vast majority, before problems occurred. The nurse would then be well placed to monitor changes;
- nurse practitioners who are GP-surgery based should ensure that inputs to the older clients are better coordinated and that older people are not 'lost in the system';
- nurse practitioners can provide continuity of care as the elderly person's needs change;
- the nurse review system should facilitate problems coming to light before medical problems which require expensive treatments, i.e. hospitalisation, occur.

So far we have advocated services for older people being locally based and GP surgery coordinated via a nurse practitioner review system. Let us now consider how speech and language therapy services would operate within this system and how they would extend through the range of care options that an elderly person might require, ranging from domiciliary service to a person who lives independently in the community to a service for highly dependent people resident in a nursing home.

Speech and language therapists would assess elderly people from medical referrals and also people referred as a result of the screening process detailed here. Self-referral should also be possible, perhaps via an accepted route such as a memory clinic. Assessment would look at language, cognition and communication. Where necessary a carer interview would be included. The speech and language therapist would report to:

- the referring agent;
- the GP via the practice nurse;
- the social worker or care manager if the client has one.

The issue of whether speech and language therapists (and other professionals) should be able to make direct referrals to social services or whether this should continue to operate through the GP needs to be evaluated. Perhaps the type of fast and efficient screening and monitoring process by a practice nurse that has been advocated above would mean that delays in referral that occur today could be avoided whilst preserving 'GP' coordination of referrals.

Speech and language therapy services would then provide the necessary management and treatment for the elderly client with psychiatric problems. Access to treatment should not be age based but should be based on needs and ultimately on proven efficacy. A code of practice for older clients with psychiatric disorders might include:

- adequate assessment;
- assessment for treatment, for example assessment of learning potential in multi-infarct dementia (see Chapter 10);
- access to direct treatment of language and communication difficulties using treatments found to be most effective;
- access to indirect treatment via (a) communication groups; (b) support groups: (c) initiatives for carers; (d) volunteer schemes;
- speech and language therapy follow up if required or a specific request to the practice nurse to follow up language and communication in subsequent general reviews.

Speech and language therapists also have an important information-giving role. This involves information carefully tailored in terms of content and method of presentation for:

- clients;
- carers;
- other professionals;
- day centre and other staff/personnel involved in aspects of community care;
- residential and nursing home managers;
- residential and nursing home staff.

The information should include a written summary encompassing specific actions that can be taken. An example might be the *Action for Dysphasic Adults* booklet specifically designed for residential care staff (Lester and Ashley, 1995). It should also include recommendations to other staff and carers for general communicative needs, for example needing to socialise or needing access to pen and paper when 'talking'.

The speech and language therapist would therefore need to maintain an input when the care provision for an elderly person changes. If home care becomes involved, then the home care workers may need help in learning how to communicate with the person. If a client subsequently enters a residential or nursing home, then a period of intervention may be needed in order to assess how the elderly person adapts to communicating in the new environment, possibly some input from the therapist to maximise this and some input to the care staff on how to manage the communication disorder and how to achieve the best possible level of effective communication with the client.

Community care recommendations for speech and language therapists

If care practices for older people with psychiatric problems are to reach the levels advocated above, it will be necessary for speech and language therapy services to change and adapt to the philosophy of care provision and to the funding method. The profession will need to initiate or take part in the following:

- There needs to be a 'national-level' agreement on the role of speech and language therapists in private sector residential and nursing care. We would advocate equal access for older people to rehabilitation irrespective of whether they have public or private sector care. For many elderly people, private residential care is the only option available to them, so this should not constitute a barrier to public sector services. Rehabilitation should be available in the 'homes' so that issues such as lack of suitable transport do not constitute a further barrier.
- The profession needs to press for a statutory requirement for the provision of rehabilitation in the private care sector.

- There should also be support for a statutory requirement for providers of residential and nursing care to include provision for staff training in their contracts.
- Speech and language therapy services need to be more involved in working in the community. The current emphasis on hospital-based services might need to be reconsidered with national guidelines agreed to promote the development of clinical specialists in the psychiatry of old age, and to recommend ways of extending services into the community, perhaps including more flexibility in working practices.
- Speech and language therapy involvement in the multidisciplinary team needs to continue to develop, again with isolated examples of practice excellency being adopted as recommended standards throughout the UK.
- Speech and language therapy clinical specialists and/or managers need to continue to be involved in local planning of all services for elderly people with psychiatric problems so that the needs of the communicatively impaired are represented and addressed.
- The profession needs to promote a clinic-based research programme to develop and evaluate working practices.

A research agenda for the future

Many changes in working practices for speech and language therapists have been advocated here, mostly based on trying to promote particular examples of good practice, which have been discussed throughout this book, as standards for national service delivery aims. All of these developments need to be supported by data from clinically based research. Some of the key areas for the future research agenda are:

- joint research initiatives with practice nurses and GPs to develop structured interview 'conversational' formats for health screening for older people;
- studies of the language breakdown in non-Alzheimer dementias where there is currently very little available information, for example multi-infarct dementia, Pick's disease, Parkinsonian dementia, progressive supranuclear palsy, multi-system atrophy, cortical Lewy body disease;
- in the absence of more specific medical diagnosis among the dementias, assessments which accurately define clients' strengths and weaknesses are needed so that therapy input can be targeted;
- more assessments for the elderly are needed; these include currently used tests which need to be standardised on older populations, specialist tests for the dementias and shorter more effective screening tests for language and cognitive functioning which might include a carer questionnaire;

- more therapies for the treatment of language and communication disabilities in the elderly mentally ill need to be developed;
- treatment interventions need to be evaluated from quantitative and qualitative perspectives;
- efficacy guidelines for intervention and management of elderly clients with psychiatric problems need to be developed.

We hope that the issues raised or highlighted here will provoke debate. Speech and language therapists and other health care professionals are committed to improving services and therapeutic interventions for older clients with psychiatric problems and this commitment should continue to provide service innovation and research.

Appendix 1: Suggested format for statistical recording of clinical services

EMI SERVICE – SPEECH/LANGUAGE THERAPY

SOURCE	REF. AND CONTACTS	LAST YEAR'S FIGURES PER QTR	APRIL– JUNE	JULY– SEPTEMBER	OCTOBER– DECEMBER	JANUARY– MARCH
Day Unit	R					
	C					
GPs	R					
	C					
Psycho-geriatrician	R					
	C					
	R					
	C					
	R					
	C					
	R					
	C					
	R					
	C					
	R					
	C					

COMMENTS

OTHER
RELEVANT
INFORMATION

Appendix 2:
Lack of Consent Form for a Legal Guardian of a Client

(A) It has been fully and carefully explained to me by:

_____

_____

(full name, description)

that if I ignore the advice given to me regarding the eating habits and/or drinking habits of

_____

_____

(full name), then he/she faces the very real and likely risk that he/she will suffer severe and potentially life-threatening consequences. The advice that has been given to me is

_____

_____

_____

_____

Patient Name:
Hospital No.
Patient/Legal Guardian Name:
Signature
Date

Speech/Language Therapist Name:
Signature
Date

Doctor in Charge Name:
Signature:
Date

Appendix 3: Lack of Consent Form for a Representative of a Client

(B) I, _____ (full name)
     _____ (address)
     _____
     _____
     _____

being the representative of

_____

_____

(patient name and hospital number)

confirm that I have given the identical advice to him/her to that given to him/her by the Speech/Language Therapist (name and designation ....) and/or doctor in charge (name and designation ....) with regard to his/her eating habits and/or drinking habits.

Signed:
Date:

SLT Name: Doctor in charge name:
Signature   and/or   Signature
Date   Date

NB.

Appendix 4: List of Addresses of Voluntary Organisations

Action for Dysphasic Adults
Northcote House
37A Royal Street
Llondon SE1

Age Concern
Bernard Sunley House
60 Pitcairn Road
Mitcham
Surrey CR4 3LL

Alzheimer's Disease Society
Gordon House
10 Greencoat Street
London SW1 1PH

Parkinson's Disease Society
22 Upper Woburn Place
London WC1H ORA
Tel: 0171 383 3513

The Stroke Association
CHSA House
Whitecross Street
London EC1

Appendix 5: Questionnaires for Staff in Residential Care Settings

LONG-STAY QUESTIONNAIRE ONE

Thank you for completing this questionnaire. We hope that it will help us to improve our teaching sessions.

Please circle the answer you feel to be correct for each statement, true or false.

1. Ways to improve your communication with residents who have difficulties understanding:
   (a) talk louder
       True/False
   (b) talk slower
       True/False
   (c) use simpler words and grammar
       True/False
   (d) reduce the amount of non-verbal communication
       True/False
   (e) increase the amount of non-verbal communication
       True/False

2. Things which limit the communication opportunities of residents in continuing care units:
   (a) the environment
       True/False
   (b) other residents
       True/False
   (c) silence
       True/False
   (d) reduced mobility
       True/False
   (e) sensory impairments, e.g. hearing/vision
       True/False
   (f) disinterest in communication
       True/False

(g)   noise
      True/False
(h)   reduced choice
      True/False
(i)   limited activities
      True/False

3.   Which of the following statements is True/False of stroke, Parkinson's disease,
      and dementia:

		Dementia	Stroke	Parkinson's disease
(e)	Speech may be affected?	True/False	True/False	True/False
(f)	Language may be affected?	True/False	True/False	True/False
(g)	Memory may be affected?	True/False	True/False	True/False
(h)	Swallowing may be affected?	True/False	True/False	True/False

4. If someone wears a hearing aid, you should:
(a)   shout?
      True/False
(b)   talk at a normal volume and speed?
      True/False
(c)   speak very, very slowly?
      True/False
(d)   make sure that they can see your face?
      True/False
(e)   talk into the ear with the aid in it?
      True/False

5. The average hearing aid battery lasts for:
(a)   a year?
      True/False
(b)   6 months?
      True/False
(c)   6 weeks?
      True/False
(d)   2 weeks?
      True/Fals
(e)   a few days?
      True/False

6. When using a standard hearing aid:
(a)   'o' = on?
      True/False
(b)   'o' = off?
      True/False
(c)   't' = tinnitus?
      True/False
(d)   'm' = mute?
      True/False
(e)   it is impossible to switch the hearing aid off?
      True/False

7.   If a resident is coughing/choking you should:
(a)   give them some water to wash it down
        True/False
(b)   get them to sit forward
        True/False
(c)   hit them on the back
        True/False
(d)   encourage them to rest before continuing
        True/False
(e)   continue to feed them to wash it down
        True/False

8.   The following are suitable ways for residents with swallowing problems or dementia to take drinks:
(a)   feeder cups
        True/False
(b)   tea cup
        True/False
(c)   spouted beakers
        True/False
(d)   straw
        True/False
(e)   syringe
        True/False

9. In general, someone with a swallowing problem will:
(a)   manage to drink tea if they can swallow ice cream?
        True/False
(b)   manage ice cream if they can swallow tea?
        True/False
(c)   need a softer, moister diet?
        True/False
(d)   need a pureed diet?
        True/False
(e)   manage iced drinks easier than hot drinks?
        True/False

Have you answered all the questions? Without the full completion of this questionnaire it will be difficult to evaluate our training and hence guarantee future speech and language therapy to your home/ward.

Thank you for completing this questionnaire

LONG-STAY QUESTIONNAIRE TWO

In order to evaluate the effectiveness of our teaching for your ward/home, please complete the questionnaire below:

Name of

Home/Ward:

Dates of Speech and Language Therapy

Training:

What were the most effective aspects of the Speech and Language Therapy training sessions?

What were the least effective aspects?

How will you be using the training to enhance patient care?

How will you measure the effectiveness of any changes made to your home/ward resulting from the training sessions, teaching file and/or videos?

Please use the space below to provide further comments on the training.

Thank you for your cooperation. Please return to Deirdre Rainbow at the address overleaf by _____ .

Appendix 6:
Extended SCCD Care Aims

ASSESSMENT

1. To determine the presence of a communication impairment.
2. To specify the nature and degree of the voice, speech, language or fluency deficit(s) and its effect on communicative efficacy.
3. To report the outcome of assessment to the patient, referring agency or other relevant person.
4. Where required to make recommendations as to prognosis, further intervention(s) or referral to another agency.

REHABILITATION

To determine impairment through assessment parameters 1–4.

2. To devise an individual patient care plan of explicit short- and long-term goals attending to those disabling, handicapping and distress factors which promote rehabilitation or optimal improvement. These might include:
   - specific technical linguistic/phonetic procedures;
   - enabling by others;
   - teaching and education of others;
   - psychosocial support;
   - behaviour modification;
   - stress management;
   - training in use of AAC.
3. To continually monitor response and gains towards rehabilitation goals against predicted change and to modify goals accordingly.

RESTORATIVE (CURATIVE) PROBLEM RESOLUTION

1. To determine the impairment through assessment procedures 1–4.
2. To determine the gap between normal competence (or milestones) and patient performance and devise a management plan which aims

to restore or achieve full voice, speech, language or communication competence. This might be achieved/delivered by a non-speech and language therapist, i.e. medical or surgical procedure, or by speech and language therapist activities. The latter might include:

- psychosocial support and counselling;
- behavioural modification;
- advice and training;
- enabling by others;
- technical speech and language therapy procedure.

3. To demonstrate at the end of a period of care that performance is within (acceptable) normal limits.

ENABLING

1. To specify and assess the nature of the communication difficulty.
2. To consider and/or determine all relevant cognitive social and educational and environmental factors contributing to communication performance.
3. To devise a management plan with short- and long-term goals attending to these patient-centred factors.
4. To train significant others in management techniques which best promote more appropriate, effective or optimal communication performance in social/family or educational contexts.
5. To regularly or continously monitor change, modify management plans and accordingly inform the enablers of these changes.

SUPPORTIVE CARE

1. To continue routine patient and carer contact at prescribed intervals within a care period.
2. To use these contacts to continually assess formally or informally all relevant linguistic, extralinguistic or communication factors in respect of:
   - communication performance;
   - communication competence;
   - readiness for other intervention(s);
   - mental or cognitive status;
   - cooperation, level of activation/initation;
   - use of AAC.
3. To provide regular ongoing status reports to relevant agencies.
4. To advise professional and family carers of modifications required to accommodate status change and implement these where appropriate.

MAINTENANCE CARE

1. To provide continued opportunity for communication in formal and/or informal settings to promote optimum communication and/or social interaction.
2. To provide social and psychosocial levels of support to specific patient groups and to their carers.

PALLIATIVE CARE

1. To continue to support and sustain contact with patients and carers by way of general welfare and concern, the technical speech and language therapy emphasis being non-essential.

Source: Walker, Gordon and Bain (1994)

Appendix 7: Elderly/Acquired Neurological Disorders

Table 7a: Distribution of Agreement on the Knowledge Base of Speech Therapy for Speech Therapists working with the Elderly/Adult Acquired Neurological Disorders

Service and Client Management

	Essential	Desirable %	Irrelevant
Theoretical and methodological bases for assessment including the following:			
Factors influencing assessment, e.g. environment related, person related	95	3	1
Differential assessments, e.g. dysphasias vs dementias	95	4	1
Standardised/non-standardised assessments	94	4	1
The therapeutic process including the following:			
Knowledge of appropriate therapies	98	–	1
Recognition of the aims and possible outcomes of therapy	97	1	1
Knowing when to refer on to another agency	96	2	1
Setting priorities	95	3	1
The role of other disciplines and how they interact	89	9	1
The role of voluntary agencies and support groups and how they interact	60	38	1
Knowledge of teaching methods and approaches including the following:			
– carers	75	22	1
– other professionals	68	28	1
– speech therapy assistants	66	30	1
– volunteers	62	34	1

Methods of supervising:

– student speech therapists	73	23	1
– speech therapists	71	26	1
– speech therapy assistants	68	29	1
– volunteers	63	35	1
Professional practice issues, e.g. code of ethics	93	5	1
Development of professional skills e.g. training needs	85	12	1
Self awareness/personal development	81	17	1
Time management	76	22	1
Health and safety issues	69	27	3
Principles of planning/organisation	61	36	1
Quality assurance indicators	56	43	–
Team dynamics	53	44	1
Clinical adult methods	45	52	3
Health Care Teams	48	50	1
Financial budgeting	17	72	10

TABLE 7B

Distribution of Agreement on the Knowledge Base of Speech Therapy for Speech Therapists working with the Elderly/Adult Acquired Neurological Disorders

Eating and Swallowing Management

	Essential	Desirable %	Irrelevant
Normal swallowing patterns	96	2	1
Anatomy and Physiology	95	3	1
Abnormal swallowing patterns	94	4	1
Health and safety issues	94	4	1
Therapy techniques	93	5	1
The role of the team	89	9	1
Ageing effects on swallowing patterns	83	15	1
Relevant equipment	83	15	1
Evaluative techniques: subjective and objective, e.g. videofluoroscopy	77	22	1
Relevant prophylactics	70	24	2

TABLE 7C

Distribution of Agreement on the Knowledge Base of Speech Therapy for Speech Therapists working with the Elderly/Adult Acquired Neurological Disorders

Policy

	Essential	Desirable %	Irrelevant
Legal aspects re speech therapy	79	20	1
Client group rights	61	36	1
Local relevance of legislation	32	61	1

Local environment and culture in			
Relation to policy implementation	29	65	5
Knowledge of terminal care agencies	29	68	2
Models of service delivery: health, education, social services	26	69	4
The NHS; structure and administration	25	71	3
DHSS policy documents and their implementation	21	74	10
Social epidemiology	14	74	10
Problems of service delivery in other disciplines	12	75	12

TABLE 7D

Distribution of Agreement on the Skills Base of Speech Therapy for Speech Therapists working with the Elderly/Adult Acquired Neurological Disorders

Teaching and Therapeutic skills

	1	2	3	4
		%		
Selecting and devising formal and informal assesments including the following:				
Making differential diagnoses	92	7	–	–
Making prognoses	87	12	1	–
Interpreting data	84	13	2	–
Administering formal assessments	83	12	4	1
Making ongoing assessments during therapy	81	9	8	1
Testing out hypotheses using a variety of assessment techniques	77	19	2	–
Recognising the client's strengths and weaknesses	24	41	22	11
Teaching skills including the following:	80	13	2	–
Train and supervise– –speech therapy assistants –volunteers –carers –other professionals				
Working within a variety of settings; institutions, homes, etc.	34	9	35	19
The application of integration of knowledge to the therapeutic process Including the following:				
Devising treatment plans	90	5	4	–
Devising management plans	75	21	2	–
Using specific diagnostic knowledge re: dementia/dysphasia/depression	75	22	1	–
Able to select appropriate intervention modes: one to one; group	72	17	8	1
Evaluate treatment effectiveness	72	15	9	2

Relate treatment tasks to functional needs	39	26	30	3
Liaise with other professionals	38	28	25	7
Using augmentative/alternative communication systems	29	18	37	13
Maintain flexibility within the treatment session	25	14	42	17
Using pacing strategies aptly	17	6	52	22
Using cueing strategies aptly	16	6	52	23
Modify own communication mode to suit client/carer	14	7	44	32
Manipulate environmental factors	13	20	37	27
Recognise variations in performance	12	17	34	34
Lip reading	4	21	35	–

TABLE 7E

Distribution of Agreement on the Skills Base of Speech Therapy for Speech Therapists working with the Elderly/Adult Acquired Neurological Disorders

The Psychological Skills

	1	2	3	4
		%		
Clinical interviewing skills	44	51	2	1
Analytical skills	32	54	8	3
Counselling skills	28	63	4	3
Problem solving skills	21	49	16	12
Logical thinking skills	19	41	20	19
Interpersonal skills– including the following:				
Explaining skills	24	25	32	16
Listening skills	21	17	31	29
Observation skills	16	21	32	28
Motivating others	10	23	34	30
Working with groups	7	15	54	22

TABLE 7F

Distribution of Agreement on the Skills Base of Speech Therapy for Speech Therapists working with the Elderly/Adult Acquired Neurological Disorders

Service and Client Management Skills

	1	2	3	4
		%		
Prioritising caseload	94	4	–	–
Recruitment/selection skills	84	13	1	–
Policy development	82	14	2	1
Report writing	77	13	5	3
Research and evaluation skills	68	28	2	–
Organisational skills	49	26	14	9
Public relations work	47	25	16	11
Recognising/giving support to staff	46	38	5	8
Time management skills	41	29	15	13

Skills of leadership	36	49	4	8
Record keeping	30	8	43	17
Managing difficult/challenging behaviour	18	50	26	4
Assertiveness skills	18	41	15	24
Management of stress	16	51	17	12
Negotiation skills including the following:				
–health authority personnel	59	37	1	1
–social services personnel	57	39	2	1
–carers	47	38	10	3

Table 7G.

Distribution of Agreement on the Attitude Base of Speech Therapy for Speech Therapists working with the Elderly/Adult Acquired Neurological Disorders

	Essential	Desirable %	Irrelevant
Respect for the client	93	4	–
Professionalism	92	4	–
Realistic	92	5	–
Flexibility	89	7	0.5
Objective	86	10	0.5
Sensitive	81	15	0.5
Positive	81	15	0.5
Empathy	80	16	–
Holistic	78	18	1.0
Tact	78	18	1.0
Self-motivated	76	20	0.5
Self-awareness	76	19	1.0
Tolerance, open-mindedness	75	20	1.0
Desire to learn	69	28	1.5
Professional self-esteem	69	27	3.0
Able to accept criticism	68	27	3.0
Understanding/awareness of ageism	67	29	–
Enthusiasm	66	29	1.5
Resourceful	63	34	0.5
Sense of humour	58	36	3.0
Self-confident	48	48	1.0
Willing to act as the client's advocate	44	43	8.0
Innovative	34	61	1.0
Creativity	34	61	1.0

Note:* Percentages do not always add up to 100% because of missing values

Appendix 8: Patient-centred procedures

MEMORY AND COMMUNICATION CLINIC: PATIENT/CARER SUMMARY

NAME: DATE: CLINICIAN:

PROCEDURE	CARRIED OUT	SCORES	QUALITATIVE	RELEVANT OR PREDOMINANT FACTORS
A				
TROG	Y N	20		
Naming	Y N	10	Sem. Phon. FAQ	
SCT	Y N	28		
Discourse (Pict)	Y N	%		
(Narr)	Y N	%		
Other				
B				
MMSE or Equivalent	Y N			
C				
Level of Disability				
D				
CCC	Y N	Frequency Severity	Rating Rating	
Communicative Burden	Y N		1 2 3 4	
Overall rating	Y N		0 1 2	
E				
Agreement Score	Y N		1 2 3 4 5 6	

TROG Test for Reception of Grammar (Bishop 1982)
SCT   Story Completion Test (Goodglass et al 1972)
MMSE Minimental State Examination (Folstein Folstein McHugh 1975)
CCC   Carers Checklist of Communication (Walker 1987)

Appendix 9: Goal Setting

ASSESSMENT

Relevant Tested Data / Whether Management Indicator	Carer reported factors (confirmed in testing) — Major	Minor	Other
Naming 6/10: Yes responds to Sem. & Phon. cues	Word finding (3:3)	Initialising	General Status
SCT 3+16:Context promotes appropriacy	Misunderstand	Non fluency	
	Word order		
	Isol. speech untelligble		
TROG incomplete: Yes Some responding to prestimulus information	Motor Speech		
	Paraphasias (3:2)		
Attempts problem solving			
Repeats for repair			
No change			
Social speech			
Word order			
Low output			
Many value judgements			
Discourse; non fluent, empty			
Conversation: deictic directed Questions			
Other			Other

MANAGEMENT

Carer reported factors (perceived)	Focus for workshop tasks	Section of workshop	Other key words
Word finding and naming errors	Use of Sem/Phon. cues and FAQ	5	Attention
		+	Registering
Comprehension loss		8a	Memory
		8b	Language Comprehension
		8c	Language production
		8d	
		8e	
		8f	

Appendix 10:
Outcome Measure

A Level of Impairment:

1   Patient-centred tasks

B Level of Disability:

0   No useful communication
1   Occasional useful/appropriate action/reaction communication with familiar or trained person
2   Occasional useful/appropriate communication action/reaction with others
3   Consistent useful/appropriate action/reaction for communication with familiar and trained person
4   Functions well with occasional assistance
5   Useful/appropriate communication generally

C Level of Communicative Burden (on Carer):

(Based on carer's checklist of perceptions in commmunication)

1   Mild level of communication burden
2   Moderate level of communication burden
3   Severe level of communication burden
4   Very severe level of communication burden

Overall Rating (from carer):   0   1   2
                        Not a struggle A bit of a struggle   A big struggle

D Agreement Score:

1   Deterioration in view of carer and therapist
2   Deterioration in view of carer or therapist
3   No change in view of carer and therapist
4   No change in view of carer or therapist
5   Change in view of carer or therapist
6   Change in view of carer and therapist

References

Action for Dysphasic Adults (1995) *Communicate*. London: ADA Publications.

Adelson, R., Nasti, A., Sprafkin, J., Marinelli, R., Primavera, L. and Gorman, B. (1982) Behavioral ratings of health professionals' interactions with geriatric patients. *Gerontologist* **22**, 277–81.

Adshead, F., Day Cody, D., Pitt, B. (1992) BASDEC: a novel screening instrument for depression in elderly in-patients. *British Medical Journal* **305**, 397.

Albert, M.L., Feldman, R.G. and Willis, A.L. (1974) The 'subcortical dementia' of progressive supranuclear palsy. *Journal of Neurology, Neurosurgery and Psychiatry* **37**, 121–30.

Amaducci, L. and Lippi, A .(1994) Dementia: risk factors. In: Copeland, J.M., Abou-Saleh, M.T. and Blazer, D.G. (Eds), *Principles and Practice of Geriatric Psychiatry*. Chichester: Wiley.

American Psychiatric Association (1987) *Diagnostic and Statistical Manual of Mental Disorders*, 3rd edn. Washington, DC: American Psychiatric Association.

Anderson, M.E. and Horak, F.B. (1984) Motor effects produced by disruption of basal ganglia output from the globus pallidus. In: McKenzie, J.S., Kemm, R.G. and Wilcock, L.N. (Eds), *The Basal Ganglia: Structures and Function*. New York: Plenum Press.

Appell, J., Kertesz, A. and Fisman, M. (1982) A study of language functioning in Alzheimer's patients. *Brain and Language* **17**, 73– 91.

Arie, T. (1979) Day care in geriatric psychiatry. *Age and Ageing* **8** Supplement, 87–91.

Arie, T. (1991) Psychogeriatric services. In: Brocklehurst, J. (Ed.), *Textbook of Geriatrics and Gerontology*, 4th edn. Edinburgh: Churchill Livingstone.

Arie, T. and Jolley, D.J. (1982) Making services work: organisation and style of psychogeriatric services. In: Levy, R. and Post, F. (Eds), *The Psychiatry of Late Life*, Oxford: Blackwell. 222–51.

Armstrong, L. (1993a) Assessing the older communication-impaired person. In:Beech, J.R. Harding, L. and Hilton-Jones, D. (Eds), *Assessment in Speech and Language Therapy*, London: Routledge. 163–74

Armstrong, L. (1993b) Differentiating fluent aphasia from early Alzheimer's disease using language and memory tests. PhD thesis, University of Edinburgh.

Armstrong, L .(1994) Differential diagnosis in older people. *Bulletin* **510**, 6–7.

Armstrong, L., Bayles, K.A., Borthwick, S. and Tomoeda, C.K. Using the ABCD in the UK. *European Journal of Disorders of Communication* in press.

Armstrong, L. and Borthwick, S. Assessing communication: do test results and carer perceptions match up? (submitted to *Age and Ageing*).

289

Armstrong, L. and Greig, L. (1992) Assessment review: elderly patients. *Bulletin of the College of Speech and Language Therapists* **484**, 6–7.

Armstrong, L. and Woodgates, S. Using a measure of communicative environment to compare two psychogeriatric day care settings. *European Journal of Disorders of Communication* in press.

Aronson, M.K., Levine, G. and Lipkowitz, R. (1984) A community-based family/patient group program for Alzheimer's disease. *Gerontologist* **24**, 339–42.

ASHA Committee on Communication Problems of the Aging (1988a) The role of speech–language pathologists and audiologists in working with older persons. *Asha* **30**, 80–4.

ASHA Committee on Communicatous Problems of the Aging (1988b) Provision of audiology and speech-language pathology services to older persons in the nursing home. *Asha* March, 72.

Asher, R. (1949) Myxoedematous madness. *British Medical Journal* **2**, 555–557.

Audit Commission (1992) *Community Care: Managing the Cascade of Change*. London: HMSO.

Ayres, A.J. (1972) *Sensory Integration and Learning Disorders*. Los Angeles: Western Psychological Services.

Bach, D., Bach, M., Bohmer, F., Fruhwald, T. and Grilc, B. (1995) Reactivating occupational therapy: a method to improve cognitive performance in geriatric patients. *Age and Ageing* **24**, 222–226.

Baines, S., Saxby, P. and Ehlet (1987) Reality orientation and reminiscence therapy: a controlled cross-over study of elderly confused people. *British Journal of Psychiatry* **151**, 222–231.

Baker, J., Borsley, D., Daniels, K., Griffiths, H. and Williams, A. (1992) Patient specific profiling. *Royal College of Speech and Language Therapists Bulletin* **479**, 6–7.

Baltes, M.M. and Lascomb, S.L. (1975) Creating a healthy institutional environment for the elderly via behaviour managemant. *International Journal of Nursing Studies* **12**, 5–12.

Bandera, A. (1977) Self-efficacy: towards a unifying theory of behavioural change. Psychological Review **84**, 191–215.

Bandera, D.A., Sala, S.D., Laiacona, M. et al. (1991) Generative associative naming in dementia of Alzheimer's type. *Neuropsychologia* **29**, 291–304.

Bandler, R. and Grinder, J. (1982) *Re-framing Neurolinguistics Programming and the Transformation of Meaning*. Moab, UT: Real People Press.

Bannister, R. (1992) *Brain and Bannister's Clinical Neurology*, 7th edn. Oxford: Oxford University Press.

Barker, M.G. and Lawson, J.S. (1968) Nominal dysphasia in dementia. *British Journal of Psychiatry* **114**, 1351–6.

Barker, P. (1986) *Basic Family Therapy*, 2nd. edn. London: Collins.

Barnett-Douglas, H. (1986) Communication needs of the elderly in the community. *RCSLT Bulletin* May, 6–9.

Barraclough, B. (1971) Suicide in the elderly. In: Kay, D.W.K. and Walk, A. (Eds), *Recent Developments in Psychogeriatrics*. London:Headley.

Baseby, A. (1989) The role of the speech therapist in care of the elderly. *Care of the Elderly* **1**, 87–8.

Battelle Memorial Institute (1984) The economics of dementia. Contract report for the Office of Technology Assessment, US Congress. Available from the National Technical Information Service (Springfield, VA) as *Losing a Million Minds, Contractor Documents. Part 2: Economics, Social Science, and Health Services Research*. Accession Number PB-87-177-598/AS.

Bayles, K.A. (1981) Comprehension deficits in several dementing diseases. Paper given at Linguistic Society of America 56th Annual Meeting, New York. Bayles, K.A. (1982). Language function in senile dementia. *Brain and Language* 16, 265–80.

Bayles, K.A. (1991) Age at onset of Alzheimer's disease: relation to language dysfunction. *Archives of Neurology* 48, 155–9.

Bayles, K.A. and Boone, D.R. (1982) The potential of language tasks for identifying senile demenia. *Journal of Speech and Hearing Disorders* 47, 210–17.

Bayles, K.A., Boone, D.R., Tomoeda, C.K. et al. (1989) Differentiating Alzheimer's patients from normal elderly and stroke patients with aphasia. *Journal of Speech and Hearing Disorders* 54, 74–87.

Bayles, K.A. and Kaszniak, A.W. (1987) *Communication and Cognition in Normal Aging and Dementia*. London: Taylor & Francis.

Bayles, K.A. and Tomoeda, C.K. (1983) Confrontation naming impairment in dementia. *Brain and Language* 19, 98–114.

Bayles, K.A. and Tomoeda, C.K. (1991) Caregiver report of prevalence and appearance order of linguistic symptoms in Alzheimer's patients. *Gerontologist* 31, 210–16.

Bayles, K.A. and Tomoeda, C. (1993) *The Arizona Battery for Communication Disorders of Dementia*. Oxford: Winslow Press.

Bayles, K.A. and Tomoeda, C.K. (1994) *Functional Linguistic Communication Inventory*. Tucson, AZ: Canyonlands Publishing.

Bayles, K.A., Tomoeda, C.K. and Trosset, M.W. (1992) Relation of linguistic communication abilities of Alzheimer's patients to stage of disease. *Brain and Language* 42, 454–72.

Bebbington, D. (1991) Speech therapy and elderly people: a study of therapists' attitudes. *Health Trends* 23, 9–11.

Bebbington, A.C. and Charnley, H. (1990) Community care for the elderly-rhetoric and reality. *British Journal of Social Work* 20, 409–32.

Beck, P. (1982) Two successful interventions in nursing homes: the therapeutic effects of cognitive activity. *The Gerontologist* 22, 378–83.

Beck, C., Heacock, P., Mercer, S., Thatcher, R. and Sparkman, C. (1988) The impact of cognitive skills remediation training on persons with Alzheimer's disease or mixed dementia. *Journal of Geriatric Psychiatry* 21, 73–88.

Bender, M.P., Cooper, A. and Howe, A. (1983) The utility of reminiscence groups in old people's homes. Unpublished (London Borough of Newham).

Benjamin, B.B. (1995) Validation therapy: an intervention for disorientated patients with Alzheimer's disease. *Topics in Language Disorders* 15, 66–74.

Bennett, D.A., Wilson, R.S., Gilley, D.W. and Fox, J.H. (1990) Clinical diagnosis of Binswanger's disease. *Journal of Neurology, Neurosurgery and Psychiatry* 53, 961–5.

Bennett, G. (1989) *Alzheimer's Disease and Other Confusional States*. London: Macdonald.

Benson, D.F. (1979) Neurologic correlates of anomia. In: Whitaker, H. and Whitaker, H.A. (Eds), *Studies in Neurolinguistics*, Vol. 4, New York: Academic Press 293–328.

Berger, R.M. and Rose, S.D. (1977) Interpersonal skill training with institutionalised elderly patients. *Journal of Gerontology* 32, 346–53.

Berne, E. (1966) *Transactional Analysis in Psychotherapy*. New York: Grove Press.

Bieliauska, L.A. and Fox, J.H. (1987) Early cognitive data in a case of Creutzfeld-Jakob disease. *Neuropsychology* 1(2), 49–50.

Bishop, D. (1983) *Test for Reception of Grammar*. Cambridge: MRC APU.

Bondareff, W. (1994) Subtypes of Alzheimer's Disease. In Burns, A. and Levy, R. (Eds), *Dementia*. London: Chapman and Hall.

Blackman, D.K., Howe, M. and Pinkston, E.M. (1976) Increasing participation in social interaction of the institutionalised elderly. *The Gerontologist* 16, 69–76.

Blanken, G., Dittman, J., Haas, J.-C. and Wallesch, C.-W. (1987) Spontaneous speech in senile dementia and aphasia: implications for a neurolinguistic model of language production. *Cognition 27*, 247–74.

Boller, F., Becker, J.T., Holland, A.L., Forbes, M.M., Hood, P.C. and McCougle-Gibson, K.C. (1991) Predictors of decline in Alzheimer's Disease. *Cortex* 27, 9–17.

Bourgeois, M.S. (1990) Enhancing conversation skills in patients with Alzheimer's disease using a prosthetic memory aid. *Journal of Applied Behavior Analysis* 23, 31–64.

Bourgeois, M.S. (1991) Communication treatment for adults with dementia. *Journal of Speech and Hearing Research*, 831–844.

Bowlby, J. (1981) *Loss, Sadness and Depression: Attachment and Loss*, Vol.3. London: Penguin.

Brayne, C.E.G. (1991) A study of dementia in a rural population. Unpublished thesis, University of London.

Brayne, C. and Ames, D. (1988) The epidemiology of mental disorders in old age. In: Gearing, B. Johnson, M. and Heller, T. (Eds), *Mental Health Problems in Old Age*. Chichester: Wiley.

Breuil, V., de Rotrau, J., Forette et al. (1994) Cognitive stimulation of patients with dementia: preliminary results. *International Journal of Geriatric Psychiatry* 9, 211–17.

BMA (1992) *Priorities for Community Care*. London: BMA.

British Medical Journal (1992) Editorial: Families of victims of Creutzfeld-Jacob disease to sue government. *British Medical Journal* 305 11 July, 73.

Brocklehurst, J. (1995) Geriatric day hospitals. *Age and Ageing* 24, 89–90.

Brodaty, H .and Peters, K.E. (1991) Cost effectiveness of a training program for dementia carers. *International Psychogeriatrics*;3, 11–23.

Brodie, J.K. (1986) Communication defects in a residential home for the elderly: their prevalence and staff perceptions of them. *Journal of Clinical and Experimental Gerontology* 8, 13–25.

Brody, E.M., Saperstein, A.R. and Lawton, M.P. (1989) A multi-service respite program for caregivers of Alzheimer's patients. *Journal of Gerontological Social Work* 14, 41–74.

Brown, R.G. and Marsden, C.D. (1984) How common is dementia in Parkinson's disease. *Lancet* ii, 1262–5.

Brown, R.G. and Marsden, C.D. (1986) Visuospatial function in Parkinson's disease. *Brain* 109, 987–1002.

Brown, R.G. and Marsden, C.D. (1988) Internal versus external cues and the control Parkinson's disease. *Brain* 111, 323–47.

Brown, R.G. and Marsden, C.D. (1991) Dual task performance and processing resources in normal subjects and patients with Parkinson's disease. *Brain* 114, 215–31.

Brumfitt, S. (1986) *Counselling*. Oxford: Winslow Press.

Brun, A. (1994) Vascular dementia: pathological findings. In: Burns, A. and Levy, R. (Eds), *Dementia*. London: Chapman & Hall.

Bryan, K.L. and Drew, S. (1987) The benefits of therapy for elderly people in care. *Speech Therapy in Practice* September, 6–8.

Bryan, K.L. and Drew, S. (1989) A survey of communication disability in an elderly population in residential care. *International Journal of Rehabilitation Research* **12**, 330–3.

Bryan, K.L. and Maxim, J. (1991) Talking and listening. In: Benson, S. and Carr, P. (Eds), *The Care Assistants Guide to Working with the Elderly Mentally Infirm*. London: Hawker.

Burnard, P. (1990) *Teaching Interpersonal Skills*. London: Chapman and Hall.

Burns, A., Luthert, P., Levy, R., Jacoby, R. and Lantos, P. (1990) Accuracy of clinical diagnosis of Alzheimer's disease. *British Medical Journal* **301**, 1026.

Butler, R.N. (1963) The life review: an interpretation of reminiscence in the aged. *Psychiatry* **26**, 65–76.

Butters, N., Sax, D., Montgomery, K. and Tarlow, S. (1978) Comparison of the neuropsychological deficits associated with early and advanced Huntingdon's disease. *Archives of Neurology* **35**, 585–9.

Button, E. (1986) *Personal Construct Theory and Mental Health*. London: Croom Helm.

Byrne, E.J. (1992) Diffuse Lewy body disease. In Arie, T. (Ed.), *Recent Advances in Psychogeriatrics*. Edinburgh: Churchill Livingstone.

Byrne, E., Lennox, G., Lowe, J. and Godwin-Austen, R.B. (1989) Diffuse Lewy body disease: clinical features in 15 cases. *Journal of Neurology, Neurosurgery and Psychiatry* **52**, 709–17.

Cameron, D.J., Thomas, R.I., Mulvihill, M. and Bronheim, R. (1987) Delirium: a test of Diagnostic and Statistical Manual III on medical in-patients. *Journal of the American Geriatrics Society* **35**, 1007–10.

Candy, J., Oakley, A., Klinowski, J. et al. (1986) Aluminosilicates and senile plaque formation in Alzheimer's disease. *Lancet* i, 1265–6.

Caplan, L.R. and Schoene, W.C. (1978) Clinical features of subcortical arteriosclerotic encephalopathy (Binswanger's disease). *Neurology* **28**, 1208–15.

Carroll, D. (1989). *When your Loved One has Alzheimer's*. New York: Harper & Row.

Carstensen, L.L. and Ericksen, R.J. (1986) Enhancing the social environments of elderly nursing home residents: are high rates of interaction enough? *Journal of Applied Behaviour Analysis* **19**, 349–55.

Carstensen, L.L. and Fremouw, W.J. (1981) The demonstration of a behavioural intervention for late life paranoia. *The Gerontologist* **21**, 329–33.

Cassel, C.K. (1994). Researching the health needs of elderly people. *British Medical Journal* **308**, 1655–6.

Challis, D., Chessum, R., Chesterman, J., Luckett, R. and Woods, R. (1987) Community care for the frail elderly: an urban experiment. *British Journal of Social Work* **18**, Supplement, 13–42.

Challis, D., Darton, R., Johnson, L., Stone, M. and Traske, K. (1991a) An evaluation of an alternative to long-stay hospital care for frail elderly patients, 1: The model of care. *Age and Ageing* **20**, 236–44.

Challis, D., Darton, R., Johnson, L., Stone, M. and Traske, K. (1991b) An evaluation of an alternative to long-stay hospital care for frail elderly patients, 2: Costs and effectiveness. *Age and Ageing* **20**, 245–54.

Challis, L. and Henwood, M. (1994) Equity in community care. *British Medical Journal* **30**, 1496–9.

Chatellier, G. and Lacomblez, L. (1990) Tacrine (Terahydroaminoacridine – THA) and ledithin in senile dementia of the Alzheimer type: a multi-centre trial. *British Medical Journal* **300**, 495–8.

Chavkin, C.F. (1990) Planning for the future: financial and legal considerations. In: Mace, N. (Ed.), *Dementia Care: Patient, Family and Community*. Baltimore, MD: Johns Hopkins University Press.

Chawluk, J.B., Mesulam, M.M., Hurtiz, H., Kushner, M., Weintraub, S., Saykin, A., Rubin, N., Alavi, A. and Reivich, M. (1986) Slowly progressive aphasia without generalized dementia: studies with positron emission tomography. *Annals of Neurology* 19, 68–74.

Chertkow, H. and Bub, D. (1990) Semantic memory loss in Alzheimer-type dementia. In: M.F. Schwartz (Ed.), *Modular Deficits in Alzheimer-type Dementia* Cambridge, MA: MIT Press 207–44.

Chertkow, H., Bub, D. and Seidenberg, M. (1989) Priming and semantic memory in Alzheimer's disease. *Brain and Language* 36 420–46.

Chui, H.C., Lyness, S., Sobel, E. and Schneider, L.S. (1992) Prognostic implications of symptomatic behaviours in AD. In: Florette, F., Khachaturian, Z. Poncet, M. and Christen, Y. (Eds), *Heterogeneity of Alzheimer's Disease*. Berlin: Springer-Verlag.

Chui, H.C., Teng, E.L., Henderson, V.W. and Moy, A.C. (1985) Clinical subtypes of dementia of the Alzheimer type. *Neurology* 35, 1544–50.

Clark, A.N.G., Mankikar, G.D. and Gray, I. (1975) Diogenes Syndrome: a study of gross neglect in old age. *Lancet* i, 366–8.

Clark, L.W. (1995) Interventions for persons with Alzheimer's disease: strategies for maintaining and enhancing communicative success. *Topics in Language Disorder* 15, 47–65.

Clark, L., Ripich, D. and Weinstein, B. (1994) Status of geriatric education in the professional education programs of speech–language pathology and audiology. Unpublished manuscript.

Clark, L. and Witte, K. (1990) Nature and efficacy of communication management in Alzheimer's disease. In: Lubinski, R. (Ed.), *Dementia and Communication*. Philadelphia, PA: B.C. Decker.

Clark, L., Witte, K. and Macchia, C. (1989) Pragmatic abilities in Alzheimer's disease: a pilot study. Unpublished research paper (Hunter College of SUNY, New York).

Cleary, T.A., Clamon, C., Price, M. and Shullaw, G. (1988) A reduced stimulation unit: effects on patients with Alzheimer's disease and other disorders. *The Gerontologist* 28, 511–14.

Cohen, D, Hegarty J. and Eisdorfer, C. (1983) The physician's desk directory of social resources: a physician's reference guide to social and community services for the aged. *Journal of the American Geriatrics Society* 31, 338–41.

Coles, R.J., von Aberdorff, R. and Herzberg, J.L. (1991) The impact of a new community mental health service team on an inner city psychogeriatric service. *International Journal of Geriatric Psychiatry* 6, 31–41.

Community Care (1994) Lodge of hope. *Community Care* 21 April, 18-19. Cook-Deegan, R.M. (1990). Changing public policy for dementia care. In: Mace, N. (Ed.), *Dementia Care: Patient, Family and Community*. Baltimore, MD: Johns Hopkins University Press.

Coons, D.H. and Weaverdych, S.E. (1986) Wesley Hall: A residential unit for persons with Alzheimer's disease and related disorders. In: Taira, E. (Ed.), *Therapeutic Interventions for the Person with Dementia*. New York: Haworth Press.

Cooper, B. (1987) Psychiatric disorders among elderly patients admitted to general hospital wards. Journal of the Royal Society of Medicine 80, 13–26.

Copeland, J.R.M., Kelleher, M.J., Kellett, J.M., Barron, G., Cowan, D.W. and Gourlay, A.J. (1975) Evaluation of a psychogeriatric service: the distinction between psychogeriatric and geriatric patients. *British Journal of Psychiatry* 126, 21–9.

Corkin, S. (1982) Some relationships between global amnesias and the memory impairments in Alzheimer's disease. In: Corkin, S., Davis, K.L., Growdon, J.H., Usdin, E. and Wurtman, R.J. (Eds), *Alzheimer's Disease: A Report of Progress in Research*, Aging. Vol.19, New York: Raven Press 149–64.

Corson, S.A. and Corson, E. (1978) Pets as mediators of therapy in custodial institutions and the aged. In: Masserman, J.H. (Ed.), *Current Psychiatric Therapies*, Vol 18, pp. 193–206. New York: Grune & Stratton.

Coupland, N., Coupland, J. and Giles, H. (1991) *Language, Society and Ageing*. Oxford: Blackwell.

Critchley, M. (1964) The neurology of psychotic speech. *British Journal of Psychiatry* 40, 353–64.

Crossman, L., London, C. and Barry, C. (1981) Older women caring for disabled spouses: a model for supportive services. *The Gerontologist* 21, 464–70.

Cummings, J.L. (1988) Intellectual impairment in Parkinson's disease: clinical, pathologic and biochemical correlates. *Journal of Geriatric Psychiatry and Neurology* 1, 24–36.

Cummings, J.L. and Benson, D.F. (1992) *Dementia. A Clinical Approach*. Boston, MA: Butterworth.

Cummings, J.L., Houlihan, J.P. and Hill, M.A. (1986) The pattern of reading deterioration in dementia of the Alzheimer type: observations and implications. *Brain and Language* 29, 315–23.

Cutting, J. (1982) Alcoholic dementia. In: Benson, D. and Blumer, D. (Eds), *Psychiatric Aspects of Neurologic Disease*, Vol 2. New York: Grune & Stratton.

Dalla Barba, G. and Wong, C. (1992) Encoding specificity and confabulation in Alzheimer's disease and amnesia. *Journal of Clinical and Experimental Neuropsychology* 3, 378–92.

Dalla Barba, G., Wong, C., Parlato, V. and Boller, F. (1992) Encoding specificity, anosagnosia and confabulation in Alzheimer's disease and depression. *Neurobiology of Aging* 13, 4–5.

Dalley, G. (1991) Beliefs and behavior: professionals and the policy process. *Journal of Ageing Studies* 5, 163–80.

Damasio, A.R., Gary, W., Van Hoesen, G.W. and Hyman, B.T. (1990) Reflections on the selectivity of neuropathological changes in Alzheimer's disease. In: Schwartz, M.F. (Ed.), *Modular Deficits in Alzheimer-type Dementia*. Cambridge, MA: MIT Press.

Danis, B.G. (1978) Stress in individuals caring for ill elderly relatives. Paper presented at the 31st Annual Meeting of the Gerontological Society, Dallas, TX.

Davies, P. and Van der Gaag, A. (1992) The professional competence of speech and language therapists I–IV. *Clinical Rehabilitation* 209–224; 311–31.

de Ajuriaguerra, J. and Tissot, R. (1975) Some aspects of language in various forms of dementia. In: E. and E. Lenneberg (Eds), *Foundations of Language Development: A Multidisciplinary Approach*, Vol 1. New York: Academic Press.

Department of Health (1989a) *Community Care in the Next Decade and Beyond*. London: HMSO.

Department of Health (1989b). *Working for Patients*. London: HMSO.

Department of Health (1990). *Community Care in the Next Decade and Beyond: Policy Guidance*. London: HMSO.

Department of Health/Social Services Inspectorate (1991) *Care Management and Assessment: Summary of Practice Guidelines*. London:HMSO.

Department of Health and Social Security (1985). *In-patient Statistics from the Mental Health Enquiry for England, 1982*. London: HMSO.

Dick, M.B., Kean, M.-L. and Sands, D. (1989). Memory for internally generated words in Alzheimer-type dementia: breakdown in encoding and semantic memory. *Brain and Cognition* 9, 88–108.

Dickson, D., Wu, E., Crystal, H., Matthiace, L., Yen, S. and Davies, P. (1992). Alzheimers disease and age-related pathology in diffuse Lewy body disease. In: Florette, F., Khachaturian, Z., Poncet, M. and Christen, Y. (Eds), *Heterogeneity of Alzheimers Disease*. Berlin: Springer-Verlag.

Diesfeldt, H.F. (1991) Impaired phonological reading in primary degenerative dementia. *Brain* 114, 1631–46.

Dietch, J.T., Hewett, L.J. and Jones, S. (1989) Adverse effects of reality orientation. *Journal of the American Geriatric Society* 37, 974–6.

Dilts, R., Grinder, J., Bandler, R., Bandler, L. and DeLozier, J. (1980) Neurolinguistics Programming, Vol. 1: *The Study of Subjective Experience*. Cupertino, CA: Metta Publications.

Dixon, J., Dinwoodie, M., Hodson, D., Dodd, S., Poltorak, T., Garrett, C., Rice, P., Doncaster, I. and Williams, M. (1994) Distribution of NHS funds between fund-holding and non-fundholding practices. *British Medical Journal* 309, 30–34.

Donaldson, C. and Bond, J. (1991) Cost of continuing-care facilities in the evaluation of experimental national health service nursing homes. *Age and Aging* 20, 160–168.

Dreher, B.B. (1987) *Communicative Skills For Working With Elders*. New York: Springer-Verlag.

Dunn, L.M. (1959) *Peabody Picture Vocabulary Test*. Circle Pines, MN: American Guidance Service.

Edelman, G. and Hughes, P.A. (1994) North West Thames Speech and Language Therapy: Staff Retention and Return to Practice Project. Unpublished report.

Egan, G. (1986) *The Skilled Helper – A Systematic Approach to Effective Helping*. Belmont, CA: Brooks/Cole.

Elliott, B. and Hyberston, D. (1982) What is it about the elderly that elicits a negative response? *Gerontological Nursing* 8, 568–571.

Emery, O.B. (1985) Language and aging. *Experimental Aging Research* 11(1), 3–60.

Emery, O.B. (1989) Language deficits in depression: comparisons with SDAT and normal aging. *Journal of Gerontology* 44, M85–M92.

Enderby, P. (1992) Outcome measures in speech therapy. *Health Trends* 24 No. 2. Health Services Division (Scotland) (1995).

Enderby, P. (1993) What makes a good service? *Therapy Weekly* 17 July.

Enderby, P. and Davies, P. (1989) Communication disorders: planning a service to meet the needs. *British Journal of Disorders of Communication* 24 (3), 301–331.

Erber, N.P. (1994) Conversation as therapy for older adults in residential care: the case for intervention. *European Journal of Disorders of Communication* 29, 269–278.

Evans, D.A. (1990) Estimated prevalence of Alzheimer's disease in the United States. *The Milbank Quarterly* 68, 267–89.

Evans, D.A., Harris Funkelstein, H., Albert, M.S., Scherr, P.A., Cook, N.R., Chown, M.J., Hebert, L.E., Hennerkens, C.H. and Taylor, J.O. (1989) Prevalence of Alzheimer's disease in a community population of older persons. *Journal of the American Medical Association;* 262, 2551–6.

Faber-Langendoen, K., Morris, J.C., Knesevich, J.W., LaBarge, E., Miller, J.P. and Berg, L. (1988) Aphasia in senile dementia of the Alzheimer type. *Annals of Neurology* 23, 365–70.

Farlow, M., Gracon, S.I., Hershey, L.A., Lewis, K.W., Sadowsky, C.H. and Colon-Ureno, J. (1992) A controlled trial of tacrine in Alzheimer's disease. *Journal of the American Medical Association* 268, 2523–8.

Fawcus, M., Robinson, M., Williams, J. and Williams, R. (1986) *Working with Dysphasics*. Oxford: Winslow Press.

Fearnley, J.M., Revesz, D.J., Frackowiak, R.S.J. and Lees, A.J. (1991) Diffuse Lewy body disease presenting with a supranuclear gaze palsy. *Journal of Neurology, Neurosurgery and Psychiatry* 54, 159–61.

Feil, N. (1982) *Validation: The Feil Method*. Cleveland: Edward Feil Productions.

Feil, N. (1985) Resolution: the final life task. *Journal of Humanistic Psychology* 25, 91–105.

Feil, N. (1992) Validation therapy with late-onset dementia populations. In: Jones, G.M.M. and Miesen, B.M.L. (Eds), *Care-Giving in Dementia*, pp. 199–218. London: Routledge.

Feinberg, T. and Goodman, B. (1984) Affective illness, dementia and pseudodementia. *Journal of Clinical Psychiatry* 45, 99–103.

Filley, C.M., Kelly, J. and Heaton, R.K. (1986) Neuropsychologic features of early and late onset Alzheimers disease. *Archives of Neurology* 43, 574–576.

Fletcher, A.E., Dickinson, E.J. and Philp, I. (1992) Review: audit measures: quality of life instruments for everyday use with elderly patients. Age and Ageing 21, 142–50.

Folstein, M.F., Folstein, S.E. and McHugh, P.R. (1975) 'Mini-mental state' – a practical method for grading the cognitive state of patients for the clinician. *Journal of Psychiatric Research* 12, 189–98.

Foster, N.L., Chase, T.N., Patronas, N.J., Gillespie, M.M. and Fedio, P. (1986) Cerebral mapping of apraxia in Alzheimer's disease by positron emission tomography. *Annals of Neurology* 19, 139–43.

Fraser, M. (1987) *Dementia: Its Nature and Management*. Chichester and New York: Wiley.

Freedman, L. and Costa, L. (1992) Pure alexia and right hernia chromatopsia in posterior dementia. *Journal of Neurology, Neurosurgery and Psychiatry* 55, 500–2.

Freedman, L., Selchan, D.H., Black, S.E., Kaplan, R., Garnett, E.S. and Nahmias, C. (1991) Posterior cortical dementia with alexia: neurobehavioural, MRI and PET findings. *Journal of Neurology, Neurosurgery and Psychiatry* 54 (5), 443–8.

Fromm, D. and Holland, A.L. (1989) Functional communication in Alzheimer's disease. *Journal of Speech and Hearing Disorders* 54, 535–40.

Fromm, D., Holland, A.L., Nebes, R.D. and Oakley, M.A. (1991) A longitudinal study of word-reading ability in Alzheimer's disease: evidence from the National Adult Reading Test. *Cortex* 27, 367–76.

Funnell, E. and Hodges, J.R. (1990) Progressive loss of access to spoken word forms in a case of Alzheimer's disease. *Proceedings of the Royal Society*.

Galloway, P.H. (1992) Visual pattern recognition memory and learning deficits in senile dementias of Alzheimer and Lewy body types. *Dementia* 3, 101–7.

George, L.K. (1986) Respite care: evaluating a strategy for easing caregiver burden. *Center Reports on Advances in Research* 10(2). Durham, NC: Center for the Study of Aging and Human Development.

George, L.K. (1988) Why won't caregivers use community services? Paper presented at the Annual Meeting of the Gerontological Society of America, Washington, DC.

Gerritsen, J.C. and van der Ende, P.C. (1994) The development of a care-giving burden scale. *Age and Ageing* 23, 483–91.

Gilhooly, M.L.M. (1984) The social dimensions of senile dementia. In: Hanley, I. and Hodge, J. (Eds), *Psychological Approaches to Care of the Elderly*. London: Croom Helm.

Gilleard, C. (1984) *Living with Dementia*. London: Croom Helm.

Gilleard, C. (1992) Community care services for the elderly mentally infirm. In: G.M.M. Jones and B.M.L. Miesen (Eds), Care-Giving in Dementia: Research and Applications, London and New York: Routledge. 293–313.

Gilleard, C.J., Boyd, W.D. and Watt, G. (1982) Problems in caring for the elderly mentally infirm at home. *Archives of Gerontology and Geriatrics* 1, 151–8.

Gladman, J., Whynes, D. and Lincoln, N. (1994) Cost comparison of domiciliary and hospital-based stroke rehabilitation. *Age and Ageing* 23, 241–5.

Gloser, G. and Deser, T. (1990) Patterns of discourse production among neurological patients with fluent language disorders. *Brain and Language* 40, 67–88.

Goate, A.M., Clartie-Harlin, M.C. and Mullan, M. (1991) Segregation of a missense mutation in the amyloid precursor gene with familial Alzheimer's disease. *Nature* 349, 704–6.

Golding, E. (1989) *The Middlesex Elderly Assessment of Mental State*. Bury St Edmunds: Thames Valley Test Co.

Goldwasser, A.N., Auerbach, S.M. and Harkins, S.W. (1987) Cognitive, affective and behavioural effects of reminiscence group therapy on demented elderly. *International Journal of Aging and Human Development* 25, 209–222.

Goodglass, H. and Kaplan, E. (1983) *The Boston Diagnostic Aphasia Examination*. Beckenham: Lea & Febiger.

Goodlove, C., Richard, L. and Rodwell, G. (1982) *Time for Action: An Observation Study of Elderly People in Four Different Care Environments*. Sheffield: Joint Unit for Social Services Research, University of Sheffield.

Gordon, E. (1976) A bi-disciplinary approach to group therapy for wives of aphasics. Paper presented to the American Speech and Hearing Association Convention, Houston, TX.

Gotham, A.M., Brown, R.G. and Marsden, C.D. (1986) Depression in Parkinson's disease. A quantitative and qualitative analysis. *Journal of Neurology, Neurosurgery and Psychiatry* 49, 79–89.

Gotham, A.M., Brown, R.G. and Marsden, C.D. (1988) 'Frontal' cognitive function in patients with Parkinson's disease 'on' and 'off' levadopa. *Brain* 111, 299–321.

Goudie, F. and Stokes, G. (1989) Understanding confusion. *Nursing Times* 85, 35–7.

Graff-Radford, N.R., Damasio, A.R., Hyman, B.T., Hart, M.N., Tranel, D., Damasio, H., Van Hoesen, G.W. and Rezai, K. (1990) Progressive aphasia in a patient with Pick's disease: a neuropsychological, radiologic and anatomic study. *Neurology* 40 (4), 620–6.

Grant, I., Adams, K.M. and Reed, R. (1984) Aging, abstinence and medical risk factors in the prediction of neuropschologic deficit among long-term alcoholics. *Archives of General Psychiatry* 47, 710–18.

Gravell, R. (1988) *Communication Problems in Elderly People*. London: Croom Helm.

Gravell, R. (1990) Assessment of the elderly. In: Beech, J.R. amd Harding, L. (Eds), *Assessment of the Elderly*, pp. 43–52. Windsor: NFER-Nelson.

Gravell, R. and France, J. (Eds) (1991) *Speech and Communication Problems in Psychiatry*. London: Chapman & Hall.

Gray, A. (1982) The challenge of multidisciplinary teamwork. *College of Speech Therapists Bulletin* 358, 1–2.

Greene, H. (1988) *Informed Carers*, General Household Survey 1985, Supplement A. London: DHSS/HMSO.

Greene, J.G., Nichol, R. and Jamieson, H. (1979) Reality orientation with psychogeriatric patients. *Behaviour, Research and Therapy* 17, 615–18.

Greene, J.G., Smith, R., Gardiner, M. and Timbury, G.C. (1982) Measuring behavioural disturbances of elderly demented people in the community and its effects on relatives: a factor analytic study. *Age and Ageing* 11, 121–6.

Greveson, G. (1994) In the community. *Age and Ageing* 23, S15–S17.

Griffith, D. (1993) Respite care. *British Medical Journal* 306, 160.

Griffiths, H. (1991) The psychiatry of old age. In: Gravell, R. and France, J. (Eds), *Speech and Communication Problems in Psychiatry*. London: Chapman & Hall.

Griffiths, H. and Baldwin, B. (1989) Speech therapy for psychogeriatric services: luxury or necessity? *Psychiatric Bulletin* 13, 57–9.

Griffiths Report (1988) *Community Care: An Agenda for Action*. London: HMSO.

Grimley Evans, J. (1989) Ageing and nutrition: questions needing answers. *Age and Ageing* 18, 145–7.

Grimley Evans, J. (1993) Hypothesis: health active life indicator (HALE) as an index of effectiveness of health and social services for elderly people. *Age and Ageing* 22, 297–301.

Grist, E. and Maxim, J. (1992) Confrontation naming in the elderly: The Build-up Picture Test as an aid to differentiating normals from subjects with dementia. *European Journal of Disorders of Communication* 27, 197–207.

Grossberg, G.T. and Nakra, R. (1988) The diagnostic dilemma of depressive pseudo-dementia. In: Strong, R. (Ed.), *Central Nervous System Disorders of Aging: Clinical Intervention and Research*. New York: Raven.

Grossman, M., Carvell, S., Gollomp, S. and Hurtig, H.I. (1992) Sentence comprehension in Parkinson's disease: the role of attention and memory. *Brain and Language* 42, 347–84.

Grossman, M., Carvell, S., Gollomp, S., Stern, M.B., Vernon, G. and Hurtig, H.I. (1991) Sentence comprehension and praxis deficits in Parkinson's disease. *Neurology* 41, 1620–6.

Gupta, S.R., Naheedy, M.H., Young, J.C., Ghobrial, M., Rubino, F.A. and Hindo, W. (1988) Periventricular white matter changes and dementia: clinical neuropsychological, radiological and pathological correlation. *Archives of Neurology* 45, 637–41.

Hachinski, V.C., Lassen, N.A. and Marshall, J. (1974) Multi-infarct dementia: a course of mental deterioration in the elderly. *Lancet* ii, 207–10.

Hachinski, V.C., Iliff, L.D., Zilkha, E. et al. (1975) Cerebral blood flow in dementia. *Archives of Neurology* 32, 632–7.

Haffenden, S. (1991) *Getting it Right for Carers*. London: DHSS Inspectorate/HMSO.

Haines, A. and Jones, R. (1994) Implementing findings of research. *British Medical Journal* 308, 1488–92.

Hall, R.G.P. and Channing, D.M. (1990) Age, pattern of consultation, and financial disability in elderly patients in one practice. *British Medical Journal* 301, 424–8.

Hallewell, C., Morris, J. and Jolley, D. (1994) The closure of residential homes: what happens to residents. *Age and Ageing* 23, 158–61.

Hanley, I.G. (1981) The use of signposts and active training to modify word disorientation in elderly patients. *Journal of Behaviour Therapy and Experimental Psychiatry* 12, 241–7.

Hanley, I. (1986) Reality orientation in the care of the elderly patient with dementia – three case studies. In: Hanley, I. and Gilhooly, M. (Eds), *Psychological Therapies for the Elderly*, New York: New York University Press 65–79.

Hanley, I.G. and Lusty, K. (1984) Memory aids in reality orientation: a single case study. *Behaviour Research Therapy* 22, 709–12.

Hanley, I.G., McGuire, R.J. and Boyd, W.D. (1981) Reality orientation and dementia: a controlled trial of two approaches. *British Journal of Psychiatry* **138**, 10–14.

Hardy, B. (1992) Hares and tortoises. *Community Care* **3** (September), 22–4.

Hardy, J. (1992) Alzheimer's disease: many aetiologies; one pathogenesis. In: Florette, F. Khachaturian, Z. Poncet, M. and Christen, Y. (Eds), *Heterogeneity of Alzheimer's Disease*. Berlin: Springer-Verlag.

Hardy, J., Houlden, H., Collinge, J. et al. (1993) Apolipoprotein egenotype and Alzheimer's disease. *Lancet* **344**, 737–738.

Harrington, J.A. (1988) Contemporary issues in psychotherapy. In: Hall, P. and Stonier, P.D. (Eds), *Perspectives in Psychotherapy*. Chichester: Wiley.

Harrison, R., Savla, N. and Kafetz, K. (1990) Dementia, depression and physical disability in a London borough: a survey of elderly people in and out of residential care and implications for future developments. *Age and Ageing* **19**, 97–103.

Hart, E. and Bond, M. (1995) *Action Research for Health and Social Care*. Buckingham: Open University Press.

Hart, J. and Fleming, R. (1985) An experimental evaluation of a modified reality orientation therapy. *Clinical Gerontologist* **3**, 35–45.

Hart, S. (1988) Language and dementia: a review. *Psychological Medicine* **18**, 99–112.

Hart, S. and Semple, J.M. (1990) *Neuropsychology and the Dementias*. London: Taylor & Francis.

Hart, S., Smith, C.M. and Swash, M. (1986) Intrusion errors in Alzheimer's disease. *British Journal of Clinical Psychology* **25**, 149–50.

Hart, S., Smith, C.M. and Swash, M. (1988) Word fluency in patients with early dementia of Alzheimer type. *British Journal of Clinical Psychology* **27**, 115–24.

Hatch, E. and Farhady, H. (1982) *Research Design and Statistics for Applied Linguistics*. Cambridge, MA: Newbury House.

Hay, J.W. and Ernst, R.L. (1987) The economic costs of Alzheimer's disease. *American Journal of Public Health* **77**, 1169–75.

Hay Group (1994) *Hay Method of Job Evaluation: the Health Service in Scotland* (Lawrence, Robertson, Eds). Hay Management Consultants (distribution restricted).

Hayter, J. (1982) Helping families of patients with Alzheimer's disease. *Journal of Gerontological Nursing* **8**, 81–6.

Health Advisory Service (1982) *The Rising Tide: Developing Services for Mental Illness in Old Age*. London: Health Advisory Service.

Health Services Division Scotland (1995) *The Scottish Community Core Dataset/EPPIC*. Health Services Division Scotland.

Hedrick, S.C., Rothman, M.L., Chapko. M., Inui, T.S., Kelly, J.R. and Ehreth, J. (1993) Overview and patient recruitment in the adult day health care evaluation study. *Medical Care* **31**(9), SS3–SS14.

Heindel, W.C., Salmon, D.P. and Butters, N. (1990) Pictorial priming and cued recall in Alzheimer's and Huntington's disease. *Brain & Cognition* **13**, 282–95.

Henwood, M. (1992a) Twilight zone. *Health Services Journal* **5** November, 28–30.

Henwood M. (1992b) *Through a Glass Darkly. Community Care and Elderly People*. London: Kings Fund Institute.

Heritage, M. and Farrow, V. (1994) Research shows the profession has a valuable role with elderly mentally ill people. *Human Communication* February, 15–16.

Heritage M. and Knaps, S. (1994) *Dysphagia Training for Nursing Staff*. Nottingham: Nottingham Community Health NHS Trust.

Herlitz, A., Adolfson, R., Backman, L. and Wilson, L.-G. (1991) Cue utilization following different forms of encoding in mildly, moderately and severely demented patients with Alzheimer's disease. *Brain and Cognition* 15, 119–30.

Heston, L. (1981) Genetic studies of dementia with emphasis on Parkinson's disease and Alzheimer's neuropathology. In: Mortimer, J. and Schuman, L. (Eds), *The Epidemiology of Dementia*. Oxford: Oxford University Press.

Hier, D.B., Hagenlocker, K. and Shindler, A.G. (1985) Language disintegration in dementia: effects of aetiology and severity. *Brain and Language* 25, 117–33.

Hing, E. (1987) *Use of Nursing Homes by the Elderly. Preliminary Data from the National Nursing Home Survey*, National Center for Health Statistics, DHHS Publication No. 87–1250. Hyattsville, MD: Public Health Service, 14 May.

Hodges J.R. (1994) Picks Disease. In Burns, A. and Levy, R. (Eds), *Dementia*. London: Chapman and Hall.

Hodges J.R., Patterson, K. and Tyler, K.T. (1994) Loss of semantic memory: implications for the modularity of mind. *Cognitive Psychology* 11(5), 505–42.

Hodges, J.R., Salmon, D.P. and Butters, N. (1991) The nature of the naming deficit in Alzheimer's and Huntingdon's disease. *Brain* 114, 1547–58.

Hodges, J.R., Salmon, D.P. and Butters, N. (1992) Semantic memory impairment in Alzheimer's disease: failure of access or degraded knowledge? *Neuropsychologia* 30, 301–14.

Hodkinson, M. (1972) Evaluation of a mental test score for assessments of mental impairment in the elderly. *Age and Ageing* 1, 233–8.

Holden, U.P. (1990) *Neuropsychology and Aging*. London: Croom Helm.

Holden, U.P. and Woods, R. (1988) *Reality Orientation: Psychological Approaches to the Confused Elderly*. Edinburgh: Churchill Livingstone.

Holland, A. (1980) *Communicative Abilities in Daily Life*. Baltimore, MD: University Press.

Holland, A.L. (1990) Research methodology I. Implications for speech–language pathology. *ASHA Reports* 19, 35–9.

Holland, A.L. and Bartlett, C.L. (1985) Some differential effects of age on stroke-produced aphasia. In: Ulatowska, A.K. (Ed.), *The Aging Brain, Communication in the Elderly*. London; Taylor & Francis.

Holland, A.L., McBurney, D.H., Moossy, J. and Rernmirth, O.M. (1985) The dissolution of language in Pick's disease with neurofibrillary tangles: a case study. *Brain and Language* 24, 36–38.

Homer, A., Honovar, M., Lantos, P., Hastie, I., Kellett, J. and Millard, P. (1988) Diagnosing dementia: do we get it right? *British Medical Journal* 297, 894–6.

Homer, A.C. and Gilleard C.J. (1994) The effect of inpatient respite care on elderly patients and their carers. *Age and Ageing* 23, 274–6.

Horner, J. (1985) Language disorder associated with Alzheimer's disease, left hemisphere stroke, and progressive illness of uncertain aetiology. In: Brookeshire, R.H. (Ed.), *Clinical Aphasiology Conference Proceedings*, pp. 149–58. Minneapolis, MN: BRK Publishers.

Horner, J., Dawson, D.V., Heyman, A. and Fish, A.M. (1992) The usefulness of the Western Aphasia Battery for differential diagnosis of Alzheimer dementia and focal stroke syndrome: preliminary evidence. *Brain and Language* 42, 77–88.

Horner, J., Heyman, A., Dawson, D. and Rogers, H. (1988) The relationship of agraphia to the severity of dementia in Alzheimer's disease. *Archives of Neurology* 45, 760–3.

Horowitz, A. and Dobrof, R. (1982) The role of families in providing long-term care to the frail and chronically ill elderly living in the community. Final Report submitted to the Health Care Financing Administration, Department of Health and Human Services.

Howard, D. and Patterson, K. (1992) *The Pyramids and Palm Trees Test*. Bury St Edmunds: Thames Valley Test Company.

Howes, D. (1964) Application of the word frequency concept to aphasia. In: de Rueck, A.V.S. and O'Connor, M. (Eds), *Disorders of Language*, Ciba Foundation Symposium. London: Churchill.

Hoyer, W.J. (1973) Application of operant techniques to the modification of elderly behaviour. *The Gerontologist* 13, 18–22.

Hoyer, W.J., Kater, R.A., Simpson, S.C. and Hoyer, F.W. (1974) Reinstatement of verbal behaviour in elderly mental patients using operant procedures. *The Gerontologist* 14, 149–52.

Huber, S.J., Shuttleworth, E.C. and Freidenberg, D.L. (1989) Neuropsychological differences between the dementias of Alzheimer's and Parkinson's diseases. *Archives of Neurology* 46, 1287–91.

Hudson, B. (1987) Collaboration in social welfare: a framework for analysis. *Policy and Politics* 15, 175–82.

Hudson, B. (1990) Social policy and the new right – the strange case of the community care white paper. *Local Government Studies* 16, 15–34.

Huff, F.J., Corkin, S. and Crowdon, J. (1986) Semantic impairment and anomia in Alzheimer's disease. *Brain and Language* 280, 235–49.

Hughston, G.A. and Merriam, S.B. (1982) Reminiscence: a nonformal technique for improving cognitive functioning in the aged. *International Journal of Ageing and Developments* 15, 139–49.

Hussain, R.A. (1981) *Geriatric Psychology: A Behavioural Perspective*. New York: Van Nostrand Reinhold.

Hutchinson, J.M. and Jenson, M. (1980) A pragmatic evaluation of discourse communication in normal and senile elderly in a nursing home. In: Obler, L.K. and Albert, M.L. (Eds), *Language and Communication in the Elderly*. Lexington, MA: D.Heat.

Illes, J. (1989) Neurolinguistic features of spontaneous language dissociate three form of neurodegenerative disease: Alzheimer's, Huntington's and Parkinson's. *Brain and Language* 37, 628–42.

Isaacs, B. and Akhtar, A.J. (1972) The Set Test: a rapid test of mental function in old people. *Age and Ageing* 1, 222–6.

Isaacs, B. and Kennie, A.T. (1973) The Set Test as an aid to the detection of dementia in old people. *British Journal of Psychiatry* 123, 467–70.

Ishii, N., Hisharara, Y. and Imamura, T. (1986) Why do frontal lobe symptoms predominate in vascular dementia with lacunes? *Neurology* 36, 340–5.

Jackson, P. (1990) A study of the speech therapy training needs of care staff working in Part Three homes for the elderly in the mid-Surrey health authority – summary. Research project carried out in conjunction with the Action Research Programme – Care in the Community (unpublished).

Jarvik, L.F. (1982) Pseudodementia. *Consultant* 22, 141–6.

Joanette, Y., Ska, B., Poissant, A. and Beland, R. (1992) Neuropsychological aspects od Alzheimer's disease: evidence for inter and intra-function heterogeneity. In: Florette, F., Khachaturian, Z., Poncet, M. and Christen, Y. (Eds), *Heterogeneity of Alzheimer's Disease*. Berlin: Springer-Verlag.

Johannson, A., Gustafson, L., Brun, A., Risberg, J., Rosen, I. and Tideman, E. (1991) A longitudinal study of dementia of Alzheimer type in Down's syndrome. *Dementia* 1(2), 159–68.

Johnson, J.A. and Pring, T.R. (1990) Speech therapy and Parkinson's disease: a review and further data. *British Journal of Disorders of Communication* 25, 183–94.

Johnson, J.B. (1986) Cris Ridge Village: a service continuum. *Provider* May, 32–4.

Jolley, D.J. and Arie, T. (1992) Developments in psychogeriatric services. In: Arie, T. (Ed.), *Psychogeriatrics*, Edinburgh: Churchill Livingstone. 117–36.

Jolley, S. and Jolley, D.J. (1991) Psychiatric disorders in old age. In: Bennett, D.H. and Freeman, H.L. (Eds), *Community Psychiatry: The Principles*, Edinburgh: Churchill Livingstone. 268–296.

Jones, D. and Lester, C. (1994) Hospital care and discharge: patients' and carers' opinions. *Age and Ageing* 23, 91–6.

Jones, D.A. and Peters, T.J. (1992) Caring for elderly dependants: effects on carer's quality of life. *Age and Ageing* 21, 421–8.

Jordan, F.M., Worrall, L.E., Hickson, L.M.H. and Dodds, B.J. (1993) The evaluation of intervention programmes for communicatively impaired elderly people. *European Journal of Communication Disorders* 28, 63–85.

Jorm, A.F. (1990) *The Epidemiology of Alzheimer's Disease and Related Diseases*. London: Chapman & Hall.

Junque, C., Pujol, J., Vendrell, P., Bruna, O., Jodar, M., Ribas, J.C., Vinas, J., Capdevila, A. and Martin-Villalta, J.L. (1990) Leuko-araiosis on magnetic resonance imaging and speed of mental processing. *Archives of Neurology* 47, 151–6.

Kaakinen, J. (1995) Talking among elderly nursing home residents. *Topics in Language Disorder* 15, 36–46.

Kaatzke, M. (1992) Swallowing difficulties in patients with dementia. Presentation to the Dysphagia/Geriatrics Interest Group, Concord, MA, April.

Kaplan, E., Goodglass, H. and Weintraub, S. (1983) *Boston Naming Test*. Philadelphia: Lea & Febiger.

Kay, D.W. and Bergmann, K. (1980) Epidemiology of mental disorders among the aged in the community. In: Berren, J.E. and Sloane, B.R. (Eds), *Handbook of Mental Health and Aging*. Englewood Cliffs, NJ: Prentice-Hall.

Kay, D.W.L., Beamish, P. and Roth, M. (1964) Old age mental disorders in Newcastle upon Tyne, Part 1: A study of prevalence. *British Journal of Psychology* 110, 146–58.

Kay, J., Lesser, R. and Coltheart, M. (1992) *Psycholinguistic Assessments of Language Processing in Aphasia*. Hove: Lawrence Erlbaum.

Kearns, K.P. (1986) Group treatment for aphasia: theoretical and practical considerations. In: Chapey, R. (Ed.), *Language Intervention Strategies in Adult Aphasia*, 2nd edn. Baltimore: Williams & Wilkins.

Kelly, G.A. (1955) *The Psychology of Personal Constructs*. New York: Norton.

Kempler, D. (1988) Lexical and pantomime abilities in Alzheimer's disease. *Aphasiology* 2, 147–59.

Kempler, D., Curtis, S. and Jackson, C. (1987) Syntactic preservation in Alzheimer's disease. *Journal of Speech and Hearing Research* 30, 343–50.

Kendrick, D.C., Gibson, A.J. and Moyes, I.C.A. (1979) The revised Kendrick Battery: clinical studies. *British Journal of Social and Clinical Psychology* 18, 329–40.

Kennedy, A. (1993) Neuroimaging in Alzheimer's disease. *Alzheimer's Review* 3, 49–53.

Kern, R.S., VanGorp, W.G., Cummings, J.L., Brown, W.S. and Osato, S.S. (1992) Confabulation in Alzheimers disease. *Brain and Cognition* 19, 172–82.

Kertesz, A. (1982) *Western Aphasia Battery*. New York: Grune & Stratton.

Kiernat, J.M. (1979) The use of life review activity with confused nursing home residents. *American Journal of Occupational Therapy* 33, 306–10.

Kinney, J.M. and Stephens, M.A. (1989) Caregiving hassles scale: assessing the daily hassles of caring for a family member with dementia. *Gerontologist* , 29, 328–32.

Kitwood, T. (1990) The dialectics of dementia: with particular reference to Alzheimer's disease. *Ageing and Society* 10, 177–96.

Knight, R.G. (1992) *The Neuropsychology of Degenerative Brain Diseases*. London: Lawrence Erlbaum.

Koh, K., Lee, R.J., Nair, T., Ho, P. and Ang, C. (1994) Dementia in elderly patients: can the 3R mental stimulation programme improve mental status? *Age and Ageing* 23, 195–9.

Kontiola, P., Laaksoner, R., Sulkawa, R. and Erkinjunsi, T. (1990) Pattern of language impairment in Alzheimer's disease and multi-infarct dementia. *Brain and Language* 38, 364–83.

Kopelman, M.D. (1986) Recall of anomalous sentences in dementia and amnesia. *Brain and Language* 29, 154–70.

Kopelman, M.D. (1991) Frontal dysfunction and memory deficits in the alcoholic Korsakoff syndrome and Alzheimer-type dementia. *Brain* 114, 117–37.

Kotsoris, H., Barclay, L.L., Kheyfets. S., Hulyalkar, A. and Dougherty, J. (1987) Urinary and gait disturbance as markers for early multi-infarct dementia. *Stroke* 18, 138–41.

Koury, L.N. and Lubinski, R. (1991) Effective in-service training for staff working with communicatively impaired patients. In: Lubinski, R. (Ed.), *Dementia and Communication*, pp. 279–91. Philadelphia, PA: Decker.

Kramer, S.I. and Reifler, B.V. (1992) Depression, dementia and reversible dementia. *Clinical Geriatric Medicine* 8, 289–97.

Kuhl, D.E., Metter, E.J. and Reige, W.H. (1984) Patterns of local cerebral glucose utilization determined in Parkinson's disease by [F18] Flurodeoxyglucose method. *Annals of Neurology* 15, 419–24.

Lahey, M. and Feier, C.D. (1982) The semantics of verbs in dissolution and development of language. *Journal of Speech and Hearing Research* 25, 81–95.

Laing and Buisson (1990) *Care of Elderly People, Market Survey 1990–91*. London: Laing and Buisson.

Laing and Buisson (1992) *Laing's Review of Private Health Care*. London: Laing and Buisson.

Lapworth, P., Sills, S. and Fish, S. (1993) *Transactional Analysis Counselling*. Oxford: Winslow Press.

Lawton, M.P. (1980) Psychosocial and environmental approaches to the care of senile dementia patients. In: Cole, J.O. and Barett, J.E. (Eds), *Psychopathology in the Aged*, pp. 265–78. New York: Raven Press.

Lawton, M.P., Brody, E.M. and Saperstein, A.R. (1991) *Respite for Caregivers of Alzheimer Patients*. New York: Springer-Verlag.

Le Brun, Y., Devreux, F. and Rousseau, J.J. (1986) Language and speech in a patient with a clinical diagnosis of progressive supranuclear palsy. *Brain and Language* 27, 247–56.

Leibovici, D., Curtis, S. and Ritchie, K. (1995) The application of disability data from epidemiological surveys to the development of indicators of service needs for dependent elderly people. *Age and Ageing* 24, 14–20.

Leng, N.R.C. (1990) *Psychological Care in Old Age*. New York: Hemisphere.

Lesser, R.R. (1989) Selective preservation of oral spelling without semantics in a case of multi-infarct dementia. *Cortex* **25**, 239–50.

Lester, R. (1994) Residential care: towards a better understanding. *CSLT Bulletin* December, 11–12.

Lester, R. and Ashley, M. (1995) *Notes for Care Staff working with Residents who have Communication Difficulties. London: ADA Publications.*

Lieberman, P., Friedman, J. and Feldman, L.S. (1990) Syntax comprehension in Parkinson's disease. *Journal of Nervous and Mental Disease* **178**, 360–6.

Lindesay, J. (1991) Phobic disorders in the elderly. *British Journal of Psychiatry* **159**, 531–41.

Lindesay, J., Briggs, K. and Murphy, E. (1989) The Guy's/Age Concern Survey prevalence rates of cognitive impairment, depression and anxiety in an urban elderly community. *British Journal of Psychiatry* **155**, 317–29.

Linsk, N., Howe, M.W. and Pinkston, E.M. (1975) Behavioural group work in a home for the aged. *Social Work* **20**, 454–63.

Linsk, N.L., Miller, B., Pflaum, R. and Ortigara-Vicik, A. (1986) The effects of an Alzheimer's disease programme on social interaction within a nursing home. Paper presented at the Gerontological Society of America's 39th Annual Scientific Meeting, Chicago.

Lipowski, Z.J. (1989) Delirium in the elderly patient. *New England Journal of Medicine* **320**, 578–562.

Lishman, W.A. (1987) *Organic Psychiatry: The Psychological Consequences of Cerebral Disorder*, 2nd edn. Oxford: Blackwell Scientific.

Lopez, M.A., Hoyer, W.J., Goldstein, A.P., Gershaw, N.J. and Sprafkin, R.P. (1980) Effects of overlearning and incentive on the acquisition and transfer of interpersonal skills with institutionalized elderly. *Journal of Gerontology* **35**, 403–08.

Loring, D.W., Meador, K.J., Mahurin, R.K. and Largen, J.W. (1986) Neuropsychological performance in dementia of the Alzheimer type and multi-infarct dementia. *Archives of Clinical Neuropsychology* **1**, 335–40.

Lubinski, R. (1981) Environmental language intervention. In: Chapey, R. (Ed.), *Language Intervention Strategies in Adult Aphasia*, Baltimore MD: Williams & Wilkins 223–45.

Lubinski, R. (1991) Environmental considerations for elderly patients. In: Lubinski, R. (Ed.), *Dementia and Communication*, Philadelphia PA: B.D. Decker 257–78.

Lubinski, R. (1995) State of the art perspectives on communication in nursing homes. *Topics in Language Disorder* **15**, 1–19.

Lubinski, R., Morrison, E.B.E. and Ridgrodsky, S. (1981) Perception of spoken communication by elderly chronically mentally ill patients in an institutional setting. *Journal of Speech and Hearing Disorders* **46**, 405–12.

Maas, M. (1988) Management of patients with Alzheimer's disease in long-term care facilities. *Nursing Clinics of North America* **23**, 57–68.

McClannahan, L.E. and Risley, T.R. (1975) Design of living environments for nursing home residents: recruiting attendance at activities. *The Gerontologist* **14**, 236–40.

McCreadie, C. and Tinker, A. (1993) Review: abuse of elderly people in the domestic setting: a UK perspective. *Age and Ageing* **22**, 65–9.

Macdonald, A. (1986) Do general practitioners miss depression in elderly patients? *British Medical Journal* **292**, 1365–7.

MacDonald, M.L. (1978) Environmental programming for the socially iIsolated aging. *The Gerontologist* **18**, 350–4.

McEvoy, C.L. and Patterson, R.L. (1986) Behavioural treatment of deficit skills in dementia patients. *The Gerontologist* **26**, 475–8.

McEnvoy, G. and Vincent, C. (1980) Who reads and why? *Journal of Communication* **30**, 134–40.

McIntosh, J.B. and Power, K.G. (1993) Elderly people's views of an annual screening assessment. *British Journal of Clinical Practice* **43**, 189–92.

Mackereth, C.J. (1995) The practice nurse: roles and responsibilities. *Journal of Advanced Nursing* **21**, 1110–16.

McNamara, P., Obler, L.K., Au, R., Durso, R. and Albert, M.L. (1992) Speech monitoring skills in Alzheimer's disease, Parkinson's disease and normal aging. *Brain and Language* **42**, 38–51.

MacPherson, I., Donald, S. and Ludbrook, A. (1992) Registered private nursing homes in Scotland: referral and assessment practice. *Age and Ageing* **21**, 429–34.

Maher, E.R. and Lees, A.J. (1986) The clinical features and natural history of the Steele–Richardson–Olszewski syndrome (progressive supranuclear palsy). *Neurology* **36**, 1005–8.

Maher, E.R., Smith, E.M. and Lees, A.J. (1985) Cognitive deficits in the Steele–Richardson–Olszewski syndrome. *Journal of Neurology, Neurosurgery and Psychiatry* **48**, 1234–9.

Mahler, M.E. and Cummings, J.L. (1991) Behavioural neurology of multi-infarct dementia. *Alzheimer's Disease Association Disorders* **5**, 122–30.

Majeed, F.A., Chaturvedi, N., Reading, R. and Ben-Shlomo, Y. (1994) Monitoring and promoting equity in primary and secondary care. *British Medical Journal* **308**, 1426–9.

Malone, R.L., Ptacek, P.H. and Malone, M.S. (1970) Attitudes expressed by families of aphasics. *British Journal of Disorders of Communication* **15**, 154–79.

Mandel, A.M., Alexander, M.P. and Carpenter, S. (1989) Creutzfeldt–Jakob disease presenting as an isolated aphasia. *Neurology* **39**(1), 55–8.

Marchant, C. (1993) Out in the cold. *Community Care* **27** May, 24–5.

Marsden, C.D. (1978) The diagnosis of dementia. In: Isaacs, A.D. and Post, F. (Eds), *Studies in Geriatric Psychiatry*. Chichester: Wiley.

Martin, A. (1987) Representations of semantic and spatial knowledge in Alzheimer's patients: implications for models of preserved learning in amnesia. *Journal of Clinical and Experimental Neuropsychology* **9**, 121–224.

Martin, A. (1990) Neuropathology of Alzheimer's disease: the case for subgroups. In: M.F. Schwartz (Ed.), *Modular Deficits in Alzheimer-type Dementia*, pp. 144–78. Cambridge, MA: MIT Press.

Martin, J., Meltzer, H. and Elliot, D. (1988) *The Prevalence of Disability among Adults*. London: HMSO.

Means, R. and Smith, R. (1994) *Community Care. Policy and Practice*. Basingstoke: Macmillan.

Martin, A., Brouwers, P., Cox, C. and Fedio, P. (1985) On the nature of the verbal memory deficit in Alzheimer's disease. *Brain and Language* **25**, 323–41.

Matison, R. Mayeux, R., Rosen, J. and Fahn, S. (1982) 'Tip-of-the-tongue' phenomena in Parkinson's disease. *Neurology* **32**, 567–70.

Mayeux, R., Stern, Y. and Sano, M. (1992) A comparison of clinical outcome and survival in various forms of Alzheimer's disease. In: Florette, F. Khachaturian, Z. Poncet, M. and Christen, Y. (Eds), *Heterogeneity of Alzheimer's Disease*. Berlin: Springer-Verlag.

Maxim, J. (1991) Can elicited language be used to diagnose dementia? *NHCSS Work in Progress* **1**, 13–21.

Maxim, J. and Bryan, K.L. (1989/1995) Talking and listening. In: Benson, S. (Ed.), *Handbook for Care Assistants*. London: Hawker (4th edn 1995).

Maxim, J. and Bryan, K.L. (1994) *Language of the Elderly*. London: Whurr Publishers.

Mawhinney, B. and Nichol, D. (1993) *Purchasing for Health: A Framework for Action* (speeches). Leeds: Department of Health/NHS Management Executive.

Meade, K. and Carter, T. (1990) Empowering older users: some starting points. In: Winn, L. (Ed.), *Power to The People*. London: Kings Fund.

Means, R. and Smith, R. (1994) *Community Care. Policy and Practice*. London: Macmillan.

Melin, L. and Gotestam, K.G. (1981) The effects of rearranging ward routines on communication and eating behaviours of psychogeriatric patients. *Journal of Applied Behaviour* 14, 47–51.

Meltzer, J.W. (1982, June) *Respite Care: an Emerging Family Support Service*. Washington, DC: Center for the Study of Social Policy.

Mendez, M.F. and Ashla-Mendez, M. (1991) Differences between multi-infarct dementia and Alzheimer's disease on unstructured neuropsychological tasks. *Journal of Clinical and Experimental Neuropsychology* 13, 923–32.

Mesulam, M. (1982) Slowly progressive aphasia without generalized dementia. *Annals of Neurology* 11, 592–8.

Mesulam, M.M. and Weintraub, S. (1992) Primary progressive aphasia: sharpening the focus on a clinical syndrome. In: Florette, F. Khachaturian, Z. Poncet, M. and Christen, Y. (Eds), *Heterogeneity of Alzheimer's Disease*. Berlin: Springer-Verlag.

Meyer, J.S., Judd, B.W., Tawakina, T., Rogers, R.L. and Mortel, K.F. (1986) Improved cognition after control of risk factors for multi-infarct dementia. *Journal of the American Medical Association* 256, 2203–2209.

Meyer, J.S., Rogers, R.L., McClintic, K., Mortel, K.F. and Lofti, J. (1989) Randomised clinical trial of daily aspirin therapy in multi-infarct dementia: a pilot study. *Journal of the American Geriatrics Society* 37, 549–55.

Milberg, W. and Albert, M. (1989) Cognitive differences between patients with progressive supranuclear palsy and Alzheimer's disease. *Journal of Clinical and Experimental Neuropsychology* 11 (5), 605–14.

Millard, S.M. (1989) Maintaining control of the Alzheimer's unit. *Nursing Home and Senior Citizen Care* 38(1&2), 13–16.

Miller, E. and Morris, R. (1993) *The Psychology of Dementia*. Chichester: Wiley.

Miller, N. (1986) *Dyspraxia and its Management*. London: Croom Helm.

Ministry of Health (1963) *Health and Welfare: The Development of Community Care*. London: HMSO.

Mishara, B.L. (1978) Geriatric patients who improve in token economy and general milieu treatment programs: a multivariate analysis. *Journal of Consulting and Clinical Psychology* 46, 1340–8.

Mishara, B.L., Robertson, B. and Kastenbaum, R. (1973) Self-injurious behaviour in the elderly. *The Gerontologist* 13, 311–14.

Montgomery, R.J. (1986) Researching respite: beliefs, facts, and questions. In: R. Montgomery, R. and Prothero, J. (Eds), *Developing Respite Services for the Elderly*. Seattle, WA: University of Washington Press.

Moriarty, J. and Levin, E. (1993) Services to people with dementia and their carers. In: A. Burns (Ed.), *Ageing and Dementia*. London: Edward Arnold. 237–50.

Morris, J.C., Edland, S., Clark, C., Galasko, D., Koss, E., Mohs, R., van Belle, G., Fillenbaum, G. and Heyman, A. (1993) The consortium to establish a registry for Alzheimer's disease (CERAD), Part IV: Rates of cognitive change in the longitudinal assessment of probable Alzheimer's disease. *Neurology* 43(12), 2457–65.

Morris, R.G., Morris, L.W. and Britton, P.G. (1988) Factors affecting the emotional well-being of the caregivers of dementia sufferers. *British Journal of Psychiatry* **153**, 147–56.

Morton, I. and Bleathman, C. (1991) The effectiveness of validation therapy in dementia – a pilot study. *International Journal of Geriatric Psychiatry* **6**, 327–30.

Mueller, D.J. and Atlas, L. (1972) Resocialization of regressed elderly patients: a behavioural management approach. *Journal of Gerontology* **27**, 390–2.

Muir Gray, J. (1988) Health and the individual. In: Groombridge, J. (Ed.), *Health Promotion and Older People*. London: HEA/CHRE.

Mulhall, D.J. (1977) The representation of personal relationships: an automated system. *International Journal of Man–Machine Studies* **9**, 315–35.

Mulhall, D.J. (1978) Dysphasic stroke patients and the influence of their relatives. *British Journal of Disorders of Communication* **13**, 127–34.

Mulhall, D.J. (1988) The management of the aphasic patient. In: Clifford Rose, F. Whurr, R. and Wyke, M.A. (Eds), *Aphasia*. London: Whurr Publishers.

Munoz-Garcia, D. and Ludwin, S.K. (1984) Classic and generalized variants of Pick's disease: a clinicopathological, ultra structural and immunocytochemical comparative study. *Annals of Neurology* **16**, 467–80.

Murdoch, B.E. (1990) *Acquired Speech and Language Disorders. A Neuroanatomical and Functional Approach*. London: Chapman & Hall.

Murphy, E., Smith, R., Lindsay, J. and Slattery, J. (1988) Increased mortality rates in later-life depression. *British Journal of Psychiatry* **152**, 347–53.

Murray, J., Marquardt, T.P., Richardson, A. and Nalty, D. (1984) Differential diagnosis of aphasia and dementia from aphsaia test battery scores. *Journal of Neurological Communication Disorders* **1**, 33–9.

Musson, N.D., Kincaid, J., Ryan, P., Glussman, B., Varone, L., Gamara, N., Wilson, R., Reefe, W. and Silverman, M. (1990) Nature, nurture, nutrition: interdisciplinary programs to address the prevention of malnutrition and dehydration. *Dysphagia* **5**, 96–101.

National Center for Health Statistics (1985) *Mental Illness in Nursing Homes*, Series 13, No. 105.

National Institute on Adult Day Care (1992) *Position Paper: Public Policy Statement*. Washington, DC: National Council on the Aging.

Navia, B.A., Jordan, B.D. and Price, R.W. (1986) The AIDS dementia complex, I: Clinical features. *Annals of Neurology* **19**, 517–24.

Nebes, R.D., Boller, F. and Holland, A. (1986) Use of semantic context by patients with Alzheimer's disease. *Psychology and Aging* **1**, 261–9.

Nebes, R.D., Martin, D.C. and Horn, L.C. (1984) Sparing of semantic memory in Alzheimer's disease. *Journal of Abnormal Psychology* **93**, 321-30.

Neill, J. and Williams, J. (1992) *Leaving Hospital: Elderly People and Their Discharge to Community Care*. London: HMSO. Nelson, J. and O'Connell, P. (1978). Dementia: the estimation of premorbid intelligence levels using the New Adult Reading Test. *Cortex* **14**, 234–44.

Nerbonne, M., Schow, R. and Hutchinson, J. (1980) Gerontologic training in communication. *Asha* **22**, 404–10.

Newkirk, J.M., Feldman, S., Bickett, A., Gipson, M.T. and Lutzker, J.R. (1976) Increasing extended care facility residents' attendance at recreational activities with convenient locations and personal invitations. *Journal of Applied Behaviour Analysis* **9**, 207.

Nocon, A. (1992) Old age benefit. *Health Service Journal* **102**, 28–9.

Norlin, P.F. (1986) Familiar faces: sudden strangers. Helping families cope with the crisis of aphasia. In: Chapey, R. (Ed.), *Language Intervention Strategies in Adult Aphasia*, Ch. 9. Baltimore, MD: Williams & Wilkins.

Norman, A. (1990) *Moving Forward to Quality in 'Caring for Quality in Services for Elderly People'*, Report of the Social Services Inspectorate. London: Department of Health.

Norris, A.D. (1986) *Reminiscence*. Oxford: Winslow Press.

Nussbaum, J.F., Thompson, T. and Robinson, J.D. (1989) *Communication and Aging*. New York: Harper & Row.

Obler, L.K. (1980) Narrative discourse style in the elderly. In: Obler, L. and Albert, M. (Eds), *Language and Communication in the Elderly*. Lexington, MA: D.C. Heath.

Obler, L.K. and Albert, M.L. (1981) Language in the elderly aphasic and in the dementing patient. In: Sarno, N.T. (Ed.), *Acquired Aphasia*, New York: Academic Press. 385–98.

O'Connor, D.W., Grande, M.J., Hyde, J.B., Perry, J.R., Roland, M.O., Silverman, J.D. and Wraight, S.K. (1993) Dementia in general practice: the practical consequenses of a more positive approach to diagnosis. *British Journal of General Practic* 43, 185–8.

O'Connor, D.W., Pollitt, P., Brook, C. et al. (1991) Does early intervention reduce the number of elderly people with dementia admitted to institutions for long-term care? *British Medical Journal* 302, 871–4.

O'Donovan, S. (1993) Call for help. *Nursing Times* 89(7), 30–3.

Office of Geriatrics and Extended Care (1994) *Continuum of Care Guide*. Washington, DC: Department of Veterans Affairs.

Office of Population and Census Studies (1987) *Population Projections 1985–2025*. London: HMSO.

O'Neill, D. (1991) Dementia and the GP. *Practitioner* 235, 644–48.

Orange, J.B. (1991) Perspectives of family members regarding communication changes. In: R. Lubinski (Ed.), *Dementia and Communication*, pp. 168–87. Philadelphia: B.C. Decker.

Orange, J.B., Ryan, E.B., Meredith, S.D. and MacLean, M.J. (1995) Application of a communication enhancement model for long-term care residents with Alzheimer's disease. *Topics in Language Disorder* 15, 20–35.

Orchard, C. (1994) Comparing health outcomes. *British Medical Journal* 308, 1493–6.

Orrell, M. and Sahakian, B. (1995) Education and dementia. *British Medical Journal* 310, 951–2.

Osborne, S. and Rees, L. (1992) Managing the transition to community care: an exploratory study of six local authorities in England. *Research, Policy and Planning* 10, 6–9.

Ott, A., Breteler, M.M.B., van Harslcamp, F., Claus, J.J., van der Cammen, T.J.M., Grobbee, D.E. et al. (1995) Prevalence of Alzheimer's disease and vascular dementia.*British Medical Journal* 310, 970–2.

Ovretveit, J. (1994) Expand your service by contracting. *CSLT Bulletin* 503, 7–10.

Parker, M. (1983) Sharing special skills. *Remedial Therapist* 5 (21), 12.

Parkes, C.M. (1975) *Bereavement*. London: Pelican.

Patterson, R.L. and Telgen, J.R. (1973) Conditioning and posthospital generalization of nondelusional responses in a chronic psychotic patient. *Journal of Applied Behaviour Analysis* 6, 65–70.

Patterson, K., Graham, N. and Hodges, J. (1994) Reading in dementia of the Alzheimer type: A preserved ability? *Neuropsychologia* 8, 395–407.

Patterson, R.L. and Teigen, J.R. (1973) Conditioning and post-hospital generalisation of nondelusional responses in a chronic psychotic patient. *Journal of Applied Behavior Analysis* 6, 65–70.

Pattie, A.H. and Gilleard, C.J. (1979) *The Clifton Assessment Procedure for the Elderly*. Windsor: NFER Nelson.

Pattie, A.H. and Heaton, J. (1990) A comparative study of dependency and provision of care for the elderly in the state and private sectors in York Health District. Yorkshire Regional Health Authority.

Peppard, N.R. (1985) Alzheimer special-care nursing home units. *Nursing Homes* 34, 25–8.

Perls, F. (1972) *Gestalt Therapy Verbatim*. London: Bantam.

Perotta, P. and Meacham, J.A. (1981) Can a reminiscing intervention alter depression and self-esteem? *International Journal of Aging and Human Development* 14, 23–40.

Perry, E.K. and Perry, R.H. (1993) Neurochemical pathology and therapeutic pathology in degenerative dementia. *International Review of Psychiatry* 5, 363–80.

Perry, R.H., Irving, D., Blessed, G. et al. (1989) Clinically and neuropathologically distinct form of dementia. *Lancet* i, 166.

Pfeffer, R.I., Afifi, A.A. and Chance, J.M. (1987) Prevalence of Alzheimer's disease in a retirement community. *American Journal of Epidemiology* 125, 420–36.

Pick, A. (1892) Ueber die beziehungen der senilen hirnatrophic zur aphasie. *Praeger Med Wochenschr* 17, 165–7.

Pickles, B. (1995) *Physiotherapy with Older People*. London: Saunders.

Pinkston, E.M. and Linsk, N.L. (1984) *Care of the Elderly: A Family Approach*. New York: Pergamon Press.

Pitt, B.M.N. (1982) *Psychogeriatrics*: An Introduction to the Psychiatry of Old Age, 2nd edn. Edinburgh/New York: Churchill Livingstone.

Podoll, K., Caspary, P., Large, H.W. and Noth, J. (1988) Language functions in Huntingdon's disease. *Brain* 3, 1475–1503.

Podoll, K., Schwarz, M. and Noth, J. (1991) Language functions in progressive supranuclear palsy. *Brain* 114, 1457–72.

Poeck, K. and Luzzatti, C. (1988) Slowly progressive aphasia in three patients. The problems of accompanying neuropsychological deficit. *Brain* 3, 151–68.

Pollock, L. (1986) The multidisciplinary team. In: Hume, C. and Pullen, I. (Eds), *Rehabilitation in Psychiatry: An Introductory Handbook*, pp. 126–48. Edinburgh: Churchill Livingstone.

Porch, B. (1971) *The Porch Index of Communicative Ability*. Palo Alto, CA: Consulting Psychologists Press.

Poulshock, S.W. and Deimling, G.T. (1984) Families caring for elders in residence: issues in the management of burden. *Journal of Gerontology* 39, 230–9.

Powell, A.L., Cummings, J.L., Hill, M.A. and Benson, D.F. (1988) Speech and language alterations in multi-infarct dementia. *Neurology* 38, 717–9.

Powell, J.A., Hale, M.A. and Bayer, A.J. (1995) Symptoms of communication breakdown in dementia: carers' perceptions. *European Journal of Disorders of Communication* 30, 65–75.

Powell-Procter, L. and Miller, E. (1982) Reality orientation: a critical appraisal. *British Journal of Psychiatry* 140, 457–63.

Praderas, K. and Macdonald, M.L. (1986) Telephone conversational skills training with socially isolated, impaired nursing home residents. *Journal of Applied Behaviour Analysis* 19, 337–48.

Quattrochi-Tubin, S. and Jason, L.A. (1980) Enhancing social interactions and activity among the elderly through stimulus control. *Journal of Applied Behaviour Analysis* 13, 159–63.

Quayhagen, M.P. and Quayhagen, M. (1988) Alzheimer's stress: coping with the caregiving role. *The Gerontologist* 28, 391–6.

Rabins, P.V. (1982) Management of irreversible dementia. *Psychomatics* 22, 591–7.

Rabins, P.V. (1986) Establishing Alzheimer's disease units in nursing homes: pros and cons. *Hospital and Community Psychiatry* 37, 120–1.

Rabins, P.V., Mace, N.L. and Lucas, M.J. (1982) The impact of dementia on the family. *Journal of the American Medical Association* 248, 333–5.

Radloff, L.S. (1977) The CES-D scale: A self-report depression scale for research in the general population. *Journal of Applied Psychological Measurement* 1, 387–93.

Raiford, C. and Shadden, B. (1985) Graduate education in gerontology. *Asha* 27, 37–43.

Ramsay, M., Winget, C. and Higginson, I. (1995) Review: measures to determine outcome of community services for people with dementia. *Age and Ageing* 24, 73–83.

Rapcsak, S.Z., Arthur, S.A., Bliklen, D.A. et al. (1989) Lexical agraphia in Alzheimer's disease. *Archives of Neurology* 46, 65–8.

Regeer, A., Boyd, J., Burke, J. et al. (1988) One-month prevalence of mental disorders in the United States. *Archives of General Psychiatry* 45, 977–86.

Reichman, W.E., Cummings, J.L.l., McDaniel, K.D., Flynn, F. and Gornbein, J. (1991) Visuoconstructive impairment in dementia syndromes. *Behavioural Neurology* 4, 153–62.

Reifler, B. (1986) Mixed cognitive-affective disturbances in the elderly: a new classification. *Journal of Clinical Psychiatry* 47, 354–6.

Reisberg, B., Ferris, S.M., de Leon, M. and Crook, T. (1982) The global deterioration scale for assessment of primary degenerative dementia. *American Journal of Psychiatry* 139, 1136–9.

Reitz, A.L. (1978) Increasing participation in recreation activities in a convalescent center. *Dissertation Abstracts International* 39, 5580B–5581B.

Riggans, L. (1992) Living with loss. *Nursing Times* 88(27), 34–5.

Ripich, D.N. (1991) Differential diagnosis and assessment. In: Lubinski, R. (Ed.), *Dementia and Communication*. Philadelphia PA: B.D. Decker. 188–215.

Ripich, D.N. (1996) *Alzheimer's Disease Communication Code: The FOCUSED Program for Caregivers*. Austin, TX: Psychological Corporation.

Ripich, D.N. and Terrell, B.Y. (1988) Patterns of discourse cohesion in Alzheimer's disease. *Journal of Speech and Hearing Disorders* 53, 8–15.

Ripich, D.N., Vertes, D., Whitehouse, P., Fulton, S. and Ekelman, B. (1991) Turn-taking and speech act patterns in the discourse of senile dementia of the Alzheimer's type patients. *Brain and Language* 40, 330–43.

Ripich, D.N. and Wykle, M. (1990a) A program for nursing assistants with Alzheimer's patients. Paper presented at the American Gerontology in Higher Education Conference, Kansas City, MI.

Ripich, D.N. and Wykle, M. (1990b) Developing healthcare professionals' communication skills with Alzheimer's disease patients. Paper presented at the Annual Meeting of the American Society on Aging, San Francisco, CA.

Ripich, D.N., Wykle, M. and Niles, S. (1991) The FOCUSED communication training program. Paper presented at the Annual Meeting of the Gerontological Society of America, San Francisco, CA.

Ripich, D.N. and Ziol, E.W. (1995a) A survey of activities in Geriatric Education Centers related to cognitively impaired elderly. Unpublished paper.

Ripich, D.N. and Ziol, E.W. (1995b) A survey of activities in the Veterans Administration Geriatric Research, Education, and Clinical Centers related to the family. *Journal of the American Medical Association* **248**, 333–5.

Rickford, F. (1993) Conflicting interests. *Community Care* **12**(August), 12–13.

Robb, S.S., Stegman, C.E. and Wolanin, M.O. (1986) No research versus research with compromised results: a study of validation therapy. *Nursing Research* **35**, 113–8.

Robertson, S.J. and Thompson, F. (1983) Speech therapy and Parkinson's disease. *CSLT Bulletin* **370**, 10–12.

Robins, P., Mace, N.L. and Lucas, M.J. (1982) The impact of dementia on the family. *Journal of the American Medical Association* **248**, 333–5.

Robbins, T.W., James, M., Lange, K.W., Owen, A.M., Quinn, N.P. and Marsden, C.D. (1992) Cognitive performance in multiple system atrophy. *Brain* **115**, 271–91.

Rochford, G. (1971) A study of naming errors in dysphasic and in demented patients. *Neuropsychologia* **9**, 437–43.

Rochon, E. and Waters, G.S. (1994) Sentence comprehension in patients with Alzheimer's disease. *Brain and Language* **46**, 329–49.

Rockwood, K. (1989) Acute confusion in elderly medical patients. *Journal of the American Geriatrics Society* **37**, 150–4.

Rogers, C. (1951) *Client Centred Therapy*. Boston, MA: Houghton Mifflin.

Rogers, D., Lees, A.J., Smith, E., Trimble, M. and Stern, G.M. (1987) Bradyphrenia in Parkinson's disease and psychomotor retardation in depressive illness: an experimental study. *Brain* **110**, 761–76.

Ross, E.D. (1981) The aprosodias: functional organization of the affective component of language in the right hemisphere. *Archives of Neurology* **38**, 561–9.

Ross, G.W., Cummings, J.L. and Benson, D.F. (1990) Speech and language alterations in dementia syndromes: characteristics and treatment. *Aphasiology* **4**(4), 339–52.

Rosser, A. and Hodges, J.R. (1994) Initial letter and semantic category fluency in Alzheimer's disease, Huntington's disease and progressive supranuclear palsy. *Journal of Neurology, Neurosurgery and Psychiatry* **57**, 1389–94.

Rossor, M. (1987) Dementia. *British Journal of Hospital Medicine* (July), 46–50.

Rossor, M. (1993) Alzheimer's disease. *British Medical Journal* **307**, 779–82.

Rossor, M.N., Kennedy, A.M. and Newman, S.K. (1992) Heterogeneity in familial Alzheimer's disease. In: Florette, F., Khachaturian, Z., Poncet, M. and Christen, Y. (Eds), *Heterogeneity of Alzheimer's Disease*. Berlin: Springer-Verlag.

Roth, M. (1981) The diagnosis of dementia in late and middle life. In: Mortimer, J.A. and Schuman, L.M. (Eds), *The Epidemiology of Dementia*. New York: Oxford University Press.

Royal College of Physicians (1981) Organic mental impairment in the elderly: a report of the Royal College of Physicians by the College Committee on Geriatrics. *Journal of the Royal College of Physicians* **15**, 142–67.

Royal College of Physicians (1992) *High-quality Long-term Care for Elderly People*. London: Royal College of Physicians.

Royal College of Physicians (1994) *Ensuring Equity and Quality of Care for Older People*. London: Royal College of Physicians.

Royal College of Speech and Language Therapists (1990) Dementia Working Party survey. Unpublished document, RCSLT, London.

RCSLT (1990) *Speech Therapy and the Elderly with Dementia. The Report of the Working Party on Dementias*. London: RCSLT.

Royal College of Speech and Language Therapists (1991) *Communicating Quality*. London: RCSLT.

RCLST (1993) *Report of the Working Party in Dementias*. London: Royal College of Speech and Language Therapists.

Royal College of Speech and Language Therapists (1993) *Speech and Language Therapy and the Elderly with Dementia*, Position Paper. London: RCSLT.

Saffran, E., Fitzpatrick-Desalme, E. and Coslett, H.B. (1990) Visual disturbances in dementia. In: Schwartz, M.L. (Ed.), *Modular Deficits in Alzheimer-type Dementia*. Cambridge, MA: MIT Press.

SantoPietro, M.J., Decotiis, E., McCarthy, J. and Ostuni, E. (1990) Conversation in Alzheimer's disease patients: implications in semantic and pragmatic breakdowns. Paper presented at the Annual Convention of the American Speech–Language–Hearing Association, Seattle, WA.

Sasanuma, S., Sakuma, N. and Kitano, K. (1990) Longterm course of cognitive abilities of patients with probable Alzheimer-type dementia and multi-infarct dementia. Paper presented at the 4th International Aphasia Rehabilitation Congress, Edinburgh, September.

Saxton, J., McGonigle, K.L., Swihart, A.A. and Boller, F. (1993) *Severe Impairment Battery*. Bury St Edmunds: Thames Valley Test Co.

Scheltens, P., Hazenberg, G.J., Lindeboom, J., Valk, J. and Wolters, E.C. (1990) A case of progressive aphasia without dementia: 'temporal' Pick's disease? *Journal of Neurology, Neurosurgery and Psychiatry* **53**, 79–80.

Schuell, H. (1973) *The Shortened Schuell Test*. Minneapolis, MN: University of Minnesota Press.

Schwartz, M.F. and Chawluk, J.B. (1990) Deterioration of language in progressive aphasia: a case study. In: Schwartz, M.F. (Ed.), *Modular Deficits in Alzheimer-type Dementia*, Cambridge, MA: MIT Press. 245–96.

Schwartz, M.F., Marin, O.S. and Saffran, E.M. (1979) Dissociation of language function in dementia: a case study. *Brain and Language* **7**, 277–306.

Schwartz, M.F., Saffran, E.M. and Martin, O.S.M. (1980) Fractioning the reading process in dementia: evidence for word specific print-to-sound associations. In: Coltheart, M., Patterson, K. and Marshall, J.C. (Eds), *Deep Dyslexia*. London: Routledge.

Schwartz, M.F., Saffran, E.M. and Williamson, S. (1981) The breakdown of lexicon in Alzheimer's dementia. Paper presnted at Lingusitic Society of America 56th Annual Meeting, New York.

Scott, S. and Caird, F.I. (1983) Speech therapy for Parkinson's disease. *Journal of Neurology, Neurosurgery and Psychiatry* **46**, 140–4.

Scott, S. and Caird, F.I. (1981) Speech therapy for patients with Parkinson's disease. *British Medical Journal* **283**, 1088.

Scott, S., Caird, F.I. and Williams, B.O. (1984) Evidence for an apparent sensory speech disorder in Parkinson's disease. *Journal of Neurology, Neurosurgery and Psychiatry* **47**, 840–3.

Seaman, J. (1990) Key issues in understanding and caring for the elderly mentally infirm people. *Speech Therapy in practice* (Suppl.) **6**, viii–ix.

Seltzer, B. and Sherwin, I. (1983) A comparison of clinical features in early and late onset primary degenerative dementia. One entity or two? *Archives of Neurology* **40**, 143–6.

Shadden, B. (1988) Education, counseling and support for significant others. In: Shadden, B. (Ed.), *Communication Behavior and Aging: A Sourcebook for Clinicians*, Baltimore, MD: Williams & Wilkins. 309.

Shadden, B. (1995) The use of discourse analyses and procedures for communication programming in long-term care facilities. *Topics in Language Disorder* **15**, 75–86.

Shulman, M.D. and Mandel, E. (1988) Communication training of relatives and friends of institutionalized elderly patients. *The Gerontologist* **28**, 797–9.

Shulman, K.I., Shedletski, R. and Silver, I.L. (1986) The challenge of time: clock drawing and cognitive functioning in the elderly. *International Journal of Geriatric Psychiatry* **1**, 35–40.

Shuttleworth, E.C. and Huber, S.J. (1989) A longitudinal study of the naming disorder of dementia of the Alzheimer type. *Neuropsychiatry, Neuropsychology and Behavioural Neurology* **1**, 267–82.

Sinclair, H. (1967) Conduites verbales et deficits operatoires. *Acta Neurologica et Psychiatrica Belgica* **67**, 852–60.

Ska, B. and Guenard, D. (1993) Narrative schema in dementia of the Alzheimer's type. In: Brownell, H.H. and Joanette, Y. (Eds), *Narrative Discourse in Neurologically Impaired and Normal Aging Adults*, San Diego, CA: Singular Publishing Group. 299–316.

Ska, B., Joanette, Y., Poissant, A., Beland, R. and Lecours, A.R. (1990) Language disorders in dementia of the Alzheimer type: contrastive patterns from a multiple single case study. *Abstracts of the Academy of Aphasia 28th Annual Meeting, Baltimore, USA*, 28 October, pp. 21–3.

Skelly, M. (1979) *Amer-Ind Gestural Code: based on American Indian Handtalk*. New York: Elsevier.

Skelton-Robinson, M. and Jones, S. (1984) Nominal dysphasia and the severity of senile dementia. *British Journal of Psychiatry* **145**, 168–71.

Sloane, P.D. and Mathew, L.J. (1991) *Dementia Units in Long Term Care*. Baltimore, MD: Johns Hopkins University Press.

Sloane, P. and Pickard, G. (1985) Custodial nursing home care: setting realistic goals. *Journal of the American Geriatrics Society* **33**, 864–7.

Smith, B.J. and Barker, H.R. (1972) Influence of a reality orientation training programme on the attitudes of trainees towards the elderly. *Gerontologist* **12**, 262–4.

Smith, S. (1989) Syntactic comprehension in Alzheimer's disease. Paper presented at the Academy of Aphasia, Santa Fe, NM.

Smith, S.R., Murdoch, B.E. and Chenery, H.J. (1989) Semantic abilities in dementia of the Alzheimer type, 1: Lexical semantics. *Brain and Language* **36**, 314–24.

Smith, W.L. (1988, May) Behavioural interventions in gerontology: management of behaviour problems in individuals with Alzheimer's disease living in the community. Paper presented at the Association for Behaviour Analysis Convention, Philadelphia, PA.

Smythe, L. (1990) *Practical Physiotherapy with Older People*. London: Chapman & Hall.

Snodgrass, J.G. and Vanderwart, M. (1980) A standardised set of 260 pictures: norms for name agreement, image agreement, familiarity and visual complexity. *Journal of Experimental Psychology: Human Perception and Performance* **6**, 174–215.

Snowden, J.S., Goulding, P.J. and Neary, D. (1989) Semantic dementia: a form of circumscribed cerebral atrophy. *Behavioural Neurology* **2**, 258–71.

Snowden, J., Griffiths, H. and Neary, D. (1994) Semantic dementia: autobiographical contribution to preservation of meaning. *Cognitive Neuropsychology* **11**, 265–88.

Speedie, L.J., Brake, N., Folstein, S.E., Bowers, D. and Heilman, K.M. (1990) Comprehension of prosody in Huntington's disease. *Journal of Neurology, Neurosurgery and Psychiatry* **53**, 607–10.

Stebbins, G.T., Wilson, R.S., Gilley, D.W. Bernard, B.A. and Fox, J.H. (1990) Use of the NART to estimate premorbid IQ in dementia. *Clinical Neurologist* **4**, 18–24.

Stengel, E. (1964) Neuropathology of dementia. *Proceedings of the Royal Society of Medicine* **54**, 911–14.

Stevens, S.J. (1985) The language of dementia: a pilot study. *British Journal of Disorders of Communication* **20**, 181–90.

Stevens, S.J. (1992) Differentiating the language disorder in dementia from dysphasia – the potential of a screening test. *European Journal of Disorders of Communication* **27**, 275–88.

Stevens, S.J. (1994) SLT – researcher or clinician? The role of memory clinics. *Human Communication* (November/December), 13–14.

Stevens, S.J., Le May, M., Gravell, R. and Cook, K. (1992) *Working with Elderly People*. London: Whurr Publishers.

Stevens, S.J., Pitt, B.M.N., Nicholl, C.G., Fletcher, A.E. and Palmer, A.J. (1992) Language assessment in a memory clinic. *International Journal of Geriatric Psychiatry* **7**, 45–51.

Stevens, S.J., Pitt, B.M.N., Nicholl, C.G. et al. (1992) Language assessment in a memory clinic. *International Journal of Geriatric Psychiatry* **8**, 175–80.

Stockwell, F. (1972) *The Unpopular Patient*. London: Royal College of Nursing.

Stokes, G. and Goudie, F. (1990) *Working with Dementia*. Oxford: Winslow Press.

Sullivan, C. (1991) Putting our patients to the test. *Therapy Weekly* (22 March), 4.

Sutcliffe, R.L., Prior, R., Mawby, B. and McQuillan, W.J. (1985) Parkinson's disease in the district of the Northampton Health Authority, UK. A study of prevalence and disability. *Acta Neurologica Scandinavica* **72**, 363–79.

Tanner, B.B. (1993) The given–new distinction: a comparative study of normal elderly, people with aphasia, and elderly people with dementia. Unpublished MLing thesis.

Tanner, B.B. and Daniels, K.A. (1990) An observation study of communication between carers and their relatives with dementia. *Care of the Elderly* **2**, 247–50.

Tanton, M. (1993) *Helping Communication in the Person with Dementia*. Published privately.

Tatemichi, T.K. (1990) How acute brain failure becomes chronic. A view of the mechanisms of dementia related to stroke. *Neurology* **40**, 1652–59.

Taylor, A.E., Saint-Cyr, J.A. and Lang, A.E. (1986) Frontal lobe dysfunction in Parkinson's disease: the cortical focus of neostriatal outflow. *Brain* **109**, 845–83.

Taylor, A.E., Saint-Cyr, J.A. and Lang, A.E. (1990) Memory and learning in early Parkinson's disease: evidence from a 'frontal lobe syndrom'. *Brain and Cognition* **13**, 211–32.

Taylor, A.M. and Warrington, E.K. (1971) Visual agnosia: a single case report. *Cortex* **7**, 152–61.

Terrell, B. and Ripich, D. (1989) Discourse competence as a variable in intervention. *Seminars in Speech and Language Disorders* **10**, 282–97.

Thompson, I. (1983) BMU Language Scales (MRC Edinburgh). *Bulletin* **378**, 1–4.

Thompson, J.M. (1986) Language pathology in Alzheimier's-type dementia and associated disorders. PhD thesis, University of Edinburgh.

Tissot, R., Duval, R.J., and de Ajuriaguerra (1967) Quelques aspects du langage des demances degeneratives du grand age. *Acta Neurologica et Psychiatricica Belgica* **67**, 911–23.

Toner, H.L. (1987) Effectiveness of a written guide for carers of dementia sufferers. *British Journal of Clinical and Social Psychology* **5**(1), 24–6.

Troster, A.I., Salmon, D.P., McCullough, D. and Butters, N. (1989) A comparison of the category fluency deficits associated with Alzheimer's and Huntington's disease. *Brain and Language* **37**, 500–13.

Trower, P., Bryant, B. and Argle, M. (1978) *Social Skills and Mental Health*. London: Methuen.

Troxel, D. (1994) Bill of Rights for Alzheimer's patients. *American Journal of Alzheimer's Care and Related Disorders and Research* (September/October).

Tweedy, J.R., Langer, K.G. and McDowell, F.H. (1982) The effect of semantic relations on the memory deficit associated with Parkinson's disease. *Journal of Clinical and Experimental Neuropsychology* 4, 235–47.

Tyrell, P.J., Warrington, E.K., Frackowiak, R.S.J. and Rossor, M.N. (1990) Heterogeneity in progressive aphasia due to focal cortical atrophy. *Brain* 113, 1321–36

UKCC (1990) *Statement on Practice Nurses and Aspects of the New GP Contract*. London: UKCC.

Ulatowska, H., North, A.J. and Macaluso-Haynes, S. (1981) Production of narrative and procedural discourse in aphasia. *Brain and Language* 13, 345–71.

United Nations (1979) *Age and Sex Composition by Country, 1960–2000*. New York: United Nations.

US Congress, Office of Technology Assessment (1987) *Losing a Million Minds: confronting the Tragedy of Alzheimer's Disease and Other Dementia* (OTA-BA-323). Washington, DC: Government Printing Office.

US Department of Commerce (1992) *Statistical Abstracts of the United States 1992*. Washington, DC: Author.

US Department of Health and Human Services, National Center for Health Statistics (1981) Characteristics of nursing home residents, health status, and care received: national nursing home survey, United States, May–December, 1977. *Vital Health Statistic*, Series 10, No. 73: DHEW, July.

US Department of Health and Human Services, Public Health Service, National Institutes of Health (1993) *Alzheimer's Disease: A Guide to Federal Programs*. NIH Publication No. 93-3635.

Utting, D. (1993) Keeping score. *Community Care* (August), 9.

Van der Gaag, A. (1988) *The Communication Assessment Profile for Adults with a Mental Handicap*. Bicester: Winslow Press (Speech Profiles).

Van der Gaag, A. (1993) *Audit: A Manual for Speech and Language Therapists*. London: RCSLT.

Van Gorp, W.G., Mitrushina, M., Cummings, J.L., Satz, P. and Modesitt, J. (1989) Normal aging and the subcortical encephalopathy of Aids. *Neuropsychiatry, Neuropsychology and Behavioural Neurology* 2(1), 5–20.

Vervoerdt, L.C.A. (1981) Psychotherapy for the elderly. In: Aris, T. (Ed.), *Health Care of the Elderly*. London: Croom Helm.

Von Behren, R. (1986) Adult day care in America: summary of a national survey. Washington, DC: National Council on the Aging.

Wade, D. (1992) *The College of Speech and Language Therapists' Response to DHA: Research Programme Epidemiologically Based Needs Assessment*. London: RCSLT.

Walker, C.G. (1992) Communication in Dementia: Evaluation of the Effect of Communication Management on Dementing Patients and Their Carer, Final Research Report (SHHD Grant). SHHD Chief Scientist's Office.

Walker, M. (1979) The Makaton in perspective. *Apex* 7, 12–14.

Walker, S.A. (1982) Investigation of the communication of elderly subjects. MPhil thesis, University of Sheffield.

Walker, S.A., Gordon, M.T. and Bain, A. (1994) Speech and Language Therapy: The Extended SCCD (work in progress). Victoria Infirmary NHS Trust (Glasgow).

Walker, S. and Williams, B.O. (1980) The response of a disabled elderly population to speech therapy. *British Journal of Disorders of Communication* 15, 19–30.

Wallace, S.P., Ingman, S.R., Snyder, J.L., Planning, M., Walker, G.K. and Phil, M. (1991) The evolving status of adult day care: evidence from Missouri. *Pride Institute Journal of Long Term Home Health Care* 1(4), 30–7.

Warrington, E.K. (1975) The selective impairment of semantic memory. *Quarterly Journal of Experimental Psychology* 27, 635–57.

Watson, P., Clark, L. and Tellegreen, A. (1988) Development and validation of brief measures of positive and negative affect: The PANAS scales. *Journal of Personality and Social Psychology* 54 (6), 1063–70.

Wattis, J. and Martin, C. (1994) *Practical Psychiatry of Old Age*, 2nd edn. London: Chapman & Hall.

Weaver, M. (1994) Adult day care: Current trends and future projections. The *Southwest Journal on Aging* 10, 19–25.

Weaver, M. (1994) Adult day care: Current trends and future projections. *The Southwest Journal on Aging* 10, 19–25.

Webb, A. (1991) Co-ordination: a problem in public sector management. *Policy and Politics* 19, 229–41.

Wechsler, A.F., Verity, M.A., Rosenschein, S., Fried, I. and Scheibel, A.B. (1982) Pick's disease: a clinical computed tomographic and histologic study with golgi impregnation observations. *Archives of Neurology* 39, 287–90.

Weeks, D.J. (1988). *The Anomalous Sentences Repetition Test*. Windsor: NFER-Nelson.

Weintraub, S., Rubin, N.P. and Marsel-Mesulam, M.M. (1990) Primary progressive aphasia: longitudinal course, neuropsychological profile and language features. *Archives of Neurology* 47, 1329–35.

Weissert, W.G., Bolda, E.J., Zelman, W.N., Mutran, E. and Magnum, A.B. (1990) *Adult Day Care: Findings from a National Survey*. Baltimore, MD: Johns Hopkins University Press.

Wells, N. and Freer, C. (1988) *The Ageing Population: Burden or Challenge*. London: Macmillan. Wells, N.E. (1979) *Dementia in Old Age*. London: Office of Health Economics.

Whitacker, H. (1976) A case of the isolation of the language function. In: Whitacker, H. and Whitacker, H.A. (Eds). *Studies in Neurolinguistics 2*. New York: Academic Press.

Whitehead, S. (1992) Support groups for the relatives or carers of aphasic adults. In: Fawcus, M. (Ed.), *Group Encounters in Speech and Language Therapy*. London: Whurr Publishers.

Whurr, R. (1974) *An Aphasia Screening Test*. London: Whurr Publishers.

Wicclair, M.R. (1993) *Ethics and the Elderly*. New York; Oxford University Press.

Williamson, J., Smith, R.G. and Burley, L.E. (1987) *Primary Care of the Elderly: A Practical Approach*. Bristol: IOP Publishing.

Williamson, S. and Schwartz, E. M. (1981) The dissolution of discourse in Alzheimer's dementia. Paper given at the Linguistic Society of America 56th Annual Meeting, New York.

Wilson, B.A. and Moffat, N. (1984) *Clinical Managemant of Memory Problems*. London: Croom Helm.

Wilson, R.S., Kasniak, A.W., Klawans, H.L. and Garron, D.G. (1980) High speed memory scanning in Parkinsonism. *Cortex* 16, 67–72.

Wirz, S., Skinner, C.S. and Dean, E.C. (1990) *Revised Edinburgh Functional Communication Profile*. Bicester: Winslow Press.

Wistow, G. and Henwood, M. (1991) *Caring for People: Elegant Model or Flawed Design?* In: Manning, N. (Ed.), Social Policy Review 1990–91. London: Longman.

Wistow, G., Knapp, M., Hardy, B. and Allen, C. (1992) From providing to enabling: local authorities and the mixed economy of social care. *Public Administration* **70**, 25–46.

Witte, K. (1986) Using the past and present to enhance family visits. Workshop presentation at the Hebrew Home for the Aged at Riverdale, Riverdale, NY.

Wolberg, L.R. (1977) *The Techniques of Psychotherapy*. New York: Grune & Stratton.

Woods, R.T., Portnoy, S., Head, D.N. and Jones, G.M.M. (1992) Reminiscence and life review with persons with dementia: Which way forward? In: Jones, G.M.M. and Miesen, B.M.L. (Eds), *Care-Giving in Dementia*, London: Routledge. 137–61.

Woods, R.T. and Britton, P.G. (1985) *Clinical Psychology with the Elderly*. London: Croom Helm.

Yesavage, J.A. (1985) Non pharmacologic treatments for memory losses with normal aging. *American Journal of Psychiatry* **142**, 600–5.

Yesavage, J.A., Brink, T., Rose, T. et al. (1983) Development and validation of a geriatric depression screening scale: a preliminary report. *Journal of Psychiatric Research* **17**, 37–49.

Zarit, J.M. (1982) Predictors of burden and distress for caregivers of senile dementia patients. Unpublished doctoral dissertation, University of Southern California, San Diego, CA.

Zarit, S., Anthony, C. and Boutselis, M. (1987) Intervention with caregivers of dementia patients: comparison of two approaches. *Psychology of Aging* **3**, 225–32.

Zawadski, R., Von Behren, R. and Stuart, M. (1992) *National Adult Day Care Census, 1989: Final Report* (HCFA Grant No. 500-89-0024). Baltimore, MD: Health Care Financing Administration.

Author Index

319

Subject Index